RABIES

RABIES

ITS PLACE AMONGST GERM-DISEASES, AND ITS ORIGIN IN THE ANIMAL KINGDOM

BY

DAVID SIME, M.D.

CAMBRIDGE:
AT THE UNIVERSITY PRESS
1903

CAMBRIDGE
UNIVERSITY PRESS

University Printing House, Cambridge CB2 8BS, United Kingdom

Cambridge University Press is part of the University of Cambridge.

It furthers the University's mission by disseminating knowledge in the pursuit of
education, learning and research at the highest international levels of excellence.

www.cambridge.org
Information on this title: www.cambridge.org/9781107456600

First published 1903
First paperback edition 2014

A catalogue record for this publication is available from the British Library

ISBN 978-1-107-45660-0 Paperback

PREFACE.

UNTIL the investigations of M. Pasteur threw light on the mystery surrounding rabies, it was not realised that there was a virus of the disease, or a rabific microbe as the *causa causans* of the virus. By keenest clinical observers the existence of either of these agents was viewed as at best problematic. Even where the germ-character of rabies was not denied, it was deemed most probable that, as surmised for untold ages, it was strictly of "spontaneous generation," or that the virus-germ underlying the disease was itself a diseased product and in reality but a virulent growth of canine morbid conditions exclusively in the salivary gland. The typical character of the canine disease, with its unvarying stability of form as an originating rabies, was never doubted; and all the modifications of rabies in other animals were taken as but the stereotyped, well-known "furious madness" and "dumb madness" of the dog. On the other hand, the phenomena of *attenuation* and of *intensification*, as induced by a transmission of rabies through the animal kingdom, were unknown. That there were an intensifying and an attenuating division of the animal kingdom was never even remotely suspected. Nevertheless, it is hardly too much to say that this disclosure was one of the most important of M. Pasteur's research. Nothing of real import was known to give any clue to the true nature of rabies, much less to its complete control. Both the clinical study of hydrophobia for centuries and the exploration of its morbid anatomy for generations had been altogether barren. The ignorance on the subject was as profound as it was universal.

But its one hopeful feature was the fact that it was by the highest authorities everywhere frankly acknowledged. This could not be better realised than by turning to the text-books of only a decade or two back, as to the great work on Surgery of the late Sir John Erichsen. There was, in consequence, in the best and most desirable quarters little or no misknowledge or misconception to clear away. From first to last M. Pasteur had the unexplored realm practically to himself, only its fringe having been traversed by his immediate predecessors or contemporaries, and in well-nigh every direction he investigated the disease.

Apart from its value in treatment, the inoculation has proved itself, as a new instrument of investigation, one of the greatest in the history of research. Nor is it too much to say that by his experimental and comparative methods of using the inoculation M. Pasteur has inaugurated a new epoch in the history of medicine, having in the realm of germ-disease originated amidst the lesions and the dry bones of morbid anatomy a very *renaissance* itself. His research of rabies is that of a master-mind which has vitally influenced and moulded every subsequent investigation of germ-disease.

It has been a merit of first importance that it has turned scientific inquiry from the charnel-house to living nature. From the *post-mortem* table M. Pasteur returned once more to a face to face investigation of the disease itself in the living organism. But his attitude and motive were somewhat different from those of the masters of antiquity, or from those of any exclusively clinical study. The clinical characteristics, *per se*, were of subordinate interest to him. The attitude of the ancient masters was at best that of a fine observer with the view to a perfect delineation. It was, however, but an investigation which was wholly confined to the crisis or final explosion of a malady. With M. Pasteur, on the contrary, the latent, evolving stages of a germ-disease, from the earliest and obscurest beginnings of this evolution, interested him much more profoundly than its explosive-point. His attitude to the disease was that, not so much of an artist, as of an investigator of superb scientific imagination who is bent on a complete reproduction, *de ovo*, of the entire natural history of the malady and of its relationships. The latent and mysterious incubation-period of a germ-disease he lit up from beginning to end with a new significance. So much so that the incubation-period of every germ-disease may be aptly termed the Pasteurian Period; for he conclusively proved it to be the only important stage alike for investigation and for treatment. From first to last M. Pasteur had a single eye, not so much to the diagnostic features of rabies or to its identification from all other diseases, as to the points wherein it resembles many diseases, but, above all, to an identification of its pathogenic micro-organism with an elucidation of its seat of germination and its *modus vivendi* in the living organism and, through such commanding knowledge, its complete control.

To the positive, face to face study of the active disease of the ancients, M. Pasteur added the experimental methods of chemistry and physics. And he accomplished this achievement with such great results that, with Harvey, Hunter, Lord Lister and the greatest masters of medicine, he succeeded in converting medicine into one of the most fruitful of the "applied" sciences, having imparted to the investigation of germ-disease a thoroughly scientific method and a genuinely creative end. The experimental investigation of the "virus" of rabies, he supplemented with the comparative methods which have yielded such magnificent results in every other field of science from embryology to anthropology and theology, from Goethe's superb generalisation on the unity of the vegetable and animal types to Darwin's still grander generalisation on evolution. Perhaps there is nothing of the research more characteristic and more invaluable than this wide-ranging comparison at every step. This use of the inoculation has imparted to it a range of light beyond even its own intrinsic brilliance. Already the experimental investigation has involved a comprehensive study of rabies as it exists, not only in man and in the dog, as for many centuries so exclusively studied, but in the rabbit, the guinea-pig, the ape, the cat, the sheep, the fox, the wolf, the hyena, the horse, the cow, the deer, the pig, even the fowl. And before the method can be said to be exhausted or its disclosures at an end, the disease has yet to be studied, if possible even more minutely, in each of these and probably other classes of animal, and likewise in its relationship to, and in the light of, every allied malady, however apparently remote.

These and many more disclosures of M. Pasteur's research are of as lasting validity in comprehending rabies as of immediate value in mastering it. For these reasons M. Pasteur's communications on rabies are invaluable as a working basis. Any explanation, not only of the preventive treatment, but of rabies itself as a germ-disease and of its relationships to other germ-diseases, much more of its possible origin in the animal kingdom, to be at all satisfactory must be grounded on the fundamental facts and the far-ranging results of the experimental research, and even built of them. Unfortunately, M. Pasteur's communications have been somewhat sparse, mere droppings, so to say, from the crucible, but of purest gold. The chief of them appeared in the *Comptes Rendus* and in *Annales de l'Institût Pasteur*. But perhaps the fullest exposition is M. Pasteur's own Address to the International Medical Congress at Copenhagen. In like manner the works of Magendie, Galtier, Bouchard, Nocard, Brown-Séquard, and, above all, of Metschnikoff, are most important and have proved of much value. Not less suggestive are the Reports of the special Commissions to the French Government, and, on the other hand, Koch's researches on tubercle and on malarial fever which are works of great genius. In England, the able investigations of Sir Victor Horsley and of Mr Dowdeswell are extremely valuable; and not less important are the various Reports to the Government. The Report in respect of the rabbit in Australia, and the Report to the House of Lords regarding the surgical treatment of rabidised wounds are as exhaustive as they are practical. But of still greater importance is the extremely interesting Report on the outbreak of deer-rabies at Richmond

Park during 1886–7. Above all, the Report on M. Pasteur's treatment of hydrophobia to the Local Government Board by a very special Committee of experts is the most masterly and the most authoritative statement which has appeared ; it has been most helpful.

On the basis of these wide researches, the following work has been grounded. It is a study of rabies in a threefold direction, its causation in the individual organism ; its place amongst germ-diseases with the end of bacterial agency in the animal economy; and, lastly, its origin in the animal kingdom. The treatment of the subject is from a series of standpoints which, in view, are far-ranging through the realm of bacterial life and activity, and which are perhaps not the least important features of the work. Thus, in the causation of the disease, the sensory rather than the motor nerve-roots of the cerebro-spinal axis are viewed as the specific nidus of the rabies-microbe, the pathogenic irritation of which is the prime lesion of the malady and underlying all the lesions. The rabies-microbe itself is described as of the simplest to the most complex structure. Far from being always simple and amorphous, it is viewed as in reality multiform, the quantity in the cerebro-spinal axis, and how it is organised, constituting the determining factor of every form of rabies. The paralytic element is taken as much the most important in canine-rabies itself, or in that of even the most attenuating division of the animal kingdom. In like manner the rabies of the sympathetic system is viewed as by far the most serious form of the disease, constituting the rabies characteristic of the intensifying division of the animal kingdom. It is taken as the sole factor of paralytic-rabies with its implication of the secreting system and of every infective form of the malady or of any paralytic element even in canine madness itself. In the consideration of the place of rabies amongst germ-diseases, the malady is treated and expounded as essentially a preventive rather than a prophylactic disease, these being described as the two great orders of the entire realm of germ-disease. Moreover, the particular

tissue which forms the exclusive germinating ground of the prophylactic order, on the one hand, and likewise of the preventive
orders, centric and peripheral, on the other hand, and as the
formative factor of the order, is carefully examined. The very
special prophylaxis of the prophylactic type of germ-disease and
the general immunity of the preventive type are discussed and explained in detail, and as indicating how far the specific germinating
tissue of the particular order of protection induces the protection.
On the other hand, the end of bacterial agency in the germinating
tissues of the living economy is also carefully examined, and its vast
importance in the origin and establishment of secreting-organs and as
a factor of evolution itself. The following study of rabies is largely
a revelation of this growth, or of the development of the pathological
into the physiological. Again, in the consideration of the origin of
rabies in the animal kingdom, the canine source of every form of the
malady which presents itself is gravely doubted; and the instability
and fading, final character of canine-rabies, as that of the entire
attenuating division, is demonstrated. The malady is viewed as,
primarily, a germ-disease of the intensifying rather than of the
attenuating division of the animal kingdom; and the universally
excellent results which follow the use of the dog-muzzle are accounted for and explained. These are problems of very profound
practical not less than of theoretic interest, which are worthy of
consideration in spite of their novelty; and the following work is
a study of rabies in this triple cycle of relationships.

Lastly, I am indebted for valuable criticisms to the scientific
expert who read the MS. for the Syndics of the Cambridge
University Press. I also desire to thank the staff of the University
Press for their aid whilst the work was being printed.

DAVID SIME.

HARRINGAY, LONDON, N.
November 1903.

CONTENTS.

CHAP.   PAGE

I.   The salivary gland, as the seat of rabies 1

II.   The bulbar substance and the lumbar-swelling, as the specific site in the nervous system 20

III.   Determination of the seat of germination from the symptoms and signs 36

IV.   Rabies of the sympathetic nervous system 50

V.   The "rabies-virus," quantitative rather than qualitative in character 64

VI.   The multiform structure of the rabies-microbe 78

VII. Mode and route of conveyance of the rabies-germ to the cerebro-spinal substance 90

VIII. The order of germ-diseases to which rabies belongs . . . 99

IX.   Pre-incubation period and incubation proper 119

X.   Rabies, a germ-disease of centric not of peripheral connective-tissue 133

XI.   The prevention and protection imparted by rabies-virus . . . 156

XII. The relation of bacterial agency to secreting organs and to the evolution of the animal organism 179

XIII. Is canine-rabies the primary form of the disease in the animal kingdom ? 204

XIV. Rabies, a germ-disease of intensifiers 222

XV. Why rabies prevails in the dog 236

XVI. How rabies arises in intensifiers 251

INDEX 275

CHAPTER I.

THE SALIVARY GLAND AS THE SEAT OF RABIES.

THE bite of a rabid animal being in every case essential to infection, it might naturally be expected, and in point of fact has been from time immemorial inferred, that the infective material of rabies lies in the salivary secretion and salivary glandular substance; or, in other words, that the salivary gland is the prime seat of the rabific microbe and the special centre of the elaboration of its "virus." Long before and up to M. Pasteur's investigation, this was a deeply rooted and widely spread idea. Now there can be no question that the "virus," or rabies-germ, or both agents, are to be obtained more constantly from the salivary secretion than from any other secreting structure in the infected organism. Why the salivary secretion should thus, above all secretions, be so frequently, and likewise invariably so *primarily* affected, is not without significance, and will receive careful attention in the sequel. Meanwhile, it is essential to point out that if the "virus" is present in the salivary gland and its secretion, when absent from all others, it by no means follows that it is invariably so. Not every mad dog, as so generally believed, is capable of imparting infection with its bite, although it be an effectual one, *i.e.* in a situation and under conditions the most favourable for infection. And, moreover, the bites of even the most dangerously rabid dog are not by any means invariably rabic, or infective, and, when this is the fact, not in every case equally rabic. There are cases of ordinary "furious" or of exclusively convulsive canine-rabies, where the salivary secretion is absolutely unaffected with "virus." The percentage of bites which never once fail to impart infection is small in the extreme and, as M. Pasteur has frequently pointed out, "altogether exceptional." Nevertheless, it is undoubted that such cases do on very rare occasions present themselves; and, moreover, there is good reason to show that they always occur at the *outset* of every extensive epidemic of the disease.

Hence, all dog bites, whether rabic or not, have hitherto been systematically treated as infective. All suspicious dogs which have bitten have been as summarily dealt with as if dangerously rabid. The custom, still well-nigh universal, but an extremely senseless one, and which has probably been handed down from the darkest of the so-called Dark Ages, has, hitherto, been to at once destroy any dog which has bitten under suspicious circumstances, not only for fear such animal should be rabid and bite others,—a reasonable enough precaution if an unreasonably excessive one,—but in case it should become rabid and, mysteriously enough, thereby doom the victims it has bitten! Not a few weird fallacies of this order still cling like cobwebs around this senile custom ; in this, if in nothing else, disclosing its extremely remote antiquity. The practice of centuries in this matter, and presumably with the object of "erring on the safe side," has been, not so much to give a dog a bad name and then hang him, as to hang the unhappy dog, and then give him a bad name! But has the error been altogether on the safe side? A little consideration will decide.

If a dog which has bitten is summarily to be destroyed on the mere suspicion of rabies, the destruction of the suspected animal cannot, in spite of all the sophistry of the most plausible optimism, prevent the development of the disease in the person so bitten; provided the bite be really a rabic one. If the man has been effectually bitten by a rabid animal, and if the salivary secretion of the latter at the moment of attack has been genuinely rabic;—but the one phenomenon by no means necessarily follows from the other,—such a procedure, however prompt and thorough, cannot prevent the development of hydrophobia, any more than summarily shooting a burglar will extinguish the burning building which he has so effectually kindled. It will not prevent the development of the disease, any more than the escape or the preservation of the dog, if not really rabid, or even when genuinely rabid if its bite be not really rabic, will by any possibility cause rabies. In either case, to precipitately destroy the animal can do no good, but to a certainty will end in the most disastrous regret, for such a procedure destroys once and for ever much valuable information, which otherwise would certainly be disclosed by the preservation (for even a week or ten days) of the animal.

Thus, if the suspicion be groundless, the person bitten, after the untimely destruction of the animal, can never be certain whether or not at the moment of attack it was really rabid. Consequently, for many months thereafter, if not years, the man, however strong-minded, will become a victim, and possibly a very needless one, to the most harassing dread and delusion; which can only become more fixed and acute as time passes, and which, there is some reason to believe, have not unfrequently ended, in neurotic subjects, in hopeless alcoholism or in genuine insanity itself. On the other hand, in the event of the victim to the dog-bite proving to be actually infected, the prostrating dread arising from the uncertainty of this fact will only have the effect of intensifying a case of, it may be, a less and even the least severe form of hydrophobia,—a convulsive hydrophobia,—and easily amenable to the Pasteurian "prevention," into one of the most deadly paralytic forms, and which probably no course of inoculations could "prevent." Of all conditions favour-able to the development of the rabific microbe, such unceasing and prostrating anguish is, there is good reason to show, the most "pre-disposing." Now if, instead of ruthlessly destroying the suspected dog, it be chained up and kept under competent observation for a few days, the nightmare dread will soon be cleared. If at the moment of attack the animal has been really rabid, on confinement it will at once reveal this fact; and all the more readily and effec-tually for the confinement and the strictest suspicion and scrutiny. But, although unquestionably rabid, it will not follow that the bite of such a dog will be infective; for it by no means follows that the salivary secretion of the ordinary "furious" canine-rabies is invariably charged with the "virus" of the disease. On the preservation of the animal, however, this important fact, or the essentially convulsive or "furious" character of the malady, could at once be disclosed. But, again, under competent observation it might and would be, sooner or later, found that, whilst not rabid at the moment of inflicting the bites, the animal, nevertheless, was unquestionably in the incubation-stage of the disease. This likewise is a revelation of the utmost value. If the animal do not exhibit rabies before a week or ten days after having inflicted the bite, it may be taken for granted that there has been no infection in the case, even although the canine-rabies, when developed, should prove to be of the most infective and deadly character, and although the wounds inflicted should be of the most extensive and dangerous kind. There is no evidence whatever to prove that a dog, or any other animal, merely in the incubation-period of the disease,—not at least until the final stages of incubation,—is capable of imparting rabies with its bite ; there being good ground to show that the salivary secretion is not in any way or to the slightest extent charged with "virus" or the rabies-germ during any such stage of the malady. What possible benefit, then, can accrue from the prompt destruction of a rabid dog merely in the incubation-stage of the disease? How, in such circumstances, can the preservation of a suspected dog, however "furious," fail to prove of inexpressible value to the victim of its bite, since, under competent examination, it has been so clearly established by the delay that the wounds inflicted could not by any possibility have been rabic, having been inflicted at a stage of the malady when infection was impossible? Lastly, if it should turn out on examination that the suspected animal is not rabid at all, merely " aggressive " and savage, and that the bite of the animal is, therefore, not in any sense rabic, as in the vast majority of dog-bites must necessarily be the case,—for canine-rabies, after all, is fortunately a very rare disease,—then, by the disclosure of such a fact, the patient's peace of mind may be at once restored. By the heedless destruction of the animal all such light is effectually ex- tinguished. If to summarily destroy a suspected animal be "an error *in the right direction*" and *"on the safe side,"* where is the particular safety? where is the wisdom of such a proceeding? It is but the blind act of panic, which is always as fatuous as it is fatal. To destroy a suspected creature, merely on suspicion and in a panic, is to destroy, not the suspicion nor the panic, but the only source of information on the subject, and the only guide to action. Is this, then, desirable?

From such facts, if there were no other, it is obvious that the infective rate of canine-rabies itself, or that of any other animal equally capable of attenuating the disease, is far from constant or invariable. All animals are not by any means alike when the rabies-germ is transmitted serially through them. The vast majority of animals *intensify* the disease on transmission. As we shall see more fully as we proceed, the entire herbivorous order, great and small, from the horse to the guinea-pig, intensify rabies, when the disease is passed serially through any given group. On the other hand, there are animals which progressively *attenuate* or lessen the disease as it is passed through them. The monkey is an excellent example of this division of the animal kingdom. But the attenuating division is very much smaller than the intensifying ; and it was a considerable time before M. Pasteur actually discovered that the monkey was capable of progressively attenuating the rabies-virus of even the most potent forms of the disease. The animal kingdom, then, may conveniently be divided into *attenuators* and *intensifiers*; or the class of animal, such as the herbivorous, which intensifies rabies on its being transmitted serially, and the class of animal, such as the monkey or the dog, which attenuates the disease on its being transmitted through a group from one to the other. In studying the disease, these two important orders must always be borne in mind ; for they are absolute contrasts.

The condition of the salivary secretion with respect to the possession of the infective material of the malady is no more uniform than any other feature of the disease, or even than any other feature of the salivary secretion itself. A dog may be most violently "furious," biting incessantly, without its bite being necessarily rabic ; just as, on the contrary,—which, however, is often ignored,—a dog may be profoundly and paralytically rabid without being at all frantic or "furious," and without any tendency to bite, and yet the salivary secretion of the animal be uniformly saturated with "virus." The salivary secretion of every animal capable of attenuating rabies, on transmission, is not precisely alike, in any group of cases, either in amount, in consistency, in liquidity, or in infectiveness, any more than all cases are precisely alike in the length of the incubation-period, in the duration and sequence of the symptoms, and in the extent and character of the lesions ; well-nigh every case, as M. Pasteur from the first pointed out, having its own set of symptoms, its own train of lesions, its own incubation-period, and its own infective rate, or a character of the salivary secretion, with respect to infectiveness, peculiar to itself. Thus, in the great majority of the exclusively "furious" or convulsive, as opposed to the convulso-paralytic, or of the pronounced paralytic and "mortal" forms, the salivary secretion is scanty in amount ; and this scanty secretion is viscid, clammy and frothy in character. In profound paralytic rabies, on the contrary, the salivary secretion is copious in amount ; and this copious secretion is, moreover, thin and liquid in the extreme and constantly dripping from the angles of the mouth. This feature has been noted, directly or indirectly, by every modern authority. M. Galtier noted it very emphatically from the outset in his admirable description of the disease in the rabbit. "There is," he says, "*always an abundant flow of saliva*[1]."

[1] *Bull. Académ. de Méd.*, January 25, 1881.

And precisely the same difference is noticeable in the churned frothiness of convulsions, epilepsy and acute mania, as contrasted with the thin, copious dribbling of idiotcy or of apoplectic paralysis. Now, if it so happened that the scanty and frothy salivary secretion of the ordinary "furious" rabies,—and this, it must be emphasised, is the most prevalent form of the disease in the dog,—*alone* contained the infective matter; were the salivary secretion of such cases not merely variously charged, but invariably saturated with the virus-germ, such cases would still be completely amenable to local surgical treatment. It would be but like wiping out the acrid insect-froth and its eggs from the interior of a flower. This, however, is far from the fact. The "furious" cases, prevalent as they are in every outbreak, are the least likely to impart infection by a bite, in spite of the fact that they are by far the most aggressive; because the viscid, churned salivary secretion, characteristic of such cases, would not, irrespective of local treatment, necessarily be absorbed, being the least absorbent of any form of secretion; and because, on the other hand, if copious in amount and highly absorbent, which is contrary to the fact, the secretion contains, there is good evidence to show, and in proportion to the amount of mere "fury" or convulsiveness, little or no virus. With respect to the essentially paralytic or "dumb" forms, on the other hand, we find that the salivary secretion is practically unlimited; and, moreover, that, far from being viscid, it is thin, liquid and absorbent in the highest degree, like the secretion of any other paralysis, and in proportion to the extent of the paralysis. So much so that, were the secretion but slightly and occasionally charged with the "virus," which, unfortunately, is diametrically opposed to the fact, it is inconceivable that any local surgical treatment, however prompt and thorough, could have the slightest effect in "preventing" its absorption in the wounded tissues. No amount of excision and cauterising, however immediate, will prevent the absorption of a hypodermic syringeful of a solution of morphia or strychnine, much less of tuberculin or of serpent-venom, or of prussic acid; yet any of these is not more easily absorbed than the thin, liquid rabic secretion of a profoundly paralytic or "dumb" canine-rabies. But these cases, where the saliva is so abundant and so easily absorbed, are likewise the very cases in which the secretion is more or less saturated with "virus," the amount of saturation being also proportioned to the amount of paralysis in the case. They are forms of the disease where the ancient surgical treatment is most wanted but of least avail;

" the cauterising," etc., when heroically done, having the effect, it may be, of sealing up the rabific microbes in the tissues rather than of destroying them. The amount of "virus" in the saliva of canine-rabies, then, far from being equal, uniform, and constant, would appear to range from zero or absolute nil up to saturation-point.

Nor is the salivary gland the only secreting organ in which the rabies-germ is to be found. Nevertheless, from the remotest ages, the "virus" has been exclusively associated with the salivary secretion; and even from the earliest of the experimental investigations it has always been, first and foremost, purposely searched for, and its presence proved, in the saliva or salivary apparatus of the infected dog. Thus, Paul Bert, Nocard of Alfort, Duboué, Galtier of Lyons, and the entire circle of French investigators,—for from the first France took the lead in the experimental investigations,—had, as their first discoveries, ascertained that the substance of the salivary and parotid glands, in severe cases, and according to their severity and the predominance of the paralytic element, is invariably rabic. In separating and differentiating the virulent and non-virulent elements of even this salivary structure itself, M. Nocard went a step further than other investigators. He ingeniously dialysed the saliva, with the result, which will be referred to again, that, whilst the solid elements of the secretion were found to be virulent, the liquid element, passed through the dialyser, when similarly injected into healthy animals, on every occasion failed to rabidise. From such experiments the impression was, if anything, but deepened that the salivary tissue was the prime seat of the rabies-germ, and the exclusive site of the elaboration of its virus.

" The saliva," as M. Pasteur justly stated, on publishing the first results of his own investigation, " was the only part where the presence of the virus had been detected with certainty[1]."

So deeply rooted was this idea in the best prevalent conceptions of the malady, that M. Pasteur himself began his great research with the salivary substance of a child who had died of hydrophobia. But hydrophobia is *par excellence* the convulsive or "furious" rabies of the dog. Is it not obvious, therefore, from this one historic "instance," that the salivary secretion of the most ordinary rabies, not less than that of the very rare "dumb" or paralytic form, is invariably rabic? It does not follow. This, as it happened, was no ordinary "instance"; and it was fortunate for humanity that it was not.

[1] *Comptes Rendus*, Dec. 11, 1882.

From the fact of being that of a young child, and more especially, as we shall see hereafter, a delicate young girl, this case was, there is good reason to show, in all likelihood of the severest form of hydrophobia to be met with, probably a case of paralytic hydrophobia. If this were so, the child's salivary substance would undoubtedly be exceptionally rabic, and, therefore, exceptionally favourable for experimentation. Be this as it may, certain it is that, if M. Pasteur began his research with the salivary substance, he by no means kept to it. He very far from adopted it even from the most pronounced paralytic forms of rabies, although the most infective, as the source whence to obtain the "virus" in its purest, most unadulterated and most "unmodified" condition, or in point of fact as a source from which to obtain it at all. It would appear that the saliva of the most profound paralytic forms of rabies to be met with, however saturated with "virus," is frequently impure and adulterated in the extreme, and not at all to be relied on for experimental purposes.

" In the saliva of rabid animals the virus is found associated with various micro-organisms; and the inoculations of this can give rise to death in one of three modes :

(*a*)   By the new microbe, which we have described under the name of 'the microbe of saliva.'

(*b*)   By the excessive development of pus.

(*c*)   By rabies[1]."

But if this holds good of the saliva of the profoundest paralytic canine-rabies, or rabbit-rabies itself, how much more is it true of the rabic saliva, when such presents itself, of an ordinary "furious" or *convulsive* rabies? If this inconstancy and uncertainty of infectiveness should exist in the case of an admittedly most virulent saliva arising, probably, from the "association" of distinctly antagonistic elements, what shall be said of the saliva of the rabid dog, *furiously* rabid, which is not virulent, and which contains no infective material at all? Such unquestionably exists, and not only on rare occasions, but in a very considerable percentage of cases. Thus, in direct opposition to the Lyons school, which had all but formally stated it as a fundamental fact of rabies, that the "virus" exists primarily and invariably in the salivary secretion, M. Pasteur deliberately asserted at the outset of his own research that "The saliva inoculated by a bite, or by direct injection, into the areolar tissue, *does not constantly give rise to rabies*[2]."

[1] *Comptes Rendus*, Dec. 11, 1882.   [2] *Ibidem.*

The saliva of the mad dog, then, is not only, *not* invariably, infective, but, as it so happens, even on the rare occasions when it is, the rabic material is by no means confined to the salivary glandular substance. According to the severity of the case, and to the predominance of the paralytic over a merely convulsive element, apparently well-nigh every secreting organ is capable of more or less eliminating the "virus." At an early stage of the experimental investigation, Paul Bert ascertained that the bronchial mucus "was to a high degree virulent." And Galtier was able to detect the "virus" "not only in the lingual glands, but in the bucco-pharyngeal mucous membrane." It has also been detected in the mucous membrane of the stomach, and in the substance of the liver itself. It has been copiously found by Galtier, Bouchard, and others in the lymphatic glands and fluids, and on very rare occasions by M. Pasteur himself even in the blood stream. Above all, it has been discovered by M. Pasteur in the richest abundance in the nervous substance of the entire cerebro-spinal substance from its centre to its remotest periphery. Still more recently, Burdoni-Uffreduzzi, of Turin, has made an extensive series of experiments on dogs and various animals, solely "to test the different degrees of virulence of the various organs." And he has found, not only that "various parts of the brain of a rabid animal show different degrees of virulence," as demonstrated so conclusively by M. Pasteur himself, but that "the pancreatic gland is nearly as virulent as the brain"; and, moreover, that "the liver and spleen, although seemingly acting much less strongly as media of the disease, are nevertheless, at times," or in the most severe paralytic cases, "highly charged and even infiltrated with the virus[1]." Thus, it is clear that there is probably not a secreting gland, any more than a mucous membrane, which, according to the paralysing virulence of the case, is not more or less charged with "virus," the amount of paralysis being a very fair index of the amount of the virus and rabific microbe in the glandular or secreting system. The salivary gland, if more constantly and intensely virulent than any other secreting organ, is by no means the only organ which eliminates "virus." The existence of the infective material in this structure is neither constant, nor, when present, is its presence in the secretion by any means unique.

The bite of a mad dog, therefore, although the animal should die of the rabies, furiously rabid, is not necessarily, and very far from

---

[1] *Nature*, Oct. 27, 1887, The Sixth International Congress of Hygiene in Vienna.

invariably, infective. The reverse of this constancy is now a well-established fact. How, under such circumstances, can the salivary gland be viewed as the specific seat of the rabies-germ, and where it alone elaborates its "virus"?

But, it may be said, and with justice, that it does not follow, because the bite of a mad dog fails to rabidise in some instances, that it is not necessarily a rabic one in any instance, or, in other words, that there is no "virus" at all in this salivary secretion. The bite may be a genuinely rabic one, and yet fail to infect. As it so happens, there are in every living animal natural *preventative* conditions of a very positive and constant character, which render the fact of infection far from certain in the most desperate and formidable attacks. These conditions may be described as of an extrinsic and an intrinsic character. The *extrinsic* preventative conditions are, so to speak, accidental to, or at least independent of, the animal or its condition, and are common to all animals. They are comprised in such natural acquisitions as fur, hair, horn, hoof, wool, clothing, etc., which at times, as in the sheep, effectually clear and clean a venomous bite of its "virus." Although more or less common to all animals, such extrinsic defence is, however, preeminently characteristic of the class of animals capable of intensifying rabies on transmission, such as the guinea-pig, hare, and rabbit; being in this entire order, the main, and in some of the class, such as the rabbit, probably the exclusive preventative conditions. The strictly *intrinsic* preventative conditions, on the contrary, are of the most vital importance to the animal, and are in reality but an expression of its vigorous vitality; this all-important refractory power, being, as we shall see, essentially physiological. This intrinsic refractory capacity is in reality pre-eminently, if not exclusively, characteristic of the class of animals capable of attenuating the disease on transmission, such as man, the monkey, and the dog; and in respect of the entire intensifying division of the animal kingdom, is reduced to a minimum, and in the most potent intensifiers is even conspicuous for its absence. Now, in nature these preventative conditions in one form or another, and often in combination, are constantly at work to ward off infection. In an attenuating animal, such as the dog, both conditions are of the most pronounced character. For refractoriness to rabies, man is certainly not less specially provided than the dog, and, probably, for the same reason. John Hunter has even noted that "dogs are *more* susceptible of the infection than the human species."

In confirmation of this opinion he gives the following very striking and conclusive case :

"Four men and twelve dogs were bitten by the same mad dog ; and every one of the dogs died of the disease, whilst all the four men escaped, though they used no other means of prevention (surgical) but such as we see every day to fail."

As the entire number of the dogs was here rabidised, there can be no question of the infecting power of the attacking animal. The bite of a rabid dog, therefore, which fails to infect, does not necessarily prove that there is no "virus" in the salivary secretion. Or, to take a more common illustration in which man himself is infected, Hunter has likewise narrated a case, where not less than twenty people were bitten by the same mad dog, "*only one of whom took rabies.*" This historic case has given rise to much criticism, and, with some ingenuity, and not a little condescension, has been explained away as an altogether "exceptional instance."

"We have failed," says Dr Suzor, "in our endeavours to find out statistics referring to rabies in the writings of John Hunter. He only states that the deaths are occasionally very few after the bite of rabid dogs ; and quotes the best case he knows of in that respect ; viz. twenty persons bitten by the same mad dog, and only one death supervening among them ; no other details are given. It would be impossible to put down a percentage *from that one exceptional and incompletely reported case*; and it is to be regretted that the old master did not think it worth his while giving figures in the course of his otherwise excellent paper[1]."

Far from the mortality of hydrophobia being only one in twenty bitten, the infective rate rises apparently, with varying authorities and from various points of view, from 15 to 25 and 30 per cent.; the Comité d'Hygiène of France, for the years 1862–72, giving even a mortality of over 50 per cent.! Clearly enough, if such estimates be accurate, Hunter's is inadequate in the extreme. But if Hunter's observation is not inaccurate and, above all, far from being "exceptional," what advantage is there in exaggerating the mortality of the disease or its infective rate? This does not magnify the efficacy of M. Pasteur's masterly treatment; it but blurs and confuses what actual preventative and protective results it is capable of, like clouds of incense. Is Hunter's observation, however, so worthless and incomplete? If so, it is very unlike the other observations

[1] *Hydrophobia ; M. Pasteur's System*, by Renaud Suzor, M.D. *Italics not Dr Suzor's.*

of this far-sighted, singularly clear-minded man of genius. "The old master" has certainly "thought it worth his while to give figures." But for this fact the observation would never have been recorded by him. If it was but a transient surmise it was a most happy one, and marvellously like an intuition of genius. That the "instance" was in reality a highly characteristic and typical one, could not be better shown than by the fact that the Committee of Experts, appointed to investigate the merits of the inoculative treatment for the Local Government Board, unanimously came to the conclusion, and after the most searching scrutiny into every kind of statistics bearing on the mortality of hydrophobia, that the average mortality of the disease from all causes is five per cent., or *one in twenty bitten by the rabid dog*[1]. But this is precisely the percentage announced by Hunter. No better proof, therefore, could be afforded, not only of the clearness and the justness of this great master's observation, but of the care and of the rare insight with which he recorded. After all, this "instance," it would appear, was the one, above all others, which was worthy of his selection. Hunter's famous group, consequently, may be taken, as without doubt he took it himself, as a tolerably typical and common one.

The rabic condition of the saliva in ordinary dog-madness, far from being constant and uniform, is, in reality, both intermittent and most unequal. So much so that, not merely five per cent., but it is possible only one out of fifty, or even out of a hundred, persons attacked by the same mad dog is at times actually infected. And this inconstancy or inequality is not less obvious in the infection of dogs themselves. This could not, perhaps, be better illustrated than by the crucial set of experiments performed by M. Pasteur before the Commission, which was appointed by the French Government. M. Pasteur sent this Commission "nineteen dogs vaccinated in succession; that is to say, dogs which had been rendered *refractory* by preventative inoculations." These nineteen "protected" dogs were divided into groups with another nineteen "unprotected" dogs, which were "brought from the pound without any sort of selection"; and both classes of animal in their respective groups were subjected together to the same tests. Summing up their observations as to the state of the thirty-eight animals so crucially tested before them, the Commission found that "out of the nineteen control (or unprotected) dogs, six were bitten; of which six, three have taken rabies; seven

[1] Report on M. Pasteur's Treatment of Hydrophobia for Local Government Board.

received intravenous inoculation, of which five have died of rabies; five were trephined and inoculated on the brain, the five have died of rabies. On the other hand, *not one of the vaccinated dogs has taken rabies*[1]."

These were certainly most triumphant results, of which the entire scientific world was proud; for they were unapproached and absolutely irrefutable. But the disclosure is of value, and hardly less so, in respect of the remarkable negative results also revealed. It is true that not one of the nineteen "protected" dogs took rabies. But, on the other hand, the entire group of unprotected dogs, "brought from the pound without any sort of selection," by no means succumbed to the disease. Undoubtedly all the "control" animals, in spite of the fact that they were as crucially experimented upon as the protected, were *not* rabidised. On the contrary, of the eighteen animals accounted for (for, apparently, one of the "control" dogs died suddenly irrespective of rabies), *not less than five escaped rabies*, *i.e.* 28 per cent. or nearly a third of the entire number. And this percentage loses nothing in significance on examining it in detail. Not less than *two* of the escapes occurred in the group of animals which had received direct intravenous inoculation itself. In this case, at all events, there could be no question of the fact that the virus, if it existed in the salivary secretion, had been directly introduced into the system. Nevertheless, nearly a third of the animals thus so adequately infected failed to take the disease. But in nature intravenous inoculation of so effective a character must be rare in the extreme. Turning, then, to the group experimented upon, which is the best imitation of nature, in other words, where the unprotected animals were *bitten* by rabid dogs, one finds that the number of escapes is actually doubled. In spite of the fact that all these "unprotected" dogs were as effectually bitten as the most absolutely unprotected circumstances would permit, and, moreover, by rabid animals whose infective capacity was sufficiently demonstrated, nevertheless, not less than one half of the animals so attacked completely escaped the disease. Thus, even of completely unprotected dogs so effectually attacked, and the salivary secretion of the attacking animal being so copiously introduced into the subcutaneous tissues, apparently not less than 50 per cent. escape. Who could have foretold that there was such a percentage of escapes under such

[1] M. Pasteur's Communication to International Medical Congress at Copenhagen, Aug. 11, 1884.

exceptionally and appallingly favourable circumstances for infection?
Where is there any evidence in such results of the saliva of the rabid
dog being uniformly or invariably rabic?

This same inconstancy was likewise revealed in Sir Victor
Horsley's equally crucial experiments on *rabbits* with ordinary dog-
virus, performed for the Committee appointed by the Local Government Board. In spite of the fact that the animals which were
bitten so effectually, *i.e.* through the bare skin, by the rabid dogs
employed for this purpose, were unprotected, if not unprotectable,
rabbits, in one set of the experiments—"nos. 4 and 5"—actually
25 per cent. escaped infection; and in another set—"no. 2"—not
less than 50 per cent. escaped[1]. If, therefore, actually 50 per cent.
escaped infection, and after the very effective bite of such undeniably
rabid dogs, it was probably at least in part due to the fact that, in
these escapes, the bite was not really a virulent one, and that, for
these particular cases, the saliva of the attacking animals contained
no "virus" whatever. What "virus" the salivary secretion of the
attacking animal was charged with was of an occasional, not of a
constant and of a uniform flow. Wherever else, or in whatever other
structure or system of the rabidised animal the rabies-germ may
be constant and never-failing, most certainly it is not in the salivary
glandular substance.

In canine-rabies then, and in that of every animal capable of
attenuating the disease,—in other words, in rabies of an essentially
"furious" or convulsive character,—the salivary secretion, far from
being constantly or uniformly rabic, is frequently enough but *intermittently* so. The flow of the rabific microbe into the secretion is,
obviously, neither constant, nor, when it occurs, uniform and unvarying in volume, but unequal, irregular and intermittent. The
salivary secretion is invariably saturated with "virus," and constantly and uniformly rabic, only in the very profoundest paralytic
canine-rabies to be met with. Such a form of the disease, however,
so far as the dog or any attenuator is concerned, is "altogether
exceptional." It would appear that the more "dumb" and paralytic
the dog-madness, and, consequently, the higher the infective rate, the
rarer it becomes.

But, again, the salivary secretion of a mad dog, and however
"furiously" mad, or of any case of essentially *convulsive*, as opposed to *paralytic*, rabies, is not necessarily even occasionally or

[1] Report for Local Government Board, Appendix A, p. 3.

intermittently infective. In a large percentage of cases the bite of the animal is not infective, the salivary secretion being wholly devoid of "virus." M. Pasteur has noted and recorded many cases where unprotected dogs, bitten by rabid dogs, and most effectually through the bare skin, and in sites the most favourable, have completely escaped infection. And that the inoculation, in spite of the most ferocious onslaught and the direct introduction of a copious supply of the salivary secretion, was no infection whatever; that, having failed to rabidise, it in no way "protected" the animals; and, more-over, that the attacked animals were, to begin with, in no sense "immunes" by nature, has been demonstrated by the fact that these same animals, when subsequently inoculated with genuine "virus" from the bulb of a rabid animal which has just died, succumbed to the disease like any other unprotected animal.

Again, and still more signal proof of the fact, the illustrious Magendie, a man of the same creative scientific foresight as M. Pasteur himself, transmitted the disease from and by one dog to another through four dogs in succession. The fourth died of rabies, "furiously mad," but it failed to impart the disease by its bite or bites to a fifth dog, the conditions of infection in this last being, nevertheless, precisely identical to those of the entire group which succumbed. Here, then, from the outset of any experimental research,—for this is the first on record,—was conclusive evidence that the dog was the most potent of attenuators, steadily and progressively diminishing the amount of "virus" in the salivary secretion itself. Not only was "the incubation-period" of the disease lengthened with every transmission, but by the time the initial rabies had been passed to the fourth dog, the virulence of the disease, or the amount of its "virus" in the salivary secretion, had been so diminished that this animal was absolutely unable to rabidise another dog with its bite. But, although the fifth dog failed to take the disease, the fourth died of genuine enough canine-rabies, "furiously mad"; and, moreover, although the salivary secretion of this latter failed to rabidise, it is certain, as shall be proved more clearly in due course, that an intracranial, or even subcutaneous, injection of an emulsion of its "bulb" would without fail have rabidised. Hence, it is beyond question that a dog may be furiously rabid, and die of the rabies, without its salivary secretion being necessarily charged with, or even at all invaded by, the "virus," and without, therefore, its bite being necessarily rabic. Is Magendie's observation, however, like Hunter's,

likewise merely a highly exceptional "instance," and not to be relied
on as an estimate?   On the contrary, one such fact is, as Lord Bacon
phrased it, "as good as a forest of facts"; a thousand, to the mind of
pre-eminent scientific foresight and imagination, not being any more
conclusive than one.   But in such an animal as the dog, which, as
Magendie's important transmission-experiments would alone indicate,
is probably one of the most potent attenuators of the disease in the
animal kingdom, such a result is even of common occurrence in every
outbreak.

And the subject, from a totally different standpoint, has been
still further experimentally investigated, by one of the ablest of the
English investigators.   The facts disclosed by Mr Dowdeswell in his
investigation of the disease,—perhaps not the least original in this
country,—strongly confirm the conclusion that the salivary secretion
of ordinary dog-rabies, *i.e.* a rabies of wholly convulsive character, or
from the beginning of the disease to death,—far from being constantly
or even intermittently infective, is, more frequently than not, wholly
devoid of "virus."   In the year 1885 there happened to be in London
and its neighbourhood a very extensive outbreak of canine-rabies,
which was so exceptionally prevalent that it necessitated on the part
of the Police Department the compulsory enforcement of the dog-
muzzle for months.   During this epidemic, which from first to last
was carefully studied by him, Mr Dowdeswell found that "experiments made by inoculation with the saliva of the rabid street-dogs
all failed to produce infection"; "thus confirming," as he justly
points out, "the reputed uncertainty of the results of the bite of
a rabid animal[1]."

Now, as it so happens, in even an extensive outbreak of dog-
madness, much the larger proportion of rabid dogs is affected with
the "furious" or convulsive, not with the "dumb" or paralytic forms
of the disease.   One can see very clearly from M. Pasteur's statistics,
as recorded in the Report for the Local Government Board in respect
of the rabid condition of the dogs which attacked and' bit his patients,
how little the pronounced paralytic forms, *i.e.* paralytic from first to
last, enter into the list of such outbreaks.   In ninety-one cases,
detailed in full, and recorded verbatim in the Report, there are not
more than *three*, or at most *four*, which can be said to strictly belong
to the class of "dumb" or pronounced paralytic rabies, completely

---

[1] For detailed report of these experiments see Mr Dowdeswell's able paper in
Trans. of Roy. Soc. 1887. Also in *Nature*, June 23, 1887, where there is an Abstract.

paralytic, *i.e.* from beginning to end of the disease[1]. It would appear, therefore, that it is exclusively in the convulsive forms of rabies, where the salivary secretion "all fails to produce infection." The very large proportion of rabid dogs in an outbreak of the disease,— probably in every case without exception which is wholly of the "furious" form, or convulsive from beginning to end,—cannot but rarely impart the disease with a bite, even when the wound inflicted is an efficient one; for their salivary secretion is not always or necessarily at all charged with the microbe of the disease. In other words, the infectiveness of the salivary or of any other secretion, or the presence of the "virus" in the salivary substance, depends upon and is wholly determined by the amount of paralysis in the case; but in dog-rabies a pronounced paralytic character is exceptional in the extreme. Most certainly, then, the saliva of a rabid dog, even when directly injected into the areolar tissue, "does not constantly give rise to rabies"; for, after such results, obviously enough it has not always the "virus" or rabies-germ to impart. How, under such circumstances, can the salivary gland be viewed as the prime and specific seat of the rabies-germ, and where it exclusively, or even mainly, elaborates its virus?

Nevertheless, it is undoubted that there are cases of canine-rabies, where the salivary secretion is copious in amount and incessant in its flow and invariably rabic, never once failing to impart infection. The English Committee in their Report for the Local Government Board refer to one such case which occurred at Deptford, where five people were bitten by the same rabid dog, "every one of whom took rabies and died[2]." Nor, unfortunately, is this appalling case unique. Other authorities have referred to cases of a like character and equally disastrous ; and M. Pasteur himself has recorded one case, that of Pantin, where, curiously enough, precisely the same number of people was bitten, every one of whom likewise took rabies and died. "On July 14, 1885, five persons were bitten by the same mad dog on the road to Pantin. The five persons took rabies and died[3]."

Fortunately, such cases in the dog are phenomenal, or, as

[1] See Report for Local Government Board, Appendix B, pp. 4—13. The cases referred to above are 15, 62, 73, and possibly 78. But even in these a persistently "dumb" or paralytic element, from first to last, is far from conclusive.

[2] Report for Local Government Board.

[3] *Comptes Rendus*, March 1, 1886.

M. Pasteur has over and over again pointed out, are "altogether exceptional[1]." It would appear then that, so far as imparting the disease by the salivary secretion is concerned, the infective rate of canine-rabies ranges from absolute *nil* up to a 100 per cent. itself; the higher the infective rate the scarcer the rabies. The disease steadily rises in infective rate with every rise of the paralytic element; and, conversely, when transmitted through the animal, it as progressively falls in infective rate, as it approaches more and more a wholly convulsive or "furious" character. For one such case as that of Deptford or Pantin in an epidemic, there are probably at least a score of cases like that of Hunter, where only one of twenty persons bitten by the same mad dog is infected. On the other hand, for one case like Hunter's, there are probably a dozen, if not a score, like those of Magendie and Dowdeswell, where, under the same circumstances, no infection takes place. It is found, then, that infection from the bite of a mad dog, of whose rabies there can be no question, may, on the rarest occasions, *invariably* occur ; less rarely, it may *frequently*, but not invariably occur ; still less rarely, it may *regularly*, every few bites, occur; still less rarely, *spasmodically*, *irregularly* and *inconstantly* ; still more common, it may *seldom* or even very rarely occur; lastly, in a considerable percentage, infection *may never take place at all*. The rabic condition of the salivary secretion, far from being invariable and uniform, is not less variable than the lesions and the symptoms of the disease, and for the same reason ; it is wholly determined by the amount of paralysis in the case, which in the dog, as in every animal equally capable of attenuating the malady, is an ever-varying and an ever-decreasing amount.

If this be so, it may be unhesitatingly asserted that, whilst it may be true that every case of hydrophobia is due to the bite of a mad dog, or of some rabid animal, yet the virus-germ of the disease cannot be primarily located in the saliva of such animal or necessarily germinated in the salivary gland at all; because, when the salivary secretion is even charged with the rabies-germ, it is by no means the only secretion which is so charged; and, not less conclusive, because the salivary secretion of a large number of rabid dogs in every outbreak "fails to produce infection"; every one of these dogs, notwithstanding, dying of rabies, "furiously mad." This, however, is a large percentage and it but increases with the dispersal of the malady through the animal, at last quite suddenly ending the epidemic. But

[1] *Comptes Rendus*, March 1, 1886.

when the salivary gland becomes so affected that its secretion is not only occasionally but invariably saturated with the virus-germ, never once failing in the longest group of cases to impart infection, it may be as unhesitatingly concluded that this implication of the gland is the effect of the general disease and secondary to it, not its cause or a primary process. The glandular system as a whole—not merely the salivary apparatus—becomes paralysed and infected in consequence of the infection and paralysis of some much more important and vital centre, on which it solely depends for its functional activity, and with which it is most intimately and structurally interwoven; the animals so affected being strictly confined to the essentially "paralytic" class. The vast importance, therefore, of the paralytic, as compared with the merely convulsive, element, characteristic and predominant as the latter is over the former, can hardly be exaggerated even in canine-rabies itself. The pronounced paralytic or "dumb" rabies of the dog, rare and exceptional though it be, is the most important form which presents itself even in this animal, and from which, as we shall see, all the others are really derived. For there is ground to show that every outbreak of dog-rabies begins as an epidemic from such paralytic forms, and from such exclusively. The notorious Deptford case, or the Pantin case, probably presented itself at the very outset of an extensive outbreak. Certain it is, from Magendie's experiments, that a simple convulsive or "furious" rabies, or even a convulse-paralytic rabies of high infective rate, would not be transmitted beyond three or four dogs in succession, before the salivary secretion, scanty in amount, and churned and frothy, would become completely devoid of "virus."

If such be the facts, it is certain that the salivary gland or its secretion cannot be the specific seat of germination of the rabies-microbe, or in point of fact its seat of germination at all. At most, it is but its main, and in some instances possibly its sole, channel of elimination.

CHAPTER II.

THE BULBAR SUBSTANCE AND LUMBAR-SWELLING AS THE SPECIFIC SITE IN THE NERVOUS SYSTEM.

THE rabies-germ being *par excellence* a micro-organism of nerve-structure, and, in certain extreme cases of the disease, of well-nigh every part of the nervous system, the question arises, what special region, if any, is its peculiar seat of cultivation? Is there one area or tract more than another where the microbe of the germ-disease habitually "resides"? Are the peripheral nerves in the infected wound this primary centre of germination? Or do the peripheral nerves of the salivary gland in their course to the spinal cord constitute the specific seat? Again, does this specific site lie exclusively in the encephalon or cerebellum, or in any particular section of such structure; or exclusively in the spinal cord itself; or in any particular area of the cord, such as the bulb or lumbar-swelling? Is there one tract more than another in the vast cerebro-spinal system to which the rabific microbe is sooner or later invariably conveyed, all through the so-called incubation-period, whatever the site or sites of infection in the periphery; and in which, in all cases of the disease, from the profoundest paralytic to the slightest convulsive forms, the rabific microbe is invariably present? This has been experimentally determined by M. Pasteur, and it has been accomplished in a two-fold direction; on the one hand, by a comparative study of the relative rabic condition of the nerve-tissue itself throughout the whole extent of the nervous system; and, on the other hand, and not less conclusively, by a comparative study of forms of rabies resulting from infection from various amounts of "virus," and at various sites in the periphery. Both methods of investigation have been exhaustive and masterly in the extreme, and, significantly enough, have led to precisely the same conclusion.

Firstly, then, what has the comparative investigation of *rabic nerve-tissue* disclosed?

Whilst it is unquestionable that the whole nervous system, to its utmost ramifications, is capable of cultivating the virus, and that the infective material is to be obtained in more or less quantity and more or less potency from every part of the nervous system, it is not less true that, so far as the disease in man or the dog or in any animal equally capable of attenuating the disease on transmission is concerned, such cases are altogether phenomenal. As there are forms of canine-rabies where the secretions, salivary or other, are so saturated with "virus" as never once to fail in imparting the disease, so there are cases where the rabific microbe is in all probability distributed over the entire nervous system. These forms of rabies, however, are characteristic only of the most potent of intensifiers, not of attenuators, or of the class of animals which intensify, not attenuate, rabies when transmitted through them. However common such forms may be in such an animal as the rabbit, it is certain that they are rare in the extreme in any outbreak of dog-rabies. In by far the large majority of cases in every outbreak, there is no such extensive dispersal of the rabific microbe in the nervous system itself, any more than in the secretions; and this holds good of the rabies of the entire attenuating division of the animal kingdom. In an animal capable of attenuating or deteriorating rabies on transmission, and in virtue of, and in proportion to, this "attenuating" power, a rabies of a relatively slight and of an essentially convulsive form is the general rule and the form normal to the animal. In this respect, likewise, the amount and the distribution of "virus" over the nervous system may be measured with tolerable accuracy by the prevalence of the paralytic element in the case; for this paralytic element in its turn is in reality solely determined by the amount and the distribution of virus-germ in the central nervous system. The more devoid the rabies of a pronounced paralytic character, or the more it approaches the simpler convulsive forms, the less copious the rabific microbe in the nervous centres, and, moreover, the less potent the virus elaborated by it. Such centres of the microbe will not only be the scantier and weaker, but their areas of activity will be the more isolated and limited. Every case of canine-rabies by no means presents the same amount of "virus" or virus-germ in the spinal-cord or brain. The disease is no more constant and invariable in this than in any other respect; such constancy holding good only of intensifiers. There is every variability in the infection of the cerebro-spinal substance, from the slightest tinge of "virus" up to saturation point; there is every variability in the distribution of the specific micro-organism from the bulb to the encephalon and the peripheral nerves. In one case, there may be simultaneously two, three, or more spreading centres in various parts of the cerebro-spinal axis which may, here and there, touch and ultimately coalesce, as in a confluent chain of fire. In another case, these centres may be strictly isolated from each other all through the disease, and, so to speak, but mere glowing sparks. Here, again, as in the so-called incubation-period, the lesions, the symptoms and the infective rate, there is nothing more characteristic of the disease —at least as it affects an attenuator—than its extreme variability and lack of uniformity. Every case of canine-rabies or monkey-rabies has its own amount of rabific microbe, and even this amount localised in its own set of nerve-centres. And it is wholly in consequence of this fact that every case has its own incubation-period, its own lesions, its own symptoms, and its own infective rate.

Whilst an experimental investigation of the rabic tissues discloses the fact that the "virus" is invariably found in the nervous substance, either of the brain, the spinal cord, the nerves, or of the salivary or other glands,—the latter being affected solely through their nervous elements,—or in extreme paralytic cases of all these regions combined, nevertheless, a *comparative* investigation of these various regions not less clearly discloses that, except in the profounder paralytic forms, the "virus" is by no means so plentiful and so uniformly diffused. The "virus" may be confined to the lower levels of the cord, or to the middle sections, or to the bulb, or to the brain; and in the very smallest centres of germination in either of these sites. In a large proportion of cases where the rabies, from beginning to end, is of convulsive character the "virus-germ," scanty in the extreme from first to last, may be strictly located in the bulb; and, far from being free, is in all likelihood as fixed in its circumscribed area, and as sessile as a fungus in a flower. On the other hand, from the outset the "virus" may have settled in large quantity, and simultaneously, in both the lumbar-swelling and the bulb; or first in the lumbar-swelling to find its way ultimately up the cord to the bulb; or, in the first instance, in the bulb, finding its way upward to the brain on the one hand, and downward to the lumbar swelling on the other; in either case producing a profound paralytic rabies. The "virus" may be met with only at one or at several of these points, whilst absent from all other parts of the cerebro-spinal axis. It may be present merely in the lumbar-swelling of the cord, whilst completely absent from the brain. It may be present in the bulb, when comparatively deficient in and, often enough, entirely absent from the brain or the lumbar-swelling ; these minute and isolated foci—only after a time, and if the condition of the nervous substance be very favourable for the cultivation of the microbe, and if the suffering animal can hold out, which, however, is rare in the extreme—will reach alike the lower levels of the spinal marrow and the very highest levels of the brain itself, having pervaded the cerebro-spinal axis from end to end.

"We have found," says M. Pasteur, "that the virus of rabies developes itself invariably in the nervous system,—brain and spinal cord, in the nerves, and in the salivary glands. But it is not present at the same moment in every one of these parts. It may, for example, develope itself at the lower extremity of the spinal cord, and, only after a time, reach the brain. It may be met with at one or at several points of the encephalon, whilst being absent at certain other points of the same region[1]."

Nevertheless, in every case without exception, various and varying as they are, when death takes place,—and death, we are assured, whatever the form of the disease, "is invariable,"—the infective material is *constantly* found, and in the richest abundance in which it exists in the case, in the bulb or medulla oblongata. The constancy of this phenomenon is unquestionable, nor without reason. In the case of death,—and this, apparently, is "inevitable,"—the rabies-germ is present in this structure, whether or not it be present in the higher or lower levels of the cerebro-spinal axis, in the brain, or in the lumbar-swelling, and whatever the peripheral site of infection, or whatever the form of the malady which has terminated in death. When the rabific microbe is copiously present in the higher and the lower levels, it is in still richer abundance and of a still higher potency in the bulb. An emulsion of the bulb of an animal which has died of the disease will never fail to rabidise, even if an inoculation of the salivary-secretion of the animal should fail to impart infection; nay, even if an emulsion of the encephalon or of the lower levels of the cord should fail to rabidise. Whatever other structure of the cerebro-spinal axis the rabific microbe may invade, and however much it may

[1] M. Pasteur's Address to International Medical Congress at Copenhagen, Aug. 11, 1884.

invade it, it will never once fail, sooner or later, to reach and settle in the bulb, and in still larger amounts. In the entire cerebro-spinal axis, only one other centre or region,—the lumbar-swelling,—will compare with the bulb for this constancy of site on the part of the rabies-germ, and for probably the same reason. In the case of the rabbit or guinea-pig, not less than in the case of attenuators, such as the dog or ape, not even the lumbar-swelling itself is a more invariable seat of the germ than the bulb. If this be so, manifestly enough the bulb, with, next to this, the lumbar-swelling, is a very constant and for some reason a very special habitat of the rabific microbe, and the most favourable of all the nerve-centres for its germination. This important fact has been absolutely established.

"We have been fortunate enough," says M. Pasteur, "to ascertain that in all cases, where death has been allowed to supervene naturally, the swelled-out portion, or bulb, of the medulla oblongata, nearest to the brain and uniting the spinal cord with it, is *always* virulent. When an animal has died of rabies (and the disease always ends in death), rabid matter can *with certainty* be obtained from its bulb, capable of reproducing the disease in other animals when inoculated into them, after trephining, in the arachnoid space of the cerebral meninges. Any street-dog whatever, inoculated in the manner described with portions of the *bulb* of an animal which has died of rabies, will certainly develope the same disease. We have thus inoculated several hundreds of dogs, brought without any choice from the pound. Never once was the inoculation a failure. Similarly also, with uniform success, several hundred guinea-pigs; and rabbits more numerous still. These two great results, *the constant presence of the virus in the bulb* at the time of death; and the certainty of the reproduction of the disease with inoculation *into the arachnoid space,* stand out like experimental axioms; and their importance is paramount[1]."

How different this constancy of the rabid condition of the bulb from the salivary secretion, or from any other part of the cerebro-spinal substance itself, yet these were but cases of ordinary "street-dog" rabies of essentially convulsive character, the most varying forms of all!

Similar results are to be noted if the cerebro-spinal substance be examined at a stage when the animal has been still suffering from

[1] M. Pasteur's Address to International Medical Congress at Copenhagen, Aug. 11, 1884. Here purposely italicised.

the malady. At such a stage the cerebro-spinal substance shows, especially in the slighter convulsive forms, if possible, even greater variability as to the centres of "virus," and as to the amount of the rabific microbe in these centres. And this variability will be the more marked the nearer the active disease to its incubation-period, or to its period of germination. If it be a slight convulsive rabies, there may be considerable difficulty in isolating the centres of virulent activity.

"If an animal is killed whilst in the power of rabies, it may require a pretty long search to discover the presence, here or there, in the nervous system, or in the glands, of the virus of rabies[1]."

This applies, however, only to the slighter forms; and even in these, nay, especially in these, if the "virus" be found anywhere, it will be found in the bulb at the source of all the morbid phenomena, such as they are. No such difficulty presents itself in a case which, from the outset of the symptoms, is of the most pronounced "dumb" or paralytic character, where not only the salivary but probably many other glands are already more or less saturated with "virus." Even at this early stage, the rabific microbe is found disseminated over the entire cerebro-spinal axis, but particularly in the lumbar-swelling and bulb; being, however, still in its maximum intensity of virulence *in the bulb*. Between these extremes, there may be any variety. Thus there may be in the substance of the cord a chain of isolated centres of more or less extent and activity, simultaneously spreading upwards and downwards. And if these centres be few and far between, and of but limited area, and if the virus-germ has been introduced into the substance of the cord in its lower levels, they may be kept isolated and relatively quiescent for a considerable time; some of them being even extinguished or their activity considerably abated, until a favourable set of conditions arises which suddenly starts the morbific process with redoubled activity. And do we not see a similar phenomenon in ague, where, although the patient has left the malarial surroundings in which he has contracted the disease, it takes, nevertheless, months before the morbific micro-organism is wholly "prevented" from starting afresh in its germination in its specific habitat? M. Pasteur has given some remarkable cases of rabies which would appear to be analogous in this *intermittent* character.

[1] M. Pasteur's Address to International Medical Congress at Copenhagen, Aug. 11, 1884.

"In my last paper on rabies I said that we had met with some dogs in whom the first symptoms of the disease subsided and disappeared, to reappear again after a tolerably long period of latency. We have, since then, met with similar cases in the rabbit. To quote one instance; on the thirteenth day after intracranial inoculation one of our rabbits showed the first symptoms of paralysis. On the following days he got better, and recovered completely. But forty-three days later the paralysis returned; and he died of paralytic rabies on the forty-sixth day."

"Such cases," M. Pasteur adds, "are very rare in the rabbit as well as in the dog. *But we have frequently noticed them in hens;* in which latter animals the recurrence of the symptoms may, or may not, be followed by death.

"I may just note here that rabies in our hens never showed any violent symptoms, but only a degree of sleepiness, loss of appetite, paralysis of the legs, and, frequently, a considerable degree of anaemia or bloodlessness, as shown by the blanching of the comb[1]."

The hen, therefore, would appear to belong to the intensifying rather than to the attenuating class; for, sooner or later, it presents the disease in a tolerably pronounced paralytic form, if somewhat chronic or subacute in its course. Such *intermittent* forms of rabies, however common in the fowl, are extremely rare in the rabbit, and probably still rarer in the dog, if not quite phenomenal in both animals; and it probably occurs, even in the hen, only where the "virus" has been received in the cord in its very lowest tract, and in the very smallest quantities. Most certainly, if introduced directly into the brain, or into the bulb, and even in the smallest amounts capable of rabidising, no such intermittent form would ensue. As this form of rabies is so rare in the animal kingdom, but particularly in mammals, it may, therefore, be taken for granted that the higher tracts of the cord, and, above all, the bulb, are the more constant sites of the rabific microbe. Nor is the *intermittent* rabies, so characteristic of the fowl, without significance; it is probably more or less characteristic of many if not all birds. As it so happens, the bulb or medulla oblongata of the fowl is a very different structure for bulk, in its relation to the spinal cord, from that of the rabbit, much more from that of the dog, or from that of any high mammal. Nevertheless, in the case of death, or when the symptoms are pronounced, the bulb is found to be invariably rabic, and more so than any other

[1] *Comptes Rendus*, Feb. 25, 1884.

structure, and not only in the rabbit and dog, but even in the hen itself.

But, again, there is reason to show that the same series of phenomena is to be disclosed even before the disease, as a manifest nerve-storm, has fairly broken out; for there is good reason to believe that, at this stage, the rabific microbe from the peripheral sites of infection has really reached the cerebro-spinal axis itself, and has become actually sown in this structure, and in the special sites where it is to germinate.

For this reason M. Pasteur soon gave up all idea of treating hydrophobia ten or twelve days before the disease could declare itself; because by this time a large part of the rabific microbe, introduced in infection, has virtually reached the central nervous system and undergone multiplication; the remainder which has not yet taken root steadily streaming towards the special sites which have already afforded settlement. The rabies-germ having not merely begun, but well-nigh finished the process of germination, no amount of preventative inoculations will now "prevent" it from sooner or later germinating to its full capacity, but, on the contrary, will possibly rather aid the process. How long anterior to the onset of the disease the rabific microbe reaches and settles and germinates in the cerebro-spinal axis, and, primarily, in what region or regions in particular, has not, hitherto, been definitely determined. But it may be safely asserted that the sections first invaded, and the amount of the invasion, and the length of time previous to the first symptoms of the disease, will depend upon the amount of rabific microbe introduced in infection, and the nearness of the peripheral site to the central nervous system, but above all to the "bulb." In a massive infection of an attenuator like the dog from the profound paralytic rabies of an intensifier like the rabbit, the rabific microbe might well be found to be more or less disseminated through the spinal cord and brain even a week or ten days before the disease has actually broken out. If so, it is certain that it will not be absent from the bulb; for the very first beginnings of the morbid process take their origin in this structure; and, from the earliest stages, the "virus" will be present and abundant in the bulb in proportion as the animal rises in the scale of organization. In such an animal as the rabbit, where profound paralytic rabies is the form normal to the animal, it is highly probable, if not certain, that the central nervous system is, here and there, crowded with the germinating rabific microbe even in the latter third of the incubation-period; and if so, particularly will be the bulb or the lumbar-swelling, or both simultaneously. So invaded will be these structures by the rapidly-multiplying micro-organism that an emulsion of the nervous substance of either of these tracts would, even at this early stage, in every likelihood. rabidise; for, as a matter of fact, it is on the point of rabidising the rabbit itself. The practical importance of the possibility of such an event in the case of the dog is manifest enough. If this be true, the bite of a dog, infected with "dumb" paralytic rabies, even a few days before the disease fairly proclaims itself, cannot be altogether free from peril. But in the case of the rabbit and of the entire class of animal capable of intensifying rabies, the theoretic, not less than the practical importance of this probability, if not certainty, is still greater.

Thus, then, it is indisputable that if the rabic tissue of the cerebro-spinal axis be examined, comparatively, through its entire extent, whether it be that of an animal which has died of rabies, or that of an animal which has been killed whilst still suffering from the disease, or even that of an animal in the later and latest stages of incubation itself, some centres of germination are found to be far more constant than others and very much richer in the rabific microbe. The sites of settlement and germination, and the amount of the rabies-germ in these sites, are as various as the various forms of the disease, even in the dog. As a matter of fact, there is no part of the cerebro-spinal axis where the rabific microbe may not take root, and where the process of germination may not primarily take place; the site determining from the first the character of the rabies induced, with the sequence of its lesions and symptoms. Not less than *clinically* or *pathologically*, rabies may be classified *anatomically*, according to the precise centre in the cerebro-spinal substance in which the disease takes its origin, or to which the rabific microbe, after infection, is first conveyed and planted. From this point of view, it may be strictly asserted that there is an essentially *lumbar* rabies, a *spinal* rabies, a *bulbar* rabies, a *cerebral* rabies, and, last and most important of all, a *cerebro-spinal* rabies, affecting uniformly one and all of these sites, and probably the entire nervous system. The last very appalling form is *par excellence* the rabies of an intensifier, and, of all the animals capable of intensifying rabies on transmission, pre-eminently the rabbit. The various other forms are characteristic of the attenuators, and, of all the animals capable of attenuating rabies on transmission, pre-eminently the dog.   But of all sites or germinating-centres the bulb is the most constant and, after infection, the earliest to be invaded.

It is clear, therefore, that rabies is not only a malady of the nervous system, but, in respect even of the nervous system itself, pre-eminently a bulbar disease ; and that in the bulb, and, next to this, in the lumbar-swelling, above all regions of the cerebro-spinal axis, the rabific microbe has, for some cogent reason, its very special seat of cultivation.   One can, accordingly, understand why, as a matter of rule, M. Pasteur at last selected and uniformly used for experimental purposes, not only nervous substance in preference to salivary or any other glandular substance, but in particular the nervous substance of the bulb.   For the rabific microbe of the smallest and scantiest infection capable of rabidising a rabbit only after 40 or 50 days, not less than that of the most potent infection capable of rabidising the rabbit after but six days, finds its way to the bulb and settles and germinates here, if nowhere else.   The bulb, therefore, must be in every case of rabies a most favourable and a very special site for the cultivation and germination of the rabific microbe.

But, *secondly*, what has a *comparative* investigation of the forms of rabies resulting from various amounts of infection, at various sites of the periphery, disclosed ?   This investigation has proved not less conclusive than the other ; and, significantly enough, has led to the same conclusion.   That the higher levels of the spinal cord, and, in particular, the highly specialised nerve-fibres, which constitute the bulbar bulk, form a very special, if not the specific, site of the " virus " is not less apparent from a comparative investigation of the various forms of rabies, arising from the various sites of infection in the periphery.   The peripheral infection is closely related to the ultimate cerebro-spinal infection itself ; and in point of fact is the determining factor of the latter.   That rabies should thus vary by a mere variation of infection, whether in quantity, mode of infection, or site, is surely very remarkable ; but of the fact itself there can be no question. Here, again, the variability of the disease, more especially as it presents itself in man, or the dog, or the entire class capable of attenuating the disease, is pronounced.   There are not two inoculations, even in the same site, varying in the least, which produce precisely the same canine-rabies ; the forms of the disease induced differing from each other, *ceteris paribus*, to the extent of the difference in the inoculations or infections.   Not only has every case its own centres of "virus" in the central nervous system, from which the bulb (if not primarily) is sooner or later invariably infected, its own set of lesions and symptoms, and its own infective-rate ; but every case would appear to have as determining factors of this nerve-infection, likewise, so to speak, its own peripheral portals and avenues in the production of this central infection.

When the infections, both in depth and in amount of "virus" inoculated, are identical in peripheral sites which are far removed from each other, the forms of rabies induced thereby are by no means identical. Again, in sites of infection, although identical, where the inoculations of "virus" vary considerably in depth and amount, the resulting forms of the disease are as unlike each other, even in the case of an intensifier such as the rabbit, as in the extremer forms to be met with in an ordinary outbreak of dog-madness. Again, in sites of infection which are far removed from each other, and where, moreover, the infections vary very materially in depth or amount, the resulting forms of rabies are as different from each other as the "dumb" and the "furious" madness of the dog, or as the most extreme forms to be met with in the most extensive epidemic. In no feature of this extraordinary and apparently Protean malady is there greater variability than in the forms of rabies arising from the mere fact of infection itself.

But various and variable as are the results of infection, even with the same "virus," nay, even with the same amount of the same "virus," this variability is no accident. An inoculation of the foot is by no means so dangerous, or so certain to rabidise, as that of the face or neck; and the rabies induced by an infection of the lower extremity is a somewhat different rabies in point of incubation and virulence from that induced by infection of even the upper extremity. The disease from the latter, much more from the former, is not to be compared for virulence with that from direct infection of the neck or face ; *e.g.* a rabid wolf-bite, or sheep-dog bite, in the face as compared with that in the calf. Why should there be any such discrepancy in the results of the same "virus"? Is this characteristic of germ-diseases as a whole? A vaccination of calf-lymph in the thigh is not any less effective than that in the shoulder ; and an infection of anthrax-virus in the lower extremity is not less serious than that in the upper extremity. An infection of syphilis in the accoucheur's finger, or in the mother's nipple, or in the infant's mouth, is not less grave in its results than in any other region. Koch's "tuberculin" is not any less searching and potent when inoculated in the shoulder than in the back, or in the foot than in either of these regions. Tetanus from a crushed thumb is not in any way different from that from a crushed toe. And is pyemia of the ankle-joint any less deadly than pyemia of the wrist or elbow? In all these cases, and many more, mere site of infection determines in no way the character or even the occurrence of the malady. What, then, is to be inferred from this remarkable fact in respect of rabies? Why should a mere variation in the site of infection modify the rabies induced, or render it more or less certain? Manifestly enough, it cannot be due to the *virus* or virulent product, as opposed to the rabies-germ which has likewise been introduced; for no amount of the virus in an infection, *per se*, rabidises. On the contrary, if in sufficient quantity, it occasions " prevention " or " protection." And could the virus, like tuberculin, be isolated from its microbe, it would be a brilliant discovery, and universally and invariably employed for this very purpose. But, again, and exactly as with tuberculin, alcohol, strychnine, and every other virulent product, mere site of infection could have no influence on the action of the bacillary product, all sites being alike. Whatever the site of infection, the virulent product would at once be taken up by the lymph- and blood-currents and thereafter borne straightway to the nerve-centres. The variation in rabies, therefore, must be due solely to the amount of rabific microbe, not to the amount of virus, in the infection. But if this be so, why should a variation in the site of infection render an equal amount, or in point of fact any amount, of rabific microbe so variable? This is not the case with the morbific microbe of tetanus, diphtheria, erysipelas, anthrax, small-pox, scarlatina, and of the vast majority of germ-diseases. In all such cases, mere site of infection in no way influences the results induced; one site being as efficient for the purpose as another.

Nevertheless, remarkable as the phenomenon would appear to be in respect of rabies, it is not unique. As we shall see hereafter, it is probably true of a distinct class of germ-diseases which, in this important feature, stand by themselves. In the meantime it may suffice to ask, is the variability not due to the fact that the microbe of rabies is not a microbe of the peripheral tissue at all, nor even of the corpuscular tissue of the blood- and lymph-streams, nervous substance, and that of the cerebro-spinal axis in particular, being its specific habitat, where it alone germinates and where it alone elaborates virus, and, on elaborating this latter product in sufficient quantity for the purpose, produces the disease?

Assuming this for the present to be the fact, one can understand why the site of infection should in itself determine the character of the rabies induced; for this site will really determine the region of the cerebro-spinal axis where the rabific microbe will settle and germinate, and therefore the amount of virus which will be elaborated in this region, and the course and the potency of the malady induced by it. Consequently, when it is said that any given rabies is more or less determined by the peripheral site or sites of infection, it is in reality tantamount to saying that it is determined by the amount of rabific microbe which is introduced in the infection, and which, from here, sooner or later gains access into the cerebro-spinal axis. But this latter amount, deducting what is aborted and absorbed on the way by intrinsic preventative power, will invariably be introduced into that part of the cerebro-spinal axis in nearest proximity to the peripheral site of infection.

Thus, it would appear that the variability of rabies from a mere variation in the site of infection is far from accidental or even incomprehensible. The irregularity is a very regular one; and the variability is invariable. And nothing could more clearly show that only the highest, the bulkiest and the most important tracts of the spinal cord, but, above all, of the bulbar substance with the lumbar substance, are the most constant and specific sites of the rabific microbe in the central nervous system itself; these sites and the amount of infection in the central nervous system being mainly determined by the sites of infection and the amount of rabific microbe in the peripheral wounds. Hence, *ceteris paribus*, rabies will be the more uncertain, and the more unequal and irregular, as the peripheral site is removed from the higher tracts of the cerebro-spinal axis; and, conversely, will be more certain and regular and rise in virulence as it approaches these tracts. In other words, the rabies will vary in character according to the amount of the peripheral rabific microbe which is allowed by the intrinsic preventative resistance of the animal to reach the cerebro-spinal axis; for the nearer the peripheral site to the latter the less distance will the rabific microbe have to traverse, and the less of its potency to lose. If the sites in the periphery, or even their depth, be at all varied, a different form of rabies, in proportion to the variation, will be the result; for a different amount of rabific microbe will, for each infection, reach, settle and germinate in the cerebro-spinal axis. And this amount will be proportioned to the proximity of the peripheral site to the higher levels of the cord, but especially to its bulbar substance.

This striking variability, although not realised by the ancients, was, however, noted before M. Pasteur's research. But the fact carried no particular significance. Why a rabic bite in the face should be more infective than a similar wound in the foot or leg was not understood. Nevertheless, of the fact itself there was no doubt. Thus, so long ago as for the years 1862—72, the French Comité d'Hygiène recorded statistics bearing on this subject. For the years mentioned the following figures are given :—

Peripheral Sites	No.	Deaths	Percentage
Bites on the face	50	44	88
,, ,, ,, hands	113	76	67·25
,, ,, ,, trunk	22	7	31·81
,, ,, ,, arms	40	12	30
,, ,, ,, legs	33	7	21·21
,, multiple (face, hands)	8	6	75
Total = 266		152	57·14

"These figures," as has been justly pointed out, "do not give an exact expression of facts[1]." They most certainly do not. Thus, the percentage of infective bites on the legs as compared with those in the hands is surely far from common. Is a bite in the leg so very rare? Admitting this divergence, however, from clothing, &c., most certainly no authority has maintained that the mortality of the disease, as a whole, is anything approaching, much less exceeding, 50 per cent.! Nevertheless, if these figures are somewhat exaggerated, as Dr Suzor has justly pointed out, "they are still of great use as indicating very fairly in what direction the truth lies[2]." From such indications, it is clear that for some cogent reason the further the peripheral site of infection from the face and the higher regions of the organism, the less likely is rabies to occur, and, conversely, that the nearer it is to the face and neck the more certain is rabies to ensue and the more severe the rabies incurred. But if it be the fact that the virus-germ of rabies is a virus-germ of nervous substance, and of this exclusively, how comes it that rabies is least likely to ensue

[1] "Hydrophobia, M. Pasteur's System," by Renaud Suzor, M.D.
[2] *Ibid.*

from the remotest peripheral infections, or that it is the least potent
of any infection for the same amount in any other site ; and invariably less potent than a much weaker infection of the same virus-
germ in the face or neck? Brown-Sequard was so impressed with the
fact that rabies was a disease of nervous substance, and of nothing
else, that he graphically described it as an "ascending neuritis," that
is to say, he assumed that the rabific microbe introduced ascended
from the site of infection through the peripheral nerves, all through
the incubation period, to the deepest nerve-centres in the cerebro-
spinal axis.   This important hypothesis will receive more attention at
a subsequent stage.   In the meantime it may be sufficient to point
out that, if this were the case, the further the site of infection from
the central nervous system the more certainly would rabies ensue,
and, moreover, the more potent would be the rabies ; and, conversely,
that the nearer the site of infection to the central nervous system
the less potent would be the rabies incurred.   If it be the fact, as
most unquestionably it is, that the rabific microbe is wholly a virus-
germ of nervous substance, why should this virus-germ, on traversing
and propagating its way through the nerves, from even the remotest
periphery, in this very fact not gain in potency?   The opposite of
any such gain, however, is the law, even in the case of intensifiers,
such as the rabbit.   And nothing could more clearly indicate the
existence of the intrinsic preventative power, so often alluded to
already.   If an animal had absolutely no refractory or attenuating
power, the same inoculation would produce practically the same
effect, whatever the site of infection.   Whether, then, the rabific
microbe propagates its way through the peripheral nerves to the
cerebro-spinal axis or not, it is certain that infection of the face or
neck is uniformly much more dangerous than infection of the lower
limbs, or of any site in the organism lower than the head.   And this
is so, because, whilst the specific microbe is *par excellence* a microbe
of the entire nervous substance from its centre to its periphery, it is
still more true that it is pre-eminently a microbe of the highest or
thickest levels of the spinal cord and, above all, of the bulbar and
lumbar substance.   Infection of the face and neck therefore is
uniformly more dangerous than that of any lower site, because the
rabific microbe introduced is nearer those higher levels of the spinal
axis which are so constantly special centres of its settlement.   On
account of this fact, the rabific microbe, having less to traverse and
less of intrinsic preventative power to meet, will have likewise less

of its potency to lose. The higher levels of the cord, consequently, but, above all, the bulbar bulk of the cord, are, it is obvious, the very special seat of the virus of the rabies microbe.

For this reason, M. Pasteur so invariably had recourse to the rabic marrow and its "bulb," in preference to all other sources of virus even in the cerebro-spinal substance. Still more important, for this reason, likewise, he instituted the subdural or intracranial inoculation for experimental purposes, and discarded every other, subcutaneous or intravenous. The idea of intracranial inoculation was no mere accident. It is perhaps without exception the most original feature of the research. Before M. Pasteur no one had dreamt of employing an intracranial inoculation, or an infection in the immediate neighbourhood of the medulla oblongata. M. Galtier had rabidised rabbits with a subcutaneous infiltration of solid rabid marrow. This was a subcutaneous infection of the most massive kind, which probably would not fail to rabidise even an elephant. But the rabies induced is by no means the rabies from whence its virus-germ has been derived. By the intracranial inoculation, on the contrary, of a couple of drops of a rabic emulsion the rabies-germ, and in the condition in which it is obtained from a rabid animal, is brought into the immediate neighbourhood of the bulb.

By this direct introduction, even in the smallest quantities, into the centres of the nervous system where it specially thrives, all disturbing factors or intrinsic preventative conditions with respect to the growth of the microbe are reduced to a minimum. In such an infection the rabific microbe cannot fail to be directly planted in the richest tracts of the cerebro-spinal substance; and since this is so, it most certainly, even in inoculations of the smallest quantities, will not fail to take root and to germinate. The inoculation in this site is as true and as uniform in its results as an inoculation of the smallpox microbe or of tetanus-bacillus or of serpent-venom in any and every site. Rabies, therefore, it is clear, is essentially a disease, not only of the cerebro-spinal axis, but pre-eminently of the bulbar substance of that axis.

CHAPTER III.

DETERMINATION OF THE SEAT OF GERMINATION FROM THE SYMPTOMS AND SIGNS.

THAT the virus-germ of rabies "resides" in nervous substance, and especially in the more substantial tracts of the spinal axis, as the bulb and lumbar-swelling where the nerve-fibre, as distinguished from the nerve-cell, is the predominant element, is established beyond question by the experimental investigation. But this conclusion is not less clearly arrived at by a study of the symptomatic characteristics of the malady in any of its modifications and "varieties." When one comes face to face with the active, actual disease itself, the symptoms and signs, if they yield little positive information as to the true nature of the malady, nevertheless afford unmistakeable evidence as to the specific seat of cultivation of the pathogenic micro-organism.

It is true that there are hardly two cases of canine-rabies or hydrophobia where the active phenomena are exactly alike. Every case shows its own symptoms and signs, not less than its own train of lesions. In spite of this fact, the clinical characteristics or symptomatic indications, such as they are, are constant enough to be of great value as evidence of the specific seat of the pathogenic micro-organism. Every symptom or sign, as it arises, points with an increasingly glowing distinctness to the central nervous system as the prime centre of the disturbance. Obviously enough, from such signs, the entire nervous system is, from beginning to end of the disease, in a state of more or less chaotic discord. Intense excitability, if it be a "furious" or convulsive case, or, if it be a paralytic-rabies, the most extreme collapse and prostration, excruciating hyper-æsthesia, on the one hand, and all over the periphery, or the profoundest analgesia and paresis, on the other hand, are from the outset, according to the gravity of the case, the fundamental features of the disturbance.   Manifestly enough, therefore, rabies is a germ-disease of the nervous system exclusively, and even more so than tetanus itself.

But what particular section of nervous substance is indicated as the specific seat of the "virus"?   Is it the same element which is so exclusively invaded by the virus of tetanus?   On the whole, tetanus, in its symptoms, signs, and lesions, is marvellously like canine-rabies of exclusively convulsive or "furious" form, as opposed to canine-rabies of a paralytic, or even partially paralytic form.   In no way does tetanus resemble the latter, there being nothing paralytic about the disease.   Like completely convulsive-rabies it is a disease of the cerebro-spinal system, and of this alone.   In both cases, as contrasted with paralytic-rabies, there is no evidence of the sympathetic nervous system being involved.   In tetanus, as in the *wholly* convulsive-rabies, there is no evidence of the virus of the specific micro-organism being eliminated in and through any of the secretions, or in point of fact of being eliminated at all.   If widely-spread, intense hyperæsthesia or an excruciating sensibility be viewed as the fundamental feature of disturbance in convulsive-rabies ; a not less widely-spread and intense spasm or cramp, as pure as from strychnine-poisoning itself, may be looked upon as the fundamental feature of tetanus.   Certainly, no one has alleged, much less proved, that hearing, seeing, tasting or feeling, or any of the special senses, in tetanus is seriously impaired, or even intensified or exaggerated.   If, then, the *motor* or anterior connections of the cerebro-spinal axis, or the efferent system of nerves and at their roots in the spinal substance, are the special structures of disturbance in tetanus, ex-cessive convulsiveness or spasm from this centric source being the most pronounced feature of irritation from first to last ; on the other hand, the *sensory* or posterior connections of the cerebro-spinal system, or the afferent nerves, and at their roots in the highest spinal nerve-centres, are from the symptoms the prime seat of dis-turbance in convulsive-rabies.   In such a case excessive hyper-æsthesia is, from the outset to the end, the most marked feature of the disease.   Both forms of disorder are essentially spinal in site ; but rabies, even convulsive-rabies, in the sensory or posterior tracts, tetanus in the motor or anterior tracts.   This would appear to form a radical distinction between the two maladies, from first to last.

But rabies is not merely a "furious" disease, whether or not this fury take rise in the motor or the sensory roots. There is also a profoundly paralytic-rabies, *i.e.* paralytic from beginning to end, which is as far removed from tetanus, and even from exclusively convulsive-rabies, as it is from strychnine-poisoning itself. From time immemorial these two marked and highly characteristic "varieties" have been recognized as the so-called "furious" or "raving," and as the so-called "dumb" or "mortal madness." But, whether of convulsive or of paralytic form, it is questionable in the extreme if rabies is ever primarily a disease of motor source or site. A grave disturbance of the *sensory* rather than of the *motor* side of the nervous system would appear to be the prime feature of the malady ; and there is ground to show that what convulsiveness or what paralysis takes place supervenes in direct consequence of this disturbance. If this be so, rabies might be aptly described as, not only of an essentially convulsive or of an essentially paralytic "variety," but, with still more justice, as pre-eminently of a hyper-æsthetic, or of an analgesic character ; the "convulsiveness," or, if it should so happen, the "paralysis," however pronounced, being essentially that of the sensory rather than of the motor centres. Be this as it may, it is undoubted that in convulsive-rabies—the rabies of attenuators—intense sensibility with excitability and "fury"; or, on the contrary, if it be a paralytic-rabies—the rabies of the intensifying class—a not less intense prostration with marked bluntness of sensibility and of every one of the special senses, is pronounced from the first. Whatever convulsiveness or whatever paralysis there may be eventually developed, this grave disturbance of sensibility would appear to be the first and the last and, all through the disease, the most pronounced feature. It is a lesion probably underlying all other disturbance.

A more headlong fury than in the "furiously" mad dog cannot be imagined. "He is in a continuous state of restlessness and agitation. In his kennel he piles up the straw, lays his chest on it, then rises in anger and scatters the litter about. In apartments he tosses the cushions and carpets, &c." "He tears everything that he meets, and swallows fragments of anything, including his own excreta, urine, earth, &c." "The sight of another dog, at once, and almost invariably, puts the mad dog in a fit of passion. This is, therefore, an easy and a valuable test-method[1]."

Again, as demonstrating the extremely excitable condition of the

[1] "Hydrophobia, M. Pasteur's System," by Renaud Suzor, M.D.

animal, the bark of the "furiously" rabid dog is so characteristic as to be diagnostic. It is most expressive of the animal's intense excitement or agitation. The bark has not the normal, full, sonorous ring, but is rather an hysterical *falsetto* screech of excitement. As Dr Suzor aptly points out, "it is not unlike the voice of dogs chasing a hare," which, it may be worth adding, is the most exciting, and possibly the most excitable, moment in the animal's existence. Along with this excitability, and everywhere underlying it, unlike tetanus, every one of the special senses is grossly exaggerated and more or less perverted. Even the sexual sense is said to be "greatly excited and increased." The animal is persistently haunted by hallucinations, illusions and distorted visions. "He barks, snaps, and growls at imaginary beings" (Youatt). It must, for example, be a spectral delusion of simply the weirdest character which will drive a rabid dog, or even a rabid cat, to spring at its master or mistress as at a fiend ; especially so in the case of the dog, which, of all animals, not excepting the horse, or elephant itself, is the most devoted and disinterested in its affection.

Or, turning to canine-rabies of a paralytic or semi-paralytic character, it is still more obvious that the disease, from beginning to end, is characterised by a corresponding vitiation in the general sensibility. The change from "furious" convulsiveness to "dumb" paralysis is solely due to this profound disturbance. No longer is there intense excitability with excruciating hyperæsthesia. The irritability has given way to prostration ; the hypersensitiveness to absolute bluntness or deadness of feeling. From the outset the paralytic-mad-dog "is analgesic; *i.e.* his general sensibility is blunted to a very considerable degree." Far from being hyperæsthetic, and aroused to overwhelming passion from the most trifling irritations,— "he now seems to feel *only the very intensest pains*. He no longer expresses pain by the usual nasal sound or the sharp cry which is so familiar. He can be beaten, pricked, and even slightly burnt, without stirring, and without uttering any sound. If severely burnt he moves to another place, but remains mute, although the face becomes expressive of pain[1]."

The poor animal has now an habitual look of dazed collapse. The mouth is permanently open, owing to the paralysis of the lower jaw; and, owing to the same paralytic affection, the saliva, which is now thin and copious, flows incessantly in driblets from the angles of

---

[1] "Hydrophobia, M. Pasteur's System," by Renaud Suzor, M.D.

the mouth, and is invariably rabic. In this it forms a complete contrast to the saliva of a completely convulsive-rabies, which, as we have seen, is invariably scanty in amount, and but seldom and very unequally rabic. Profound as the disturbance of sensibility is in convulsive-rabies, and important as it is as a factor of all the morbid phenomena, it is vastly more profound in paralytic-rabies. The wide-spread analgesia and paresis are not merely a negation of sensibility, as in ordinary paralysis from a spinal accident or from apoplexy. Associated with this there is also a positive vitiation of feeling. The senses are, one and all, blunted and perverted; much more so than in the case of convulsive-rabies, and are abso-lutely falsifying. If the "convulsiveness" of furious rabies is a convulsiveness of sensibility more than of motion, the paralysis of "dumb" rabies is likewise a paralysis of sensibility much more than of motion; and in both cases the affection of the motor tracts is, in every likelihood, secondary, and determined by the affection of the sensory tracts. This disturbance is particularly noticeable in every one of the special senses. The animal's sight, his hearing, his taste, and all his other senses are blighted to the point of collapse and completely vitiated.

"The eyes are open, without expression; constantly fixed in the same direction. The animal is constantly lying down or sleepy; and he has neither the will, *nor the power to bite*[1]."

If he moves at all it is but for an instant, and with a staggering, dragging gait, and with an expression of utter helplessness and apathy.

These indications are, of course, more pronounced in the rabbit, where paralytic-rabies of a still more prostrating character is the form of the disease normal to the animal.

"The rabbit in which rabies is developing itself," says M. Galtier, in his admirable description of this form of the disease, "remains quiet and low-spirited, often sleepy, more rarely agitated, and frightened by the slightest sound. From the very outset there is well-marked weakness, sometimes localised in the first instance to the lumbar region, the hind limbs, and even the cervical region; soon it creeps and invades the whole body, and then it is gradually replaced by paralysis. All the movements of the animal are difficult, irregular, ill-defined, and soon become impossible[2]."

[1] "Hydrophobia, M. Pasteur's System," by Renaud Suzor, M.D. Italics not Suzor's.

[2] Galtier, *Bull. Acad. de Méd.* January 25, 1881.

Along with this "low-spirited" prostration with irregular, creeping paralysis of movement, the disturbance and perversion of the sensory side of the nervous system are still more definite and still earlier phenomena.

"General sensibility is gradually dulled; and is sometimes quite lost; so that it becomes quite possible to thrust a pin into the animal without giving rise to any reaction on its part. *Sight is lost* or *perverted*; the eye becoming gradually less and less sensitive. The conjunctiva is congested, and the cornea and the aqueous and vitreous humours dull and cloudy[1]. The sense of taste," continues M. Galtier, "appears to be also *perverted*; for the rabid rabbits are to be seen swallowing fragments of straw and of faecal matter, and to lick the floor of their cage. As a rule, *they do not try to bite*, and there is *an abundant flow of saliva.*"

"Finally, even the thirst and hunger, vitiated as they are, likewise disappear; or when the subject tries still to drink or to eat there soon supervenes a moment when deglutition is quite impossible[2]."

Or, lastly and not less clearly, if we turn to hydrophobia itself, the same indications of sensory disturbance present themselves as the fundamental lesion of the malady. The paroxysmal excitement with convulsiveness; or, in the worst but extremely rare paralytic cases, the profound nervous prostration with ill-defined, creeping paralysis, is not less marked than the widely-spread intensely disturbed sensibility which is so early a feature of canine-rabies. In the convulsive-hydrophobia, which is the normal form of the disease, nervous excitability with restlessness and intensest agitation is conspicuous from the first; the sensibility, both general and special, but particularly the latter, being grossly exaggerated and falsifying. Manifestly enough, from the outset of the disease, the cerebro-spinal system, from centre to periphery, is under the blighting effect of one of the most deadly of irritants. And the experimental demonstration on another animal of the existence of this irritant in the cerebro-spinal substance "renders it easy," as M. Pasteur has remarked, "to explain the nervous excitement which is so often present in rabies, and which in man gives rise to the strange symptom known as aërophobia[3]." But why should merely the slightest draught of air, or the very thought of such a draught, shake a man with

---

[1] Galtier, *Bull. Acad. de Méd.* January 25, 1881. Italics not M. Galtier's.

[2] Galtier, *Bull. Acad. de Méd.* Feb. 25, 1881.

[3] *Comptes Rendus*, Feb. 25, 1884.

terror and throw him into a paroxysm of convulsions? Simply because the cerebro-spinal system is so intensely overstrung on its sensory side, and in this overstrung condition so appallingly irritated, that every impression from the periphery or even from the brain, objective and subjective, however trivial, is exaggerated in the extreme; there being no such thing as a slight irritation; and this impression, with its exaggeration and excess, is violently thrown on the motor tracts to produce the convulsive storm. Thus, the merest draught of air or the rustling of his bed-clothes is excruciating to the patient, and never fails to excite a paroxysm of convulsions. Even the touch of a feather on any part of the skin, particularly in the angles of the mouth, is, there is reason to believe, as startling as the touch of a hot iron. Could any symptom or set of symptoms more clearly reveal the terrible condition of the general sensibility, and how important a lesion this disturbance constitutes from the outset? There is no such lesion of the sensory system in tetanus, or from strychnine-poisoning. Nor is it the mere general sensibility that is thus so affected. Every one of the special nerves of sense is still more so. Hearing, sight, taste, and even smell itself, are intensely acute, being exaggerated to the point of pain, and but broken and falsifying media to the mind. The sudden opening or shutting of a door, a brusque tone of talk, a sip of water or beef-tea, a sudden flash of light as from the opening of a hunter's watch or from the light of a mirror, the merest sniff of ammonia;—any of these trifling irritants of sensibility never fails to bring on convulsions. Enormously exaggerated delusions and illusions of a spectral character occur, varied with transient fits of frenzy, based on such illusions. Abject terror, with a look of anguish, hardly less pronounced than in the worst delirium tremens itself, is marked from the beginning. But all such signs may be referred to the acute and profoundly vitiated sensation. The patient appears as if overwhelmed with the most gigantic and distorted sensations; and from the beginning to the end of the disease he has a scared, hunted look, which is pathetic in the extreme. There is no more pathetic face in the wide realm of disease. Amidst this chaotic disturbance of sensibility there is, however, no evidence of the higher mental faculties being impaired. There is evidence only of the deranged framework of sensation. A profoundly exaggerated sensibility is at the root of every subjective as well as of every objective sign or symptom. Thus, in the well-known case of the Duke of Richmond, Governor of Canada, one of the memorable symptoms of hydrophobia (from rabid fox-bite) which presented itself was the persistent fancy that some poplars, adjoining his bed-room window, were gigantic men peering in on him! Had there been no poplars there would have been something else to have served as the same falsifying basis of horror;—a solitary boulder or two, perhaps, in a field, like a weird head and shoulders cropping up through the soil! From such indications it is clear that the entire reflex-nervous apparatus of the cerebro-spinal axis, both in its sensory and in its motor connections, but pre-eminently and primarily in the former, is overstrung to the point of collapse; and in the case of the paralytic forms, where the quantity of virus and virus-germ in the central nervous system is so vast, collapse is invariably reached. The signs and symptoms are everywhere referable to a reflex disturbance from an intensely irritated cerebro-spinal axis, whose afferent and efferent connections from the centre of disturbance, upwards to the brain as well as downwards to the remotest periphery, are jangled and completely out of tune. The "virus," not only in the worst but in the least severe forms of the malady, is obviously a "virus" of the central nervous system, not of the periphery; and, from the first symptoms of the disease, of the sensory centres of the cerebro-spinal axis rather than of the motor.

If, however, the signs and symptoms be followed more narrowly, the special seat of the rabific microbe, even in the substance of the cerebro-spinal axis itself or, in what special sensory tracts above others, is indicated with a precision which leaves little room for doubt. When the disease has once broken forth the signs and symptoms from every part of the convulsed, or, if it be an extreme case, of the paralytic organism, point to the disturbed medulla oblongata and its immediate structures, but particularly to its great sensory centres and tracts, as the capital source of the disorder. The more special the signs and symptoms the more directly do they point to the bulb and its immediate neighbourhood as the central seat of the disease.

Thus, much the most intense sensibility and convulsiveness; or, if it be a profound paralytic-rabies, by far the most pronounced analgesia and the most constant paresis or paralysis, are to be found, not in the hands or feet, not in the face, not in any of the normal tracts of emotion, but in the throat, gullet and larynx, the tongue and palate. But this is a region whose network of nerve-distribution, both sensory and motor, particularly the former, takes its origin solely in the substance of the "bulb" or medulla oblongata. It is true that the hyperæsthesia of the entire surface of the body in hydrophobia or convulsive-rabies is excessive. Nevertheless, in such a case, the hyperæsthesia of the tongue, palate, throat and pharynx— and in the dog and cat in all probability likewise even of the stomach, itself—is still more intense. The sensibility of this special region with its accompanying convulsiveness, and, in pronounced paralytic cases, the analgesia with its accompanying paresis or para-lysis, are much more intensified, and at an earlier stage of the disease, than in any other part of the body. The maximum of disturbance and distress always centres in this region above all regions. Could there be a clearer indication of the essentially bulbar character of the malady, and, moreover, of the sensory side of the bulb as the prime seat? In hydrophobia or convulsive-rabies any attempt to swallow at once induces reflex convulsive movements in this whole region. The bare suggestion of such an attempt in-variably ends in the same violent paroxysm of convulsions. Hence the mere act of swallowing is the greatest agony which the sufferer has to endure. For this reason the disease, from time immemorial, has been aptly termed a *hydrophobia*. For the swallowing of even the blandest liquids is the invariable starting-point of a convulsive storm which never fails to sweep over the system. Anything which remotely suggests the thought of swallowing is distressing in the extreme. The sound, for example, of water being poured from one vessel into another, as from a jug into a basin, is excruciating. The sight of water, or of a sheet of water, is, if possible, even still worse. In the Duke of Richmond's case, already referred to, the friends of the patient had the greatest difficulty in getting him to enter a boat to cross a lake, in order the sooner to reach his home. For a long time he insisted upon being driven round the lake at whatever cost of fatigue or loss of time, and was only at last persuaded to submit through sheer exhaustion. The dread of water is a terribly real one, and probably is the fruit of a very complex set of disturbed sensations. Be this as it may, it is certain, as the late Sir John Erichsen long ago stated, that the recollection of the special sufferings and convulsions in the act of swallowing, in itself, constantly "makes the subject of hydrophobia afraid to repeat the attempt; hence, the fear of liquids, from which the disease derives its name[1]." The patient has a dread, not only of water, but of all liquids; it

[1] *Science and Art of Surgery*, by John E. Erichsen, Vol. I. p. 149.

is, however, not so much of liquids as of the act of swallowing. For as a matter of fact the throat and gullet have to contract much more, whether the contraction be spasmodic or harmonious, well or ill done, on liquids than on soft solids; and this convulsive contraction invariably involves in its wake by far the most agonizing of the sufferings of rabies.

To what, then, is due the excessive sensitiveness with its corresponding convulsiveness, or the excessive analgesia with its corresponding paralysis of this special region over that of any other, or of all other regions combined? It is due to the very specially rabidised condition of the nerve-supply of this particular region, as compared with that of any other; and, moreover, not in its peripheral distribution over throat and gullet, but in its highest and deepest centres in the cerebro-spinal axis itself. What are the nerves which so specially supply this region? They are the *glosso-pharyngeal*, filaments of the *spinal-accessory*, the *pneumogastric*, the *hypoglossal* and the *gustatory*. But every one of these great nerves,—not excepting the *gustatory*,—one of the most important branches of the *fifth*, and not less a special sense than the pneumogastric or ophthalmic itself, rises in and proceeds directly from the inmost substance of the medulla oblongata.

Every one of these nerves in its ultimate distribution over throat, tongue, palate, pharynx, larynx, salivary and parotidean glands, &c., is intimately interwoven with every other of the group; the filaments of one blending in its progress with the filaments of all. Now, if the rabies-microbe were present in any large quantity, or even at all, in any one of these nerves, it could find its way to every one of them. One nerve of the group could not be seriously invaded without ultimately the entire group being invaded, and every part of this delicate network to its finest subdivisions. And this would be the fact were rabies, like tetanus and diphtheria, and many other germ-diseases, exclusively of peripheral cultivation; and the "virus" of the malady solely elaborated at the periphery. This, however, in respect of rabies, as shall be shown more clearly as we proceed, is by no means the fact. Far from rabies being an "ascending neuritis," there is every reason to believe, on the contrary, that it is in reality a *descending neuritis*, and that both the micro-organism and its virus (the virus preceding the germ) descend to the periphery from the central nervous system through the nerve-roots. Now, assuming this centric origin of the "virus," an invasion from above of the entire network of nerves which so specially supply the glosso-pharyngeal region would be much more certain and thorough than any invasion from below or from the periphery. For the group of nerves, constituting this glosso-pharyngeal network, would from the outset of the disease have, one and all, become invaded at their point of origin in the medulla oblongata; in this way causing the disease and accounting for its suddenness in the remotest periphery. The sensory and motor tracts of this nerve-supply, wide as it is, would everywhere be just as acutely irritated as if the irritation were solely in the periphery itself; and they would be none the less seriously impaired in function and structure for being already irritated and injured beyond all recovery in their very origin in the medulla oblongata.

But is it the fact that the special nerve-supply of throat, tongue, gullet, salivary and parotid glands, so exclusively takes its origin in the bulbar substance? If so, the fact is of prime importance in the causation of the malady. What are the anatomical disclosures in respect of this connection?

"According to the observations of Stelling, part of the grey matter at the back of the medulla forms special deposits of nuclei, which are connected with the roots of the *spinal-accessory*, the *vagus* or *pneumogastric*, the *glosso-pharyngeal* and the *hypoglossal* nerves. Of these nuclei, the first or lowest is concealed in the substance of the medulla, whilst those which are situated higher up gradually appear in the floor of the fourth ventricle as small angular eminences pointing downwards near the apex of the calamus scriptorius. The *first* nucleus, proceeding from below, is that for the *spinal-accessory* nerve; it reaches some way down in the cord, and is there lost in the intermedio-lateral tract. Above this nucleus, and close to the middle of the medulla, is another, the *second*, commencing higher up and connected with the *hypoglossal* nerve; the roots of which, coming forward between the anterior pyramid and the olivary body, appear at the surface in the depression between these parts. Continuing to ascend, these two nuclei reach the back of the medulla, and then make their appearance in the floor of the fourth ventricle. Higher up, the nucleus for the spinal-accessory nerve is succeeded by a *third* in the same line which is connected with *the nervus vagus* (or pneumogastric) and is also placed to the outer side of that for the hypoglossus. Further out, a *fourth* nucleus begins to be observed, belonging to the *glosso-pharyngeal* nerve[1]." These, however, are the

---

[1] Quain's *Anatomy*, Part II. sect. v., *Neurology*, pp. 519—20.

special nerves, along with the *gustatory*, or the lingual branch of the fifth, which so materially supply the throat, tongue, and pharynx. And even the gustatory nerve itself, there is reason to show, also takes its deepest origin in the bulb.

"The greater root of the fifth, the fibres of which are *sensory*, and constitute the whole of the first and second and the greater (or gustatory) part of the third division of the nerve, runs behind the transverse fibres of the pons towards the lateral part of the medulla oblongata at the back of the olivary body. Some anatomists trace it into the floor of the fourth ventricle between the fasciculi teretes and the restiform bodies. By some it is considered to be continuous with the fasciculi teretes and lateral columns of the cord; whilst others connect it *with the grey mass* which is regarded by Stelling as the nucleus of the glosso-pharyngeal nerve[1]."

From the signs and symptoms of the disease, therefore, it is sufficiently obvious that the bulbar substance is the central and specific site of the "virus" of rabies; and that its sensory, even more than its motor roots constitute the most favourable germinating-ground of the rabific microbe. The rabies-germ, however feeble in potency, or, which is the same thing, however small in amount in the central nervous system, elaborates, even in the simplest convulsive form of the disease, still so potent an irritant that it attacks in the most limited area of the bulb both sensory and motor roots. Neither one species of nerve-fibre nor the other, it would appear, can resist its virulence; in this the "virus" of rabies being very different from the "virus" of tetanus or from strychnine, which wholly impairs the motor roots. But in respect of rabies the sensory, even more than the motor roots are in all probability involved, or, in other words, constitute from its entrance into the cerebro-spinal substance the more fitting germinating site for the rabies-microbe. Why should this necessarily be so? Is there any inherent property or characteristic in the sensory root or tract as compared with the motor which should render the former a more favourable germinating-medium than the latter?

Assuming that the "virus" of rabies is exclusively a "virus" of nervous substance, even when it presents itself in secretions and secreting organs, and for this very reason of nerve-fibre rather than of nerve-cell; assuming, consequently, that the sensory and the motor roots of the bulb or of the lumbar-swelling or of any other section

---

[1] Quain's *Anatomy*, Part II. sect. v. p. 586.

of the cerebro-spinal substance constitute a specially fitting soil for the growth of the micro-organism; nevertheless of the two structures, the sensory roots would still be the earlier and the more seriously invaded. And this is so for the same reason that the bulb or the lumbar-swelling or both are more early and invariably more seriously invaded than any other part of the cerebro-spinal substance. Significantly enough, all over the cerebro-spinal system the sensory roots are distinctly larger and bulkier than the motor. Still more important this disproportion, even if the sensory and motor nerve-fibres are equally favourable media for the cultivation of the rabies-germ—which is questionable—is the more marked *the nearer they approach the bulb* or medulla oblongata. If this be so, on the arrival of the rabific microbe into the cerebro-spinal substance after infection, whether it be into the bulb or the lumbar-swelling or both structures, the sensory rather than the motor roots would constitute the richer cultivating-ground for the settlement of the microbe, and the fitter medium for the elaboration of its virus. The sensory roots, being the larger of the two, and therefore the richer in the elements necessary for the germination of the micro-organism, would in this fact prove from the first the better pasture-ground, and be the more promptly invaded. Is it, however, the fact that the sensory roots and the sensory tracts are distinctly larger than the motor, *all over the cerebro-spinal axis?*

"The posterior (or sensory) roots of the nerves are distinguished from the anterior roots *by their greater size*, as well as *by the greater thickness* of the fasciculi of nerve-fibre of which they are composed. Each (sensory) spinal nerve is furnished with a ganglion. The size of the ganglion is in proportion to that of the nerves on which they are formed.

"The anterior (or motor) roots of the spinal nerves are, as will be inferred from what has been already stated, *the smaller of the two*. They are devoid of ganglionic enlargement; and their fibres are collected into two bundles near the intervertebral ganglion, as in the posterior root[1]."

This difference in bulk between the two sets of nerves, as just stated, is characteristic of the entire cerebro-spinal axis; but it is much greater and still more pronounced between the sensory and motor roots of the bulbar substance than those of any other part of the spinal cord. Whilst this is true of the higher sections of the cord,

[1] Quain's *Anatomy*, Part II. p. 631.

in the inferior or the lower one descends, the anterior or motor roots become more important in size, although never quite so pronounced as the posterior or sensory roots.

"The roots of the lower lumbar and of the upper sacral nerves are the largest of the spinal nerves. Of these, however, *the anterior roots are still the smaller;* but the disproportion between the anterior and posterior roots is not so great as in the cervical nerves[1]."

Nowhere is this disparity greater than in the medulla oblongata, which, as it happens, is the capital centre of the rabific microbe. The great sensory nerves,—such as the pneumogastric, the glosso-pharyngeal, the gustatory of the fifth, &c.—which take their origin directly in the bulbar substance itself, are their largest nerve-roots.

Now, on the assumption that both the sensory and the motor root and tract are equally favourable media for the cultivation of the rabific microbe and the elaboration of its virus, which by no means follows, the disease is for this reason, in all probability from the first, rather more sensory than motor in character, and consequently rather more bulbar in site than lumbar: for the sensory roots are much more pronounced in the former than in the latter. All over the cerebro-spinal axis the sensory root and tract are in amount of nerve-fibre a very different structure from the motor. They are distinctly larger; and this disparity greatly increases the nearer they approach the bulb.

Hence, it follows that the "nidus" or specific seat of the germina-tion of the rabies microbe is not only in the bulbar and lumbar substance above all sections of the spinal axis, but, preeminently, amidst its sensory roots. The onset of the malady and the progress of the rabies-germ with its virus will, therefore, be from the first in a sensory rather than in a motor direction. Thus, the widely-spread hyperæsthesia, or, as the case may be, the marked analgesia and bluntness of sensibility are no accident. They arise from the prime and fundamental lesion of the disease, and are invariably of centric and bulbar source.

[1] Quain's *Anatomy*, Part II. p. 631.

CHAPTER IV.

RABIES OF THE SYMPATHETIC NERVOUS SYSTEM.

FROM the clinical, not less than from the experimental evidence, then, it is safe to affirm that, of all the nerves in the entire cerebro-spinal axis, the special set which supplies the glosso-pharyngeal region, and at their root in the medulla oblongata, not in their peripheral terminations, is the constant centre of virulence in every case of rabies. The rabific micro-organism germinating and elaborating its virus in such a site, the entire train of morbid phenomena characteristic of rabies could not fail to follow; and if the virus elaborated be particularly virulent or, which is the same thing, be particularly copious, involving even still more than the sensory and motor roots in the bulb, it could not fail to induce rabies of the most infective and the most pronounced paralytic form. When rabies is essentially convulsive as opposed to paralytic, *i.e.* convulsive from first to last, it is indicative of the fact that the rabific microbe of the case is but of a minimum amount compatible with the disturbance produced, and that it is exclusively confined in its germination and virulent action to but a very limited area of the bulbar substance. When, however, the disease is from the outset of paralytic character, *i.e.* profoundly paralytic from beginning to end, it is indicative of the fact that the rabific microbe, far from being scanty in amount or strictly circum-scribed in its morbific action to the sensory or motor roots of the bulb, is copious in the extreme and practically unlimited in area, the cerebro-spinal substance from bulb to cauda equina being more or less invaded with the micro-organism. If this be so, a "furious" rabies is merely a localised irritation of the sensory and motor roots of the bulb, acute and terrible enough from the vital importance of the site to invariably induce convulsive-rabies and death. A very different state of things, however, is revealed in a profoundly paralytic-rabies. Here, the irritation of the sensory and motor roots is on so extensive a scale and is of so massive a character that in the widely-spread virulence involved, the normal function of the nerves is not merely exaggerated or intensified, as in convulsive-rabies, but perverted to paralysis. If it be a very profound paralytic-rabies, every part of the cerebro-spinal system will be more or less charged with the micro-organism, and the amount of virus elaborated may be measured with precision by the extent of the paralysis induced. Or, lastly, if a small amount of rabific microbe, a quantity equivalent to the induction of merely a convulsive-rabies when settling in the bulb, should primarily settle in the lumbar swelling or the lower instead of the higher levels of the cord, long before death should take place, the micro-organism will have slowly and steadily germinated and multiplied up through the cord, producing a prolonged, creeping, intermittent paralytic-rabies. Thus, it may be stated that there are three distinct forms of the malady : completely *convulsive-rabies*, of strictly bulbar site and source ; *ascending* or prolonged and *intermittent paralytic-rabies* of lumbar source ; and *acute* or *profoundly paralytic-rabies*, which is, from the first, simultaneously of both bulbar and lumbar site, and practically germinating over the entire cerebro-spinal axis. Simple, convulsive-rabies, therefore, may be viewed as a purely localised affection of the cerebro-spinal substance, being exclusively a bulbar disease. Its virulence, if directly limited to this vital structure, through this structure, covers the entire glosso-pharyngeal region ; and the exclusively convulsive character of the malady is due to the fact that the virus is so scanty and sparse and of so strictly limited a range that it extends no further than this localised area, with its sensory and motor roots, which it so "furiously" irritates. Paralytic-rabies, on the other hand, whether partial or complete, prolonged or rapid, creeping or simultaneously universal, is a widely-diffused rabies, with its prime and capital centres of activity in the bulb and lumbar-swelling. Its virus-germ is of such massive amount and of such appalling potency that it invades nervous substance wherever it exists, and far beyond its primal sources ; beyond even the cerebro-spinal axis itself, down to the remotest peripheral nerve, whether sensory or motor. As a matter of fact, no nervous substance in the entire organism can withstand the virulence of the virus of a profound paralytic-rabies, or resist its progressive invasion. A convulsive-rabies would appear, then, to differ from a paralytic-rabies, only in the amount of virus-germ in the cerebro-spinal axis. But the entire cerebro-spinal axis might be practically disseminated with the micro-organism, without necessarily the secretions being charged with it. Were the micro-organism invariably confined to the cerebro-spinal system, through however large an extent of its substance, it would not necessarily follow that the secretions would thereby become implicated, or that rabies would be any more infective than such a disease as tetanus. As a matter of fact, however, a paralytic-rabies is invariably infective, for, as we have seen, the salivary secretion in such a case is invariably charged with the "virus." Why should this be so?

When canine-rabies is, from first to last, solely of convulsive character, which in a certain percentage of cases in an outbreak of dog-madness is unquestionable, it is so because the virus-germ is strictly limited in range and area in the central nervous system. The secretions in such a case are unaffected, because the nervous supply of the secreting organs is unaffected. The rabific microbe received in infection, small in amount to begin with, simply fixes in a still smaller amount in the bulbar substance amidst the nerve-roots, and becomes in this structure practically as sessile as a fungus. But, although thus strictly confined to the bulbar nerve-roots, all the signs and symptoms of a convulsive or "furious" rabies would still ensue and be present from the outset; and the seat of irritation being in so vital a centre, death would in the long run be as "inevitable" as in the most pronounced paralytic case. Nevertheless, in spite of the paroxysms of pharyngeal convulsions, with the intense glosso-pharyngeal hyperæsthesia, nay, in direct consequence of these facts, the salivary or any other secretion of such a case would be in no way affected by the bulbar disturbance, the nervous structures of such secreting organs being in no way involved, except functionally and indirectly. If the bulbar irritation which induces the hyperæsthesia and convulsiveness characteristic of hydrophobia or convulsive-rabies has any direct influence whatever on the salivary or other secretions, it is in a direction precisely the opposite from that of paralytic-rabies. It will decrease rather than increase secretion, the centric irritation influencing the secreting structures and their vascular supply precisely in the same spasmodic manner in which it influences other structures. Hence, thirst and a persistently parched condition of throat and palate are so characteristic of hydrophobia or of "furious-madness," in spite of the dread of all liquids. In consequence of the convulsive character of the malady, the salivary secretion is diminished in amount and rendered churned and clammy. Moreover, this diminished, viscid and frothy saliva, so characteristic of completely convulsive-rabies, is devoid of "virus" or infective material, and incapable of rabidising, also in consequence of the wholly centric nerve-site of the disease and in proportion to its limitation. Hence, it becomes explicable how the bite of a mad dog, however "furious" or "raving" the animal, and when the bite is effective, is by no means invariably rabic, or, at times, even infective at all. Contrast such a state of the salivary secretion with that of a completely paralytic case, where there is invariably "an abundant flow." But why should the secretion of a paralytic case be so enormously increased, and rendered so liquid and absorptive? Above all, why should this increased amount be so invariably charged with the rabific microbe? Mere paralysis of the centric nervous system will not account for this phenomenon. Certainly, paralysis, according to its extent, will increase the amount of salivary secretion and liquify it. But a localised, rabific irritation of the cerebro-spinal axis, whether of the bulb exclusively, or of the lumbar-swelling exclusively, or of both simultaneously, or even of the entire cerebro-spinal substance itself, an irritation amounting to absolute paralysis of the sensory and motor nerve-centres affected, would not necessarily mean a positive vitiation of the secretions, or involve the existence of the centric paralysing virus and virus-germ in the secretions. In such a case, although the specific micro-organisms would be much more copious and potent than in any convulsive case, it would still be strictly confined to the cerebro-spinal substance. As, however, in paralytic-rabies the salivary secretion is invariably more or less rabic, according to the extent of paralysis, clearly enough its rabific microbe is not confined even to the cerebro-spinal axis itself, and is determined in its spread through the organism by the paralytic character of the malady. In other words, in profound paralytic-rabies, but only in this form of the disease, it is obvious that the sympathetic (ganglionic) system, not less than the cerebro-spinal system, is invariably more or less invaded by the rabific microbe.

How is this invasion from the one nervous system to the other occasioned? What is the link between the two systems by which, at times, a well-nigh universal spread of the micro-organism from the central nervous system takes place even to the secreting organs and their secretions? The signs and symptoms of paralytic-rabies point as conclusively as the experimental investigation itself to a virulent paralysis, not only of the cerebro-spinal system proper, but likewise of the adjoining sympathetic system. And in this invasion, secreting glands have become rabic through their sympathetic nervous elements; and the salivary secretion of such a case will never fail to rabidise. Once the sympathetic system has become seriously invaded and spreading channels of the rabific microbe, the outermost and coarsest centres, so to speak, of the nervous system have at last been overcome, and the virus, followed by its micro-organism, may now stream in an increased volume through every such nerve to the peripheral secreting structures, and charge to saturation point the salivary secretion with the infective material. The invasion of the sympathetic system, therefore, which however is so constant a feature only of paralytic-rabies, is a most appalling complication. There is no disease of the nervous system more complete and disastrous. There is no part of the entire nervous system, motor, sensory or sympathetic, which is not capable of being pervaded and perverted and destroyed by the "virus" of such a rabies. The salivary secretion, with probably many other secretions, cannot fail to be more or less constantly charged with the virus-germ. It cannot, consequently, fail to infect, and, in the very worst cases, such as that of Deptford or at Pantin, to invariably infect. This is a very different virus-germ, both in quantity and quality, and in range of attack or area of cultivation, from that which induces merely a convulsive or "furious" rabies.

Clearly enough, then, the nervous system is not everywhere or in all its branches or sections alike sensitive to the virulence of the virus of rabies, or an equally favourable soil for the germination of the micro-organism. Otherwise, the simplest convulsive case, or the smallest possible amount of the rabies-germ introduced in an infection, and capable of rabidising, would invariably affect, not merely the bulbar substance or the cerebro-spinal axis, but likewise the sympathetic ganglionic system. Every case of rabies without exception would, therefore, sooner or later become a paralytic, infective rabies, the salivary-secretion being invariably rabic. This would follow were the disease always primarily centric and bulbar in its seat of cultivation; for, if the sympathetic system were an equally favourable medium as a germinating-ground, it would, sooner or later, be likewise involved. This would still more certainly follow if the disease were really peripheral, not centric, in its seat of cultivation. The virus-germ, in its ascent through the nervous-system from the periphery, would, in every case, find its way to all nerves, sympathetic not less than cerebro-spinal. But in a considerable percentage of cases the sympathetic system is not invaded, nor, hence, is the salivary secretion charged with infective material. Far from the nervous structure of every part of the nervous system being an equally favourable medium for the cultivation of the micro-organism, or equally sensitive to the virulence of the virus, there is reason to show that the sympathetic system will tolerate with comparative impunity, if not with absolute immunity, a virus which will irritate the cerebro-spinal system, but, above all, the sensory roots of the bulb itself,—perhaps the most specialised point in their entire extent,—into convulsive rabies of the most "furious" character. But in consequence of this toleration on the part of the sympathetic system as compared with the early collapse of the bulbar motor and sensory centres, the secretions in such a case will be in no way implicated. A sympathetic nerve of the ganglionic system,—perhaps the most important relic of invertebrate life in the vertebrate kingdom, including even the lymphatic system itself,—is much less highly specialised than either a sensory or a motor nerve, and, consequently, to this extent more capable of resisting the virulence of any virus, or the germination of any micro-organism, and, therefore, much less easily invaded and injured by that of rabies.

When the sympathetic system is materially invaded, it is only by a "virus" of rabies of the most massive kind to be met with, and which has already been disseminated to overflowing through the entire cerebro-spinal field. When the "virus" in the central nervous system is sufficiently copious, and consequently sufficiently virulent, not only to irritate functionally the bulbar centres, and through these in the same way sympathetic ganglionic centres, which, from the increased temperature, and from the scanty, frothy, salivary-secretion is probably the case in convulsive-rabies, but likewise to impair and paralyse the ganglionic system itself, there is a very different condition of things to meet.

In connection with these widely-spread, disastrous effects of a paralytic-, as opposed to merely convulsive-rabies, it has to be borne in mind that it is the sympathetic, not the cerebro-spinal system, which regulates all secretion, and mainly, if not solely, through its vascular mechanism ; for the secreting glands are, one and all, built on a network of sympathetic nerves, and well-nigh of these exclusively. The virus, therefore, which irritates the cerebro-spinal axis through its sensory and motor roots into wide-spread peripheral hyperæsthesia and convulsiveness, will stimulate the sympathetic system, if it will stimulate it at all, through its ganglia into merely a still fainter peripheral spasmodic affection ; which, as already stated, will practically have the effect of diminishing rather than of increasing secretion.   And it will diminish it, because the vascular supply of the glands, if not the glandular tissue itself, will everywhere be under the influence of the same spasm.   The nervous elements of the glands being almost wholly sympathetic will be solely influenced by the morbid condition of the ganglia.   But, on the other hand, the virus which not only acutely irritates but absolutely paralyses even the ganglionic sympathetic system itself with a corresponding paresis or paralysis of the glandular structure and of its vascular supply, will, *ipso facto*, have the effect of enormously increasing secretion ; for the vascular supply, under the blighting influence of the paralysing irritant, will everywhere be paralysed, and there will be no control on the secretion whatever ; it will simply flow passively and incessantly.   Moreover, the virus-germ which is located in the ganglia, controlling the nerve-supply of the gland, will find its way in steady streams through the sympathetic nerves to the nervous elements of the gland itself ; with the result that the unchecked, flowing secretion will be, in proportion to the amount of paralysis, charged and saturated with the virus and its micro-organism.

Now, this is precisely the set of morbid conditions which one finds in, respectively, convulsive- and paralytic-rabies.   The secretion is diminished in the former, but enormously increased in the latter ; and the diminished secretion of the former is deficient in, and at times wholly devoid of, infective material, whilst the thin, overflowing secretion of the latter is, sooner or later, saturated with virus-germ. It may, consequently, be probably taken as a rule that the more a secreting organ depends upon the sympathetic nervous system for its nerve-supply, and, therefore, for the amount of its secreting power, or the more the sympathetic nervous system enters into its structure and composition, the more certainly, in the event of a rabic infection of the sympathetic nerve-centres, may the rabies-microbe be looked for in the thin, unchecked secretion of these secreting organs.

And this is pre-eminently true in respect of the salivary gland and the salivary secretion above all other secretions in the economy.   So true is this that the paralytic element may be taken as an absolute surety of the existence of a rabic secretion in the salivary glands, and, therefore, which is of the greatest practical moment, of a capacity on the part of the paralysed or partially-paralysed victim to infect with a bite. As we have already seen, every important secreting organ is always more or less involved in paralytic-rabies, but only in paralytic-rabies, and in proportion to the amount of paralysis induced. There is probably no extent of paralysis, however apparently insignificant, which is not accompanied by a corresponding implication of secretion. But whilst so many important secreting organs are involved in every paralytic case, it nevertheless still remains the fact that the salivary gland with its secretion is the most involved of any, or, from first to last, invariably the *most* virulent. Not only is it the most intensely rabic of any, but it is likewise the first and the earliest to be invaded by the micro-organism.

Why, however, should the salivary-secretion be so early involved of any, and always the most seriously and thoroughly? Is it to be inferred from this fact that the rabies-germ is, after all, like that of tetanus and diphtheria and many other germ-diseases, 'of peripheral, not of centric, cultivation, and that its prime peripheral seat is really in the salivary gland itself? There would be considerable force in such an argument were the secretions in the case of tetanus, as in paralytic-rabies, saturated, or even at all charged, with the micro-organism of the germ-disease ; or, on the other hand, in respect of paralytic-rabies itself, were the salivary gland the only gland which yielded the rabies-germ. This, however, as we have seen, is not the case. Consequently, the salivary gland is not the specific seat of germination of the rabific micro-organism, any more than the pancreas or liver, and the micro-organism arrives hither, as it arrives in all the other excretory glands, only in its normal progress through the nervous tracts from above.

Why, however, it may be insisted, should the salivary gland, as compared with any other, be necessarily so early invaded in the course of the paralytic form of the disease ; and why should it be so invariably and so inevitably rabic, even if no other secretion should be so? Clearly enough, it is at least the prime channel of elimination. Turning once more to the immediate scene of the more pronounced signs and symptoms, particularly of paralytic-rabies, *i.e.* to the glosso-pharyngeal region, where the paresis and analgesia are most marked, we have a very distinct clue to the solution. Assuming that rabies is centric in its cultivation, and that there is a progress of the rabific microbe from the bulb or cerebro-spinal substance through the nerve-tracts to the very periphery itself, it is not surprising that so massive an invasion, from above, should be more pronounced and more thorough in this particular region than in any other in the affected organism. Under such circumstances the bite of a rabid dog, suffering from "dumb madness," should never fail to infect, as its salivary-secretion would never fail to be rabic.

As it so happens, the important group of nerves, already specified, which constitutes the cerebro-spinal nerve-supply of the glosso-pharyngeal region proceeds directly from the substance of the bulb. As we have already seen in their distribution over throat, tongue, palate and pharynx, parotid and salivary glands, &c., these nerves are most intimately blended with one another ; but, still more important, each nerve of this group,—pneumogastric, the gustatory, the glosso-pharyngeal, &c.—is likewise not less intimately interwoven with filaments of the sympathetic nerve-system to its finest subdivisions. This same series of nerves is more intimately interwoven with the ganglionic sympathetic system than is any other nerve or group of nerves in the entire cerebro-spinal system, from the brain to the cauda equina. This is surely a fact of deep significance, and a most important consideration in the causation of the disease ; for if this be so, the anatomical connection is an all-important factor in the pro-duction, not merely of the paralytic form of the malady, but through this of the infective or rabic condition of the salivary secretion of every such case. Under such circumstances it is inconceivable that the salivary secretion could ever fail to be rabic ; and, moreover, since the bulb is the head-centre of the germination of the rabies-germ, that it should not invariably be the earliest to be charged with the infective material and, from first to last, the most virulent of any secretion in the economy. If a rabic paralysis of the glosso-pharyngeal sympathetic system of ganglia, from a progressive invasion of the rabific microbe from the bulbar substance into these ganglia, be at the root of the most pronounced paralytic and infective phenomena of rabies ; here is a special network of sympathetic nerve-tissue which, given a progressive, paralysing "virus" from the bulb, could not fail to induce the most paralytic and, at the very earliest stages, the most infective form of the disease. If the ganglionic, not less than the cerebro-spinal, centres be not rabidised and paralysed, and crowded centres of the germinating rabies-germ, it is difficult to see why the salivary-secretion should ever be charged with the micro-organism. But, conversely, the ganglionic centres, not less than the cerebro-spinal, being invariably more or less rabidised and paralysed, and active foci of the rabies-germ, in the profoundest paralytic-rabies, the salivary-secretion, sooner than any other, cannot fail to be implicated; and it is inconceivable that infection could fail to take place from the saliva of such a case.

Nor is the progress of the rabific microbe from the cerebro-spinal axis to the sympathetic.ganglionic system a mere accidental invasion. The path to the sympathetic system is a direct and inevitable one, and invariably through the *sensory*, not the *motor* side of the cerebrospinal system. In this connection it is worth recalling, and surely not without significance, that the fundamental feature of rabies, whether it be of convulsive or of paralytic character, is the disturbance of sensibility rather than of motion; it is the widely-spread hyperæsthesia or, as the case may be, the pronounced analgesia rather than the convulsiveness or the paresis and paralysis. Even on the assumption that the motor and sensory roots are equally favourable media for the cultivation of the rabies-germ, as we have already seen, the distinctly greater size of the latter all over the cerebro-spinal axis would determine the sensory roots as the more special germinating-ground, and render the sensory disturbance the more pronounced in every form of the malady. Now, if this be the fact, in its invasion through the bulkier sensory roots and tracts, the rabific microbe of a paralytic-rabies would not only gain in activity, but, still more disastrous, with this multiplication and increase of activity, it would likewise, in migratory colonies, pass from the cerebro-spinal axis to the sympathetic ganglionic system; and both systems would become simultaneously raging centres of paralysing virulence. For not only are the sensory nerves, all over the cerebro-spinal axis, larger and bulkier than the motor, but, still more important, in respect of the production of infectiveness, it is the sensory, not the motor roots, which are provided with sympathetic ganglia.

" The posterior (or sensory) roots are distinguished from the anterior by their greater size. *Each sensory nerve is furnished with a ganglion. The size of the ganglion is in proportion to that of the nerves on which they are formed.* The anterior or motor roots are the smaller of the two, and *they are devoid of ganglionic enlargement*[1]."

And for this reason strychnine or such a virus as that of tetanus, as opposed to that of rabies, being so exclusively a motor irritant, never affects the ganglionic system, or therefore the secretions. The fact that tetanus and strychnine-poisoning are wholly

---

[1] Quain's *Anatomy*, as above. Here, purposely italicised.

spinal diseases, and mainly in the inferior tracts of the spinal substance, would, in itself, point to the exclusively motor character of the maladies ; for the further down the cord (from the "bulb") the more prominent are the motor fibres.

Be this as it may, the entire sensory side of the cerebro-spinal system is most intimately intermingled with the ganglionic sympathetic system. It is so organically incorporated that they cannot be separated from each other ; and this, moreover, is the more marked the higher up the cerebro-spinal axis we proceed. The posterior spinal nerves have each their ganglion, down to the cauda equina itself, nay, further, it is important to note that "the size of the ganglion is in proportion to that of the nerves on which they are formed." So that the larger the sensory root and the more favourable as a "nidus" for the rabific microbe, the larger likewise will be the annexed sympathetic ganglion, and the more favourable as a fresh "nidus" of germination. It is the motor roots which are so destitute of ganglia ; they have none at all. The great sensory nerves of the bulb and brain are still more intimately blended with them ; and here, too (even more than in respect of the spinal nerves), the size or number of the ganglia is "in proportion to that of the nerves on which they are formed." Thus, the fifth or trifacial nerve, "the largest cranial nerve," "is analogous to the spinal nerves, in respect that it consists of a motor and sensory part, and that the sensory fibres pass through a ganglion, *while the motor do not*" ; the sensory division being likewise much the larger and bulkier[1]. But, so far as the production of the most active and characteristic phenomena of acute paralytic-rabies is concerned, the all-important set of bulbar sensory nerves which so specially supply the glosso-pharyngeal region, is, as already demonstrated, more intimately incorporated, not only with each other, but with the ganglionic system, than perhaps any other group of nerves of the spinal axis. Every one of these great sensory nerves has two or more ganglia incorporated in its structure, and the sympathetic nerves from these ganglia run side by side with the sensory fibres to their utmost distribution over the tongue, palate, throat, pharynx, parotid and salivary glands.

Nor is this complete incorporation of the sensory, as opposed to the motor, side of the cerebro-spinal axis with the ganglionic system a mere anatomical accident. It is much too constant and thorough to be any fortuitous union. It is perhaps hardly too much to say

---

[1] See Quain's *Anatomy*, p. 595.

that the incorporation is probably as old as the genesis and evolution of the cerebro-spinal system itself, and, in reality, but an abiding trace of the stage when the cerebro-spinal system was but a simple offshoot of the sympathetic in process of differentiation. It was an offshoot, however, whose ultimate differentiation has transcended the relatively simple structure from which it has been derived more wonderfully than even the most beautiful flower or fruit has transcended the simple leaf, or cluster of leaves, of which it is still so essentially constructed. Whether this be so or not, the sensory nerve, and at its very root in the cerebro-spinal substance, is still as intimately interwoven with the ganglionic system, as if it had dragged the latter along with it to the very cerebro-spinal axis, itself.

They are so completely incorporated at their point of union, and in so many features so closely allied to each other, that the sensory nerve may be said to stand functionally, not less than anatomically, midway between the voluntary motor nerve and the simple sympathetic. The anatomical connection is by no means merely apparent.

"The fibres of the posterior roots in man and the mammalia appear to pass through the ganglion without union with its cells. The cells are both unipolar and bipolar; but the fibres connected with them all pass to the periphery (Kölliker); so that beyond the ganglion the posterior root of the nerve has received an additional set of fibres besides those which it contains before reaching the ganglion.

"But in fishes, on the contrary, *all the fibres of the posterior root are connected with the opposite extremities of the bipolar cells of the ganglion*[1]."

With so demonstrated a connection in the fish and the lower vertebrates, and probably the lower one searches the more obvious will be the union, the apparent isolation of the fibres in man, or the highest vertebrates, might well be a mere appearance. In respect of the nature and the origin of the connection between the two systems of nerve, their proved union in the lowest vertebrates is a much more significant fact than if the union had been actually demonstrated in man, and were but an apparent one in the fish. The anatomical connection, such as it is, is therefore, clearly enough, a very profound one; being as old as the cerebro-spinal system of the fish or lowest vertebrate, itself.

[1] Quain's *Anatomy*, Part II. p. 631.

And the functional character of the sensory nerve is not less closely and intimately blended with that of the sympathetic. A sensory nerve will not long seriously suffer without, sooner or later, a sympathetic nerve or a sympathetic ganglion and the region which they supply more or less suffering. The lesion of the one tract is transferred directly to the other. And, conversely, a sympathetic nerve or ganglion or the region which it supplies will not long be irritated without a corresponding irritation in some of the sensory fibres which accompany it to its remotest distribution. Thus, an hepatic lesion involving some ganglionic centre,—say, cancerous or even inflammatory infiltration of the ganglion,—gives rise to persistent pain in the right shoulder; the disturbance affecting some sensory tracts of the region. Again, a carious tooth not only induces widely-spread neuralgia, but long-continued neuralgia of intense character will induce a corresponding irritation of the ganglionic system with which the sensory fibres are incorporated; and this, in its turn, may induce ophthalmia, spasmodic croup, or the acutest gastritis. Or, again, tubercular infiltration of the base of the lung may induce a ganglionic lesion which will result in herpes zoster; or pneumonic condensation of the lung will induce a ganglionic disturbance which will result in herpes labialis, in both cases, probably, through fibres of the pneumogastric.

No such relationship to the sympathetic system is characteristic of the motor nerve, voluntary or involuntary. The motor system of nerves would appear to be absolutely independent of the ganglionic system, and to owe their function and very integrity solely to their connection with the cerebro-spinal axis.

In the light of these considerations it is obvious why in rabies of the sympathetic system, or, in other words, in every profound paralytic form of the malady, the salivary secretion should be exceptionally rabic, and the earliest of all the secretions to be invaded by the rabific micro-organism. The salivary gland is pre-eminently supplied with the sympathetic nervous element and with the largest sensory nerves; and both arise in the bulb itself, which, however, is the specific seat of germination of the rabific micro-organism. These bulbar sensory nerves are, one and all, incorporated with the largest sympathetic ganglia, and also with the greatest number of them, in the entire cerebro-spinal axis. In the event of paralytic-rabies, or of a paralysing "nidus" of virus-germ in the sensory roots of the bulb, and likewise, simultaneously, in the sympathetic ganglia of these sensory roots, how could the salivary secretion fail to be the first to be involved of any secretion, and from first to last to be the most thoroughly invaded with the rabific microbe? If, to begin with, the rabific microbe be at all copious in the cerebro-spinal axis,—and in no structure will it be more copious or potent than in the bulb,— assuming that, in consequence of bulk, the rabies-germ invades in all probability sensory even more than motor strands, to a certainty the sensory tracts will be the first paths of its germinating progress ; and this, again, with a cumulative germination, will inevitably lead to the ganglionic system. The invasion of this ganglionic system, however, with its paralysis of secreting structures, is a fundamental factor in the causation of infective rabies. The micro-organism, still multiplying and accumulating in these ganglionic centres, will, ultimately, overflow them, and with its virus in copious streams will find its way down the sympathetic nerves to the remotest secreting organs, but before all to the salivary, the parotidean and bucco-pharyngeal secreting glands. The abundant, ever-flowing secretion resulting therefrom, salivary and parotidean, will at last, literally, be saturated with the virus-germ. So much so, that an animal, whether a dog or a rabbit, suffering from this profoundly paralytic-rabies, will, as a matter of fact, never fail to impart infection with its salivary secretion.

CHAPTER V.

THE RABIES-VIRUS QUANTITATIVE RATHER THAN QUALITATIVE IN CHARACTER.

It would appear, then, that one form of rabies differs from another,—the completely convulsive, for example, from the convulso-paralytic, and this in its turn from the exclusively paralytic,—in the amount rather than in the intrinsic nature of the rabies-microbe, which settles and germinates in the central nervous substance. After infection, the rabies-germ will, sooner or later, settle in some part of the cerebro-spinal substance, and induce the disease. But the amount which will reach and be deposited in this structure will not necessarily be the exact amount received in infection. This will be determined by the distance of the peripheral site from the cerebro-spinal substance, and by the amount of refractoriness to the rabific microbe possessed by the infected animal. In every case of the disease, the rabies-germ in the infected wound will in some amount ultimately reach the cerebro-spinal substance; and, having settled in this most fertile germinating ground of the entire animal economy, the due germination of the microbe will ensue, and nothing thereafter "prevent" its growth. But this accounts merely for the occurrence of the disease. It does not explain the extraordinary, protean variability of the malady, particularly in the dog, or the class of animal capable of attenuating or deteriorating rabies. Since in every case without exception the rabies-microbe in some amount reaches and germinates in nervous substance,—for it can germinate in no other structure,—why should rabies vary so much, or even at all?

From the outset of the malady, the variations would appear to depend upon the variations in the amount of the rabies-microbe introduced in infection. This will really determine the quantity which will at last settle in the central nervous axis, itself; and the character of the rabies induced will be often enough irrespective of that of the rabies from which it was derived. Even the typical "specific" character of any given form of rabies, however characteristic of whole races of animals, as dog-rabies, monkey-rabies, cat-rabies, or rabbit-rabies, the experimental investigation has proved to be solely determined by the specific quantity of rabies-microbe, of which its virus-germ is constituted. And as this quantity may vary with every possible variation of infection, the rabies induced will likewise vary, and to a corresponding extent.

For this reason, of two inoculations of precisely the same infective material, and, of even the same amount, injected into two totally different sites, for example, in the face and in the foot, by no means the same amount of the rabies-germ will have reached the central nervous system in the diseases resulting therefrom; and the difference in this amount may be exactly measured by the difference in the rabies induced. If this be so, it is obvious that the amount of the rabies-microbe received in infection, and which ultimately reaches and settles in the cerebro-spinal substance, is the sole cause of every form of rabies which occurs. As this amount varies with precisely the same inoculations in different sites, or different inoculations in precisely the same site, the resulting rabies, according to the site, or according to the variation in the amount of rabies-microbe involved in the site, will invariably be a form equivalent to the amount of infective material which reaches the cerebro-spinal axis. This would appear to be a fundamental law in the causation of the disease; and it is a fact of paramount importance in the elucidation of the malady.

A graduated series of rabic bites or of inoculations of the rabies-virus in even the same site in a group of the same animals,—the wounds in the areolar tissue but varying in depth and extent,—will reveal a series of rabies, varying in virulence, not only from each other, but from the rabies from which they are derived, and strictly in proportion to the amount of rabific microbe in the respective wounds. In spite of their common origin in one and the same rabies, the varying rabic wounds (although in the same vicinity) will yield a group of rabies, ranging from a form of the disease so essentially convulsive in character that the salivary secretion may be practically unaffected, up to the severest convulso-paralytic or even wholly paralytic rabies of highest infective rate. The initial rabies may be unlike any one of the group, being either severer or feebler. This phenomenon was well illustrated by M. Galtier's experiments on rabbits, already referred to. In spite of the "virus," which was used, being only a canine-virus, it induced in the massive form in which it was inserted into the subcutaneous areolar lymph-sacs, not a convulsive-rabies, but a pronounced paralytic-rabies. No such phenomenon would result from the most massive inoculation of any small pox-virus, or anthrax-virus, or even of tetanus-virus, or of that of many more germ-diseases. In such germ-diseases, on the contrary, neither the site, nor the amount of infection, determines the character of the resulting malady; one amount of the same virus-germ, and one site being as effective as another. But varying quantities of the same rabic medulla, whatever its intrinsic rabific quality, whilst they will undoubtedly rabidise the rabbit or any intensifier, even irrespective of site, will by no means induce in each case the same rabies, or necessarily reproduce the rabies from which they have, one and all, been derived. The rabies induced will in every case be strictly commensurate with the quantity of rabific microbe in the subcutaneous infiltration. Progressively smaller quantities of the infective material will, in spite of the original rabies being of the severest form, yield progressively feebler forms of the disease with longer incubation-periods. Conversely, larger and larger quantities of the rabic medulla, in spite of the original rabies being of the feeblest form, will yield severer and more complicated forms of the disease. The disease will change with every change in the amount of infection, and will be irrespective of the special rabies from which it was derived. If this be so, it follows that rabies in every form, from the feeblest to the severest, depends, not so much upon the special virulence of the rabies from which it is derived, as upon the special quantity of the rabific microbe introduced in infection; its special potency, as a rabies, being determined by the special quantity of the rabific microbe settling in the cerebro-spinal axis; and this again by the extent and depth of the rabic wounds or, in other words, by the amount of the peripheral infection.

But, if it be the fact that mere quantity of the virus-germ is the sole determining factor of every form of rabies, is it so very certain that a rabific microbe exists; or, assuming the existence of the microbe, that it so invariably reaches the cerebro-spinal axis to elaborate its virus; or that, in point of fact, it ever leaves the peripheral site? Since a varying quantity of virus-germ is so essential to the production of the varying forms of rabies, without which there never probably would be any variation in the disease at all; since the virus-germ of rabies is a quantitative one, and induces a rabies strictly proportioned to the amount employed; is it not probable that the virus or poisonous product of the rabific microbe, itself, apart from the quantity of the micro-organism, is the direct and exclusive cause of all the morbid phenomena? The pathological effects of strychnine, morphia, alcohol, arsenic, and of every other virulent product, organic or inorganic, are strictly proportioned to the amount of the product injected or administered. The pathological effects of the virus or virulent product of such germ-diseases as have proved capable of being separated from their productive micro-organisms, such as Koch's tuberculin, the bacillary product of diphtheria and of tetanus, and of many others, are in like manner strictly proportioned to the amount of the virus employed. They are quantitative viruses. This quantitative relationship is absolute. So, apparently, is it with respect to rabies-virus; the train of morbid phenomena set up is strictly commensurate with the amount of the virulent product elaborated in the disease. From this circumstance, therefore, it may be unhesitatingly asserted that the virulent product ultimately evolved by the rabific microbe, and not the rabific microbe, is, *per se*, the cause of every form of the disease to be met with; and that without such virulent product, and suddenly secreted in the nerve centres, there never would be rabies, however much rabific microbe might be cultivated in the tissues. But although the virulent product evolved in the disease solely induces it, it by no means follows that the rabific microbe which elaborates this virus does not invariably accompany or precede it even to the deepest centres of the cerebro-spinal axis. Were this not so, mere change of site would make no difference whatever in the action of the toxic product or virus. As with strychnine, alcohol, morphia, tuberculin, all sites of infection would be equally effective. Consequently, it is not so much a variation in the amount of virulent product *as a variation in the amount of rabific microbe introduced*, which accounts for the variation of any given series of rabies; for in reality the amount of virus evolved will solely depend upon the amount of rabific microbe in the case.

But this fact by no means involves that this poisonous product is elaborated only at the peripheral site, or, indeed, even in the peripheral tissues at all. It does not preclude the possibility of the rabific microbe being constantly conveyed to the central nervous system, where it exclusively elaborates its virus. If the rabies-microbe were, like the tetanus-bacillus, strictly confined to the periphery, or its virus or pathogenic product solely elaborated in the peripheral tissue, and poured into the blood-stream to do its remote deadly work, all peripheral sites would be equally effective. The smallest amount of any given virus-germ, capable of inducing the disease, would be in any and every site, as effective as the largest amount; and, as in tetanus, all forms of the disease from the same virus-germ would be practically alike. But in respect of rabies this is not the fact. The amount of the individual rabific microbes in an infection, not of the virus or virulent product which they, ultimately, in nervous substance elaborate, is, therefore, the real factor of any given form of rabies.

Fortunately, M. Pasteur's research in the elucidation of this subject leaves no room for doubt.

"We have found," says M. Pasteur, as one of the earliest of his discoveries, "that by inoculating small quantities of virus, the duration of incubation was considerably increased. And the same (virus), if diluted beyond a certain limit, which (in the dog) is not very far, remains without effect when inoculated[1]."

Or, again,

"We have as a matter of fact recognized that it is possible, experimentally, to produce 'furious' rabies from 'dumb' rabies, and, inversely, 'dumb' rabies from 'furious' rabies[2]."

How is this remarkable transformation effected? Simply by a variation in the amount of the same virus-germ in the infection. A large copious injection of the virus-germ of a furious rabies will induce a dumb or paralytic rabies, as in Galtier's experiments on the rabbit, or as in paralytic-hydrophobia from extreme cat-bite or wolf-bite of the face and hands; and, on the contrary, a very small injection of the virus-germ of this dumb-rabies will as certainly induce a merely furious or convulsive-rabies. Here, then, was clear evidence of the general fact that the strength or weakness of rabies wholly depends upon the amount of the rabific microbe introduced in infection. And this variation into the extreme forms of the disease from one and the same infective material will occur, whatever the site, or whatever the mode of inoculation, intracranial, intravenous, or subcutaneous, provided the amount of rabific microbe in the infection be correspondingly varied. But, it is important to note, the paralytic-rabies induced, when the amount of rabific microbe

[1] *Comptes Rendus*, Dec. 11, 1882.   [2] *Ibidem.*

injected is very large, will be all the more pronounced the nearer the peripheral site of infection to the central nervous system; and, conversely, the "furious" or convulsive-rabies induced, when the amount of rabies-germ is very small, will be all the more pronounced the further the site of infection from the central nervous system. In other words, the paralytic- or the convulsive-rabies will be determined by the amount of rabific microbe which, in a potent and active condition, will reach and be sown in the cerebro-spinal axis; and this, in its turn, by the amount of rabific microbe in the infection, and its proximity to the central nervous system.

If this be so, the intracranial inoculation ought to be the most unfailing in producing *the paralytic form* of the disease, even in such an alternator as the dog. ' This, however, would appear to be by no means the fact. The intracranial inoculation in the dog, or any animal equally capable of attenuating rabies or transmission, is almost always followed by merely a convulsive or *"furious rabies,"* whereas the intravenous or even subcutaneous inoculation, so very much further removed from the medulla oblongata, is as frequently followed even in the same class of animal by a paralytic or "dumb rabies."

"It is well known," says M. Pasteur, "that the bitten dog, if he takes the disease at all, shows in the majority of cases symptoms of furious rabies with a propensity to bite and the special rabid voice. In the habitual run of our experiments, when we inoculate the rabies-virus into a vein, or into the subcutaneous areolar tissue, *we more often give rise to the dumb* or *paralytic form* of madness, voiceless and tame. By intracranial inoculation, on the other hand, *the rule is that furious madness is produced*[1]."

Is this, then, an exception to the general rule, that the nearer the peripheral site of infection to the cerebro-spinal axis the more rabific microbe will reach the cerebro-spinal substance, and the more potent and active will be the microbe? The exception is only an apparent one, and but proves the rule. What is the character of this *intracranial inoculation*; and wherein does it differ from the subcutaneous and intravenous? In the former, as it so happens, *only two drops of* the "*supernatant liquid*" of a rabid emulsion are used. Any larger injection than this in the neighbourhood of such vital structures would probably kill outright, without respect to the production of rabies. The intracranial inoculation from its very

---

[1] *Comptes Rendus*, Feb. 25, 1884. Purposely italicised.

site must, therefore, if it is to rabidise at all, be extremely limited in amount. But there is no such limit in an intravenous or a sub-cutaneous inoculation. The rabific microbe in such an infection may be of the largest amount, without necessarily being lethal. Thus, it will not be maintained that the intravenous or the subcutaneous inoculation which produces a dumb- or paralytic-rabies contains but the "two drops" of an emulsion which, on intracranial inoculation, produce in the same class of animal merely a furious or convulsive-rabies. And if this be the fact, it will not be contended that the massive subcutaneous inoculation, if borne, when injected under the meninges, or directly into the neighbourhood of the medulla oblongata itself, will produce merely a furious rabies. No one has shown more clearly than M. Pasteur that the very contrary of this is the invariable law.

"It might be asked," he says in discussing this subject, "why intracranial inoculation invariably produces rabies, and never the refractory state? It would not be a sufficient answer to say that by that process the virus is in all cases brought at once in immediate contact with the encephalon. For, as a matter of fact, the massive hypodermic inoculations must in a large number of cases have, quite as directly as by the intracranial inoculation, conveyed the virus and its figured elements to the encephalon by the venous or lymphatic channels. The real difference between the two modes of inoculation appears to me to consist in this circumstance, that subdural inoculation never introduces into the system more than *a very minute quantity of virus*; whereas for hypodermic injections *the quantities used have always been much more considerable.*"

And, again, in alluding to the "dogs bitten by mad dogs," he adds,—

"Dogs bitten by mad dogs do not always take rabies. This is a well-known fact. Such bites, *like the subdural inoculation,* can only introduce into the system *very small quantities of virus*[1]."

If, then, the quantity of rabific microbe in an infection be the determining factor of every form of rabies; and if the intravenous or the subcutaneous inoculation which produces a paralytic-rabies has invariably a much more considerable quantity of virus-germ than the intracranial inoculation, it is not surprising, not only that the rabies resulting from such very different infections should vary so

[1] *Annales de l'Institut Pasteur.* Note by M. Pasteur, Dec. 27, 1886. Italics not M. Pasteur's.

considerably ; but that the rabies from intravenous or subcutaneous inoculations should be so much more pronounced and paralytic.

If there were no such difference in the quantity of virus-germ for each of these inoculations, an injection into the popliteal vein,— the usual intravenous site which was used by M. Pasteur,—is, as it so happens, nearly as favourable a site for effective infection as the intracranial inoculation itself ; and, without question, a much more favourable site for the ultimate development of a paralytic-rabies of the prolonged, creeping, intermittent character. Such a site is very closely and directly related, through the lymphatic even more than the venous channels, to the lumbar-swelling of the chord itself, which is probably the invariable starting-point of every case of ascending and intermittent paralytic-rabies. Virus-germ introduced into this structure in the smallest quantity, providing the bulb be not simultaneously or soon invaded, would to a certainty germinate and multiply up the cord, invading a very large tract of the spinal axis before the bulb would be seriously affected and death take place. And in such cases of what one may term *inferior* as opposed to *superior* primary invasion of the spinal axis, the rabies, simple to begin with, is probably always paralytic in the end, however protracted, and however intermittent from first to last. That in this *inferior* invasion, particularly from an intravenous inoculation, the lumbar-swelling is an all-important centre in the settlement of the rabies-germ has been experimentally demonstrated by M. Pasteur. Thus, in alluding to the particular form of paralytic-rabies, resulting from the intravenous inoculation, he says,—

"We sacrificed several dogs on the appearance of the first symptoms of paralysis ; and, then, by a comparative study of the spinal cord,—*in the lumbar-swelling* in particular, and *of the medulla oblongata*, we discovered that the former was occasionally virulent when the latter was not so[1]."

Or, again,

"The details of our experiments would tend to show that after inoculation of the poison in the way we have indicated" (that is, from intravenous or massive subcutaneous infection) "the spinal marrow is the region first attacked; the virus locating itself and multiplying there before spreading to other parts[2]."

But if the intracranial inoculation produces merely a furious rabies, on the other hand, it will not be asserted that every intra-

[1] *Comptes Rendus*, Feb. 25, 1884.   [2] *Ibidem*, Dec. 11, 1882.

venous injection of even "purest virus," or of the most potent rabific microbe, invariably produces a paralytic-rabies. Such is by no means the fact. Any form of rabies, a purely furious rabies itself, may be induced by an intravenous infection according to the quantity of the rabific microbe in the injection, and even when the rabies from which the injection has been obtained has been of the profoundest paralytic character.

"We have also ascertained that it is possible to give rise to *furious* madness"—in addition to the "dumb" paralytic madness— "by intravenous or subcutaneous inoculation, *provided that very small quantities only* of the virus be used. The smaller the quantity of virus or disease-material used in the intravenous or hypodermic inoculation, the more certainly is the *furious form* of rabies reproduced[1]."

It is obvious, therefore, that if the usual intracranial inoculation be always followed by a furious rabies, it is solely because it always contains the very smallest possible quantity of the rabid material; and that, could the site tolerate, till the disease was matured, a very much larger and more virulent inoculation of even the same virus-germ, a still more pronounced paralytic-rabies would be produced than by any intravenous or hypodermic injection, however massive the latter.

It follows from such results that, broadly speaking, any given form of rabies is determined by the quantity of the rabies-germ, which ultimately settles and multiplies in the cerebro-spinal substance; and that the nearer the site of peripheral infection to the central nervous system the greater the quantity of the peripheral rabific microbe which will settle in the latter, and the more potent and active the micro-organism. With a minimum quantity in any infection, intracranial, intravenous or subcutaneous, a *furious* or convulsive-rabies is the result. With a maximum quantity, whatever the mode or site of infection, providing it does not kill outright or produce a condition of "protection," a *paralytic*-rabies is the invariable result. With an *inferior invasion* of the spinal axis of minimum quantity, where the lumbar-swelling is the prime seat of germination, a prolonged or sub-acute, creeping, *intermittent paralytic-rabies* will ensue. With, on the contrary, a *superior invasion* of the spinal axis of a minimum quantity of the rabies-germ, and where the bulb is the prime seat of germination, a *furious*

[1] *Comptes Rendus*, Feb. 25, 1884. Italics not M. Pasteur's.

or *convulsive*-rabies, with death, will invariably ensue. With a *superior* and *inferior* simultaneous invasion of the spinal axis of maximum quantity, where the bulb is the central seat of the microbe settlement, an *acute, general, paralytic-rabies* probably as certainly ensues.

As illustrating this fundamental quantitative principle in the causation of the malady a few typical groups of M. Pasteur's experiments may be cited, as absolutely conclusive.

"On May 6, 1883," says M. Pasteur, "we inoculate into the vein of the right popliteal space (behind the knee) of three dogs portions of a rabid medulla diluted in sterilised broth. To the first dog, we give *half a cubic centimetre* of the turbid liquid; to the second, *one-hundredth part of that quantity;* to the third, *the two-hundredth part only.* As early as the tenth day, the first dog begins to lose his appetite, and on the eighteenth he is completely paralysed; he dies two days later without having at any time had the peculiar bark of mad dogs *or tried to bite.* On the thirty-seventh day after inoculation, the second dog still eats well. On the thirty-eighth day he begins to look suspicious. On the thirty-ninth day, he has the rabid voice; and is found dead the next day—*i.e.* the fortieth. The third dog has not taken the disease at all[1]."

Here, then, we have three inoculations, in animals of the same race, where, nevertheless, simply on account of a diminution in each case of the amount of the disease-material used,—for, otherwise, the conditions of infection were absolutely identical,—we have for each inoculation a very different rabies produced. This is surely a most remarkable variability; nevertheless, it is a very uniform and exact one, and depends wholly on the quantity of rabific microbe received in infection, which in this set of experiments has been just as mathematically exact. No such law as this, no such quantitative relationship, holds good of the morbific microbe of smallpox or scarlatina or anthrax, or even of tetanus and many germ-diseases.

Such results are still more pronounced when double the amount of the "virus" is used. Take such an instance.

"Another experiment consisted in inoculating into a popliteal vein *one cubic centimetre* of rabid matter"—the same "rabid matter" as used in the set of experiments just examined,—"in sterilised broth for the first dog; *one-twentieth of that quantity* for a second dog; and *one-fiftieth* for a third dog. The incubative periods were, respec-

[1] *Comptes Rendus*, Feb. 25, 1884.

tively, *seven, twenty*, and *twenty-five days*. The two first dogs took paralytic-rabies; the third had the *furious*, barking, and biting form[1]."

Of what special form the initial rabies was in this double set of experiments has been omitted to be mentioned. But from the results obtained it was probably of very pronounced paralytic character. Although the conditions of infection are again so similar, the varying results obtained, if on a much larger scale, are exactly parallel to the differences in the quantities in the inoculations. Thus, in spite of the first inoculation being so saturated with rabific microbe that it actually rabidised a dog in *seven days*, the lumbar-swelling and the bulb being, in all probability simultaneously, invaded by the infective material, nevertheless, an inoculation, possessing the $\frac{1}{20}$th part of this "virus" does not rabidise another animal of the same race for *twenty days*; and as it was likewise a paralytic-rabies, it was, from its duration, probably the sub-acute, creeping paralytic-rabies of inferior or lumbar invasion. The same "virus," or virus-germ, when reduced to $\frac{1}{50}$th of its original quantity, imparts the disease only after *five-and-twenty days*, and in so wholly a convulsive or furious form that there is reason to believe that the salivary or any other secretion was unaffected, and that the animal would fail to impart the disease with a bite. There is not one of the forms of rabies here produced which is the same as the original rabies, or the same as any other of the group. Even in so limited a set of experiments there is as great a difference between the extreme forms, as there is between the extreme cases to be found in the most extensive epidemic of dog-rabies. And this extraordinary variability, fortuitous as it looks, is no accident.

The special character of each of these forms has been determined solely by the special quantity of the rabies-germ which, after infection, has reached and settled in the cerebro-spinal substance.

Let, now, another group of experiments be examined with an initial rabies of known strength; and, this time, instead of a paralytic-rabies, a convulsive-rabies or the ordinary canine madness of the streets, whose "virus" is as a rule equivalent to an incubation-period, in the rabbit, of 15 or 16 days; a profoundly paralytic or "dumb" canine-rabies being equivalent to an 11 or 12 days' incubation in this animal. And the "ordinary" canine-virus will be the more suggestive because M. Pasteur, himself, has insisted upon this as the most stable

[1] *Comptes Rendus*, Feb. 25, 1884.

and unvarying of any "virus," not only in the dog, but in the entire animal kingdom. If this be so, no better rabies could be found to test the principle before us. Here, at all events, if in no other form of the disease, one might expect some considerable constancy under every condition of infection. What, however, is the fact?

"An emulsion was prepared by crushing a portion of the bulb of a dog, *which had died of ordinary canine-madness*, in three or four times its volume of sterilised broth.

"On May 10, 1882, we injected into the popliteal vein of a dog ten drops of this liquid; into a second dog we injected the $\frac{1}{100}$th of that quantity; into a third, the $\frac{1}{200}$th.

"Rabies showed itself in the first dog on *the eighteenth day* after the injection. Rabies showed itself on the *thirty-fifth day* in the second dog. The third dog did not take the disease at all"; "which means," as M. Pasteur adds, "that for that last animal, with the particular mode of inoculation employed, the quantity of virus injected was not sufficient to give rabies[1]."

The "virus" of even ordinary canine-rabies, therefore, in spite of its extreme prevalence over the animal kingdom, would appear to vary very considerably in potency and virulence, according to the quantity of the rabies-germ of which it is composed. This is surely singularly conclusive evidence that even in the most prevalent forms of rabies known, the special quantity,—rather than the special quality,—of the individual rabies-microbe is the factor of the special form of rabies produced.

That in this particular set of experiments the "virus" used was that merely of an *attenuator*, and in point of fact one of the most powerful in the animal kingdom ; and, moreover, that this "virus" was exclusively experimented with *on attenuators*, or on the class of animals capable of attenuating rabies on the transmission of the disease, may be taken as an objection. No such result, it may be alleged, would have occurred in respect of *intensifiers* or the order of animals capable of intensifying rabies. True ; the virus-germ of an attenuator, when passed through an attenuator, such as the dog or monkey, as we shall see, can never be a steady one. So far as the dog is concerned, the intrinsic, preventive power which it possesses above most animals will render an inoculation which is primarily weak even still weaker, and a virus-germ which is primarily

[1] M. Pasteur's Address to International Medical Congress at Copenhagen, Aug. 11, 1884.

potent and relatively unvarying, if not less virulent, certainly less stable and steady. In the case of an intensifier, on the contrary, such as the rabbit or guinea-pig, the reverse of this phenomenon is the invariable law.

Take, then, lastly, and as the most crucial test of all, the "virus" of the most pronounced paralytic rabbit-rabies to be met with even in the laboratory, and employed, not in the dog or any attenuator, but in the rabbit itself, perhaps the most pronounced intensifier known. Still more crucial, let the inoculations be, one and all, intracranial, not subcutaneous, nor intravenous.

"I now take another example," says M. Pasteur, "bearing on rabbits, and by a different mode of inoculation. This time the bulb of a rabbit which has died of rabies, after inoculation of an extremely powerful virus, is triturated and mixed up with two or three times its volume of sterilised broth. The mixture is allowed to stand a little; and then *two drops of the supernatant liquid* are injected, after trephining, into a first rabbit; into a second rabbit $\frac{1}{4}$th of that quantity; and, in succession, into other rabbits $\frac{1}{16}$th, $\frac{1}{64}$th, $\frac{1}{128}$th, and $\frac{1}{152}$nd of that same quantity. All these rabbits died of rabies, the incubation having been (respectively) eight days for the second; nine and ten days for the third and fourth; twelve and sixteen days for the last ones[1]."

Here, likewise, and in spite of the fact that the experiment has been conducted on the most potent of intensifiers, we have conclusive proof that in every form of rabies the special quantity of the rabific microbe in infection is the main factor in its production. In this most crucial set of experiments, as in the others examined, the form of rabies induced is, in one and all of the inoculations, in strict conformity with the quantity of virus-germ employed. Here, likewise, the rabies produced is irrespective of that which has originated the group. And it is surely most noteworthy that whilst with a "canine-virus," or in all the other sets of experiments examined, the initial rabies is frequently exceeded in virulence in the induced disease; here, on the contrary, in not one of the inoculations is the original form reproduced, much less exceeded in virulence. For stability of form and steadiness of potency, the initial rabies has commanded one and all of the inoculations. If persistency in virulence and stability of character are to be taken as the test of a "typical" rabies,—and there is no more infallible test,—then, this

[1] M. Pasteur's Address at the International Medical Congress at Copenhagen.

acute and extremely profound paralytic rabbit-rabies, not the
"ordinary" canine-rabies, would appear to be the most "typical"
and specific of all. The very appalling potency of the virus-germ of
the initial rabies of this group, and its stubborn stability, may be
gathered from the fact, that the rabies of the second inoculation,
which, however, possessed but a fourth part of its infective material,
nevertheless yielded an incubation of *eight days*,—in itself a most
deadly form of even the acutest paralytic rabbit-rabies of the
laboratory. An inoculation which possessed but the one-sixty-fourth
part of the initial infective material nevertheless yielded a rabies of
ten days' incubation, or a form of the disease still so extremely potent
that it was equivalent to the *normal* or characteristic rabbit-rabies,
and more than equivalent to that of the worst "dumb" paralytic
canine-madness in an epidemic. An inoculation which possessed but
the one-hundred-and-twenty-eighth part of the initial "virus," nevertheless yielded a rabies of *twelve days'* incubation, or a form of the
disease still so potent that it was equivalent to the "dumb" paralytic
canine-madness which is so phenomenally rare in an epidemic.
Lastly, an inoculation which possessed but the one-hundred-and-
fifty-second part of the initial rabific microbe was still of such
potency that it actually yielded a rabies of *sixteen days'* incubation;
or a form of the disease, which, as we have already seen, is exactly
equivalent to that of the ordinary or *normal* canine-rabies.

From such results two conclusions of prime importance may be
deduced. On the one hand, alike the most potent and the least
potent and transient forms of the disease are solely determined by
the quantity of the individual rabific microbe, which is introduced
in infection; the virus-germ is quantitative rather than qualitative
in character; its specific quality, as a "virus," depending on its
specific quantity. On the other hand, and not less important, an
acute, complete, profoundly paralytic-rabies, not a convulsive-rabies,
however prevalent the latter in attenuators, is the initial rabies of
every known form, even in the dog; its virus-germ including and
involving that of every known "variety" of the malady.

CHAPTER VI.

THE MULTIFORM STRUCTURE OF THE RABIES-MICROBE.

FROM the very varying results of the inoculations of rabies-virus just examined, whether in respect of intensifiers or of attenuators, and under every condition of infection, it is warrantable to infer that the variation in the forms of rabies to be met with is due to a variation in the quantity of the rabies-micro-organism in the infection. From the outset, the character of any rabies would appear to be settled by the amount of the peripheral infection, or by the quantity of rabific microbe which thereby is introduced into the system. The exact form of the induced rabies is rarely, in attenuators, determined by that of the rabies from which it has been derived, but very much a reproduction of the peripheral amount of the rabies-germ.

Nevertheless, in commenting on by far the most crucial of the above groups of experiments, *i.e.* in respect of the most potent "laboratory" rabbit-virus, and as inoculated into rabbits or intensifiers, M. Pasteur states that "the variations in the length of the incubation in these cases were *not the result of any weakening or diminution of the intrinsic virulence of the (initial) virus*, brought on possibly by dilution"; "because," as he adds, and surely very conclusively demonstrates, "the incubation of seven days,"—or that of the initial rabies,—"*was at once recovered, when the nervous matter of all these rabbits was inoculated into new animals*[1]."

This is a somewhat startling revelation; but the significance of which can hardly be overestimated; for, whilst apparently in opposition to the experimental results which have just been examined, it gives a distinct clue as to the "specific" form and constitution

[1] M. Pasteur's Address at the International Medical Congress at Copenhagen. Italics not M. Pasteur's.

of every "rabies-virus." It is no exceptional phenomenon. It is a fundamental, elemental fact, which, in the interpretation of the disease, cannot be ignored, and is an admirable working basis. The constancy of the phenomenon is absolutely irrefutable.

Take, *e.g.* the last inoculation of the last group. The 16 days' incubation of this experiment is likewise the incubation-period of the "ordinary," convulsive canine-rabies of the street. It is surely a startling fact that a "virus" which rabidises a rabbit in 16 days, and but consisting of the $\frac{1}{152}$nd part of a virus-germ which rabidises another rabbit in seven days, should, on re-inoculation into a fresh animal of the same species, and as a 16 days' rabies, nevertheless, rabidise the latter also in seven days! How is this? It is certain that ordinary, convulsive canine-rabies of 15 or 16 days' incubation would never, on re-inoculation, induce even in a rabbit such a rabies, and however massive the infection. Before a rabies of such overwhelming potency could be developed, the canine-virus would require to be transmitted, serially, through scores, if not hundreds, of rabbits, or the most potent of intensifiers. Yet, here, we have two "viruses" of precisely the same incubation-period, and therefore of, presumably, precisely the same quantity of the individual rabific microbe, producing under the same conditions of infection such very different results! But there is this vast difference between these "viruses." The one is a normal complete canine virus-germ, of ordinary convulsive character, yielding in a fresh rabbit a rabies of 16 or 15 days' incubation. The other is but *a fractional* or fragmentary "rabbit" virus-germ, which in its completed form yields a rabies of seven days' incubation, or a form of the disease which is probably not less than many hundred times as potent as the former.

Is, after all, the length of the incubation-period no such reliable index of the potency of a rabies as has been so frequently insisted upon? It is unquestionable that the length of the incubation-period of every form of rabies is, inversely, as its potency and virulence. This relationship may be taken, as M. Pasteur has over and over again taken it, as a fundamental law of the malady. But, in spite of the very varying forms of rabies produced by a systematic dilution, the fact of the *instant recovery* of the initial rabies on the retransmission of even its most fractional rabies into an intensifier, such as the rabbit, would seem to show that, after all, the inherent quality of any given "virus," and not the quantity of rabific microbe of which it is composed, is the determining factor of any given rabies;

that in every case it is not a matter so much of the special quantity as of the specific quality or potency of the rabific microbe itself. Is this the fact?

How can two "viruses" of alike 16 days' incubation, and presumably, therefore, of the same potency or possibility of germination, produce such very different forms of rabies? Was the recovery of a seven days' incubation in this case an accidental and altogether exceptional one? On the contrary, in an intensifier, such as the rabbit, such recovery is not only a common event, but "*the invariable rule*"; and the restoration is probably all the more immediate and complete,—always on a second transmission, however fractional the "virus,"—the higher the virulence of the initial rabies.

"Suppose, for instance," says M. Pasteur, "we take some virus from rabbits with protracted incubation-periods,—protracted to one month and even more" (*i.e.* from a fractional virus),—"and inoculate it, by trephining, into healthy live rabbits, we, in all cases, *at once reproduce* our 7 days' incubation. *The rule is absolute*[1]."

The immediate restoration, then, of the original 7 days' rabies was by no means unique. And M. Pasteur accounts for the phenomenon as follows:—

"Experimentation shows, I believe, that the delays in the time of incubation are a result of the diminution in the quantity of the rabies-virus which is dying out, *rather than a diminution in the degree of its virulence.* In practice, it does not seem that we have to deal with weaker and then with progressively stronger viruses (or vice versa), *but rather with a virus of unvarying intensity,* ruled, indeed, by the law, which will have it so, that the duration of the incubation varies inversely with the quantity inoculated, *the virus remaining the same.* Thus, the smaller the quantity used the longer the incubation, and vice versa. The facts agree better with the notion of a vaccinal matter which we may suppose associated with the rabies-microbe, the latter preserving *its own virulence intact in all the drying marrows*[2]."

According to this view, it would appear that the *special virulence of any initial virus-germ* is maintained intact even in the most fractional amount. But if the variations in rabies, resulting from a quantitative variation of the rabies-microbe in a series of inoculations,

---

[1] *Annales de l'Institut Pasteur.* Letter from M. Pasteur to Professor Duclaux, Dec. 27, 1886. Italics not M. Pasteur's.

[2] M. Pasteur's Letter to Professor Duclaux, as above.

be not the result of diminishing the special amount or special virulence of the initial disease-material, or of any "diminution in the degree of its virulence," why, in the cases examined, should there have been any variation at all? There was not one of the fractional inoculations which produced a rabies of the same form as that from whence it was derived. There was rabies-microbe, and, moreover, the same rabies-microbe, in one and all of the inoculations, and in the last as in the first. Under such circumstances, the pathogenic micro-organism of smallpox, or of anthrax, or of scarlatina, or of any prophylactic germ-disease whatever, or even of many of the preventive germ-diseases would, even in the most fractional amounts capable of inducing the disease, always and "at once" produce the form of the malady induced by the *initial* disease: there would be no variation. In such cases the quantity of the specific micro-organism received in infection has nothing to do with the quality or character of the malady produced, this being determined by the special quality or potency of germination of the individual micro-organism itself, which, *per se*, unlike that of rabies, far from being "unvarying," would appear to be variable and modifiable in the extreme. That the virus-germ of dog-rabies, or of rabbit-rabies, or of any other form of the disease, is "intrinsically one in virulence," and "always one and the same" in nature, there can be no question. In the group of experiments examined, the virus-germ which yielded an incubation of 16 days is none the less a virus-germ than that which yielded an incubation of 7 or 8 days, because it happened to possess but the $\frac{1}{152}$nd part of its virulence. Precisely because it was the *same* virus-germ and virus with the *same* intrinsic virulence, but in so different an amount, it produced so different a form of the very same disease. But that dog-rabies, any more than rabbit-rabies, or any other "special" rabies of any other race of animal is "sensibly one" in *its* virulence; or that the amount of virulence which constitutes it a special form over any other is "always one and the same" in this amount and for all conditions of infection, is surely quite in opposition to the experimental evidence just examined, or to any of the results obtained by research. If this were the fact, ordinary dog-madness and, on the other hand, ordinary or normal rabbit-madness could never, under any conditions of infection capable of rabidising, induce any other forms of the disease than, respectively, a convulsive-rabies or a paralytic-rabies. But, as we have already frequently seen, the one form may produce the other, or either both, according to the quantity of virus-germ introduced in infection. If the special amount of the "intrinsic virulence" of the initial rabies, whatever this may have been, were not lessened by the process of dilution, and in a very definite relationship to this dilution, to what other cause could any variation be assigned? The "special" amount of virulence characteristic of any specific "variety" of the disease is by no means retained intact for even one transmission, much less for a second or third, especially and invariably through an attenuator. This is still more true if the virus-germ of the special rabies be subjected to a process of dilution or desiccation. True; in these cases, however much variation may have been produced in the initial rabies, the virus-germ is from first to last "intrinsically" the same virus-germ. The particular potency of the original rabies has varied, because the special amount of its "intrinsic" virulence has in each case varied. Hence, every form of rabies, however characteristic of entire races of the animal kingdom, depending for its particular virulence upon the special quantity of the micro-organism which it happens to possess in the central nervous system, cannot, although the virulence is essentially "one and the same" in nature in all forms, fail to be different in every form. The variations, therefore, in the length of the so-called incubation-periods, character-istic of all known forms of rabies, of canine-rabies, feline-rabies, vulpine-rabies, monkey-rabies, or rabbit-rabies, &c.—of convulsive, convulso-paralytic, and paralytic rabies—are to be assigned not to any "intrinsic" difference in the virulent product of the rabies or its virus-germ, for this, indeed, like the individual rabies-microbe itself, never varies, but to a variation in the special quantity of this unaltering virus-germ, this, alone, constituting it a "special" form of rabies. Consequently, *the fractional virus* of a 7 days' rabies which produces a 16 days' rabies, contains in reality no more indi-vidual rabies-microbes than the virus-germ of an ordinary convulsive-rabies which yields the same incubation-period; in spite of the fact that the former on being transmitted through a fresh rabbit will at once restore a 7 days' rabies, whilst the latter will not develop such a rabies before hundreds of transmissions.

If this be so, the immediate recovery of a 7 days' rabies, on the re-inoculation of a virus-germ of even 35 days' incubation, could only have occurred, either because, from without or artificially in the process of infection, there was suddenly superadded an amount of virus-germ equivalent to that of a 7 days' rabies, or because, from within or naturally after infection, there was suddenly evolved an amount of rabific microbe, which practically rendered the inoculation in the last as in the first instance equivalent to a 7 days' rabies. It is certain that there was no such sudden increase in the amount of virus-germ in the mere process of re-inoculation. The inoculation in the last as in the first instance was an intracranial one of merely two drops. The nervous matter of the rabbit which had succumbed to a 16 days' rabies was introduced, "after trephining, into the subdural space," precisely as was the nervous matter of the initial rabbit which had succumbed to a 7 days' rabies. Consequently, the amount of rabies-microbe which was so suddenly developed in the case as to at once recover a 7 days' rabies was in reality evolved in virtue of the character of the fractional virus, and of the extraordinary intensifying property of the infected animal. It was so suddenly evolved, and such restoration of an initial rabies is so immediate and invariable, because the virus-germ of such a case is in reality only *a fractional* one. An ordinary convulsive canine-rabies of 16 days' incubation will never induce such a rabies on one transmission, because it is in reality *a complete virus-germ*, and a specific entity. It is, as a matter of fact, only a *fractional virus-germ* which will so suddenly develop into the most potent ; nor will it ever develop in one transmission a higher virus-germ than that of which it is but a part ; and, moreover, so far as has yet been determined, it is significant in the extreme that it will so develop, and the integral initial form be so suddenly reproduced, only in an intensifier, or in the order of animal capable of intensifying rabies on transmission.

Why, then, should two inoculations of the same amount of this unvarying micro-organism produce such very different results ? There must be some inherent, structural difference between the two amounts, precisely similar in quantity though they may be. What is this difference ? Is it not essentially a difference of form, and therefore of force ? Does not the immediate restoration of every *fractional virus* to its initial, completed form prove that every modification of the disease which is sufficiently pronounced and sufficiently persistent to be viewed as a normal or "specific" rabies, such as canine, feline, monkey, or rabbit-rabies, has not only a special quantity of the rabies-microbe in the central nervous system to constitute it the special rabies, but that, from the outset of infection, it contains this special quantity in a, more or less, highly specialised form or composition as its determining factor ? Hence, when rabies is transmitted through a series of animals, intensifiers or attenuators, the form of the virus-germ, inducing the rabies, will rise or fall with the amount of the specific micro-organism evolved, or, as the case may be, aborted by the process of transmission. In an intensifier, such as the rabbit, the special virus-germ will gain in fulness of form and in persistency of structure with every fresh passage of the disease, or with every increase of the rabies-microbe. In an attenuator, on the contrary, such as the dog or ape, the virus-germ will lose in magnitude and in persistency of form and force with every transmission. Even the most pronounced, paralytic rabies, in such an animal, not only progressively diminishes in its amount of the rabies-microbe, but this amount as progressively disintegrates and deteriorates to the simplest and loosest forms ; the individual micro-organisms still maintaining, *per se*, in the loosest condition, their unvarying potency as individual monads or units. If such be the fact, it follows that the special, as opposed to the intrinsic, virulence of a rabies is determined by the special quantity of the individual rabies-microbes, and how this quantity is differentiated and organised, this specialised amount constituting it a special rabies.

There is reason, then, to show that the unit rabific-microbe, whatever the "variety" of rabies from which it is obtained, is, intrinsically, of one and the same force, and, invariably, of one and the same activity as a microbe. This, however, is far from the fact in respect of the pathogenic microbe of the vast majority of germ-diseases. The individual or unit pathogenic microbe of such germ-diseases as small-pox, anthrax or scarlatina, and the entire prophylactic order, is by no means of the same potency or germinating-capacity in every form of the disease. Hence, a mere quantity of the pathogenic microbe, introduced in infection, in no way determines the character of the induced disease ; one quantity of the same pathogenic micro-organism, and one site of infection, being as effective as another. For every change in the form of the malady the individual morbific microbe has, *per se*, changed in its potency or capacity of germination ; one may produce thirty, one fifty, one a hundred fold.

But this is not the fact in respect of the rabies-microbe. In this disease the quantity of the rabies-germ introduced in infection alone determines the character and form of the induced rabies. Consequently, the individual rabies-microbe is, probably, unvarying, and in every modification of the disease invariably of the same form and force. Hence, every "variety" or modification will be dependent for its particular form, as a rabies, exclusively upon the number of such elemental units as are combined together and organised into a complex whole, and into one special but by no means permanent form, as the characteristic unit in the case, and the special factor of the form of the disease induced. Thus, according to this view, one form of rabies, an exclusively-convulsive rabies, the simplest of all, would be wholly constituted of what one may term the elemental units, or of individual rabies-microbes. As a virus-germ, it may be simply of, so to speak, but *a one-microbe form and force*, and the rabies-micro-organisms practically loose and amorphous. Take, *e.g.* an extreme case, cited by M. Pasteur, of a canine-rabies of 58 days' incubation. What rabific-microbe there was in this case was probably strictly confined to the bulbar substance, producing a wholly convulsive-rabies. It was not only slight in amount and strictly limited in area, but probably likewise of the simplest conformation, and practically *amorphous*, or a rabies of a one, or 1-microbe form and force. But a second may be, so to say, of a 2- or 3-microbe form and force ; whilst a third may be of a 5-microbe form; a fourth of a 10- to a 15-microbe form ; and a fifth, or extreme "variety," may be of a 25- up to a 50- and possibly even 100-microbe form and force ; and so on. And between the morbific action of the first or amorphous and simplest and of any of the latter or multiform "viruses," there may be, in reality, as much difference as between the tumult of an amorphous crowd, and the organised, specialised force of systematically-formed bodies of troops.

Or, to represent the subject diagrammatically, something like the subjoined scheme might be permissible.

Now, according to this view, on a rabies, however simple to begin with, being transmitted, serially, through an intensifier, such as the rabbit, its rabific-microbe will not only materially increase in quantity with every transmission, but, even if it be wholly amorphous in the first instance, this increasing quantity will likewise gain in com-position, form and force. It will gradually rise from a virus-unit of a lower and simpler to that of a higher and a much more complex structure ; multiplying and developing from the simplest amorphous condition into a rabies-unit of a 2-microbe form, a 5-microbe form, a 10-microbe form, a 20- to 50-microbe form and force, and so on. Not that these particular rabies-units, here hypothetically repre-sented, exhaust by any means all the special forms of the disease, much less the possible forms which may yet be evolved in intensifiers.

Unfortunately, as yet, the rabies-micro-organism itself has not been

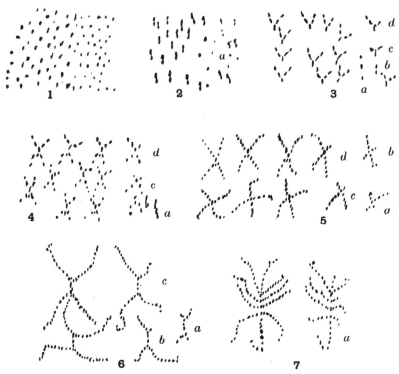

CONFORMATION OF THE RABIES-VIRUS.

1. Virus of 1-microbe form, amorphous = simplest rabies of 35 to 40 days' incubation in rabbit.
2. Virus of 2-microbe form, organised = furious canine madness of 25 days' incubation in rabbit.
3. Virus of 5-microbe form, organised = convulso-paralytic (infective) of 15 days' incubation in rabbit.
4. Virus of 10-microbe form, organised = dumb or paralytic canine-rabies of 12—11 days' incubation in rabbit.
5. Virus of 20-microbe form, organised = ordinary rabbit-rabies of 10 days' incubation in rabbit.
6. Virus of 50-microbe form, organised = profoundest known paralytic rabbit-rabies of 8—6 days' incubation in rabbit.
7. Virus of 100-microbe form, organised = a possible rabbit-rabies of 4—3 days' incubation in rabbit.

a, *b*, *c*, and *d*, virus in process of intensification or attenuation.

conclusively identified. Some investigators—Fol of Geneva, for example—have claimed to have discovered it. M. Pasteur also imagined that at times he detected it in amorphous clouds. But the micro-organism must be most minute to have eluded detection so long; much more infinitesimal than even Pfeiffer's microbe of influenza. That, as a special virus-germ, it is always so simple and unvarying in structure, as alleged by those who have claimed to have discovered it, is questionable in the extreme[1].

If the rabies-microbe progressively increases in quantity when transmitted through intensifiers, and this quantity as progressively gains in structure and form, then a special rabies-unit may be looked upon as one where the special quantity of rabies-microbe, of which it is structurally composed, is as fully specialised and organised as the quantity is capable of; this complete development and differentiation constituting a fully formed, specific or typical rabies. But this holds good only in respect of the process of intensification, and, therefore, only of the intensifying division of the animal kingdom. In the figured representation above, there is a sketch of what possibly takes place in an intensifier, such as the rabbit, on the continuous transmission of any rabies through the animal. And, on retracing the sketch from its severest, multiform rabies-microbe, to its simplest and distinctly amorphous " viruses," one may see what takes place in an attenuator, such as the dog or monkey. Hence, it becomes comprehensible why a very large quantity of the simplest rabies-germ, even in its amorphous condition, is capable of inducing not merely a convulsive, but a paralytic-rabies; and why, likewise, the smallest fractional virus-germ of the profoundest paralytic-rabies known is capable of inducing only the simplest convulsive-rabies, in spite of its origin, and in spite of the very complex, special rabies-unit of which it is a fragment.

Now, as just stated, were the rabies-microbe, individually, like that of smallpox, anthrax, scarlatina, or of any strictly prophylactic germ-disease, there would be a somewhat different result, from mere infection. An effectual inoculation of 10 drops of smallpox "virus" in an active condition, or even one drop, will yield a not less severe smallpox than an inoculation of 100 drops of the same "virus"; or 100 drops prove not one whit more malignant or prophylactic than 10. If the rabies-microbe were, *per se*, such a micro-organism, the smallest fractional virus-germ capable of rabidising would yield the same rabies as the most massive inoculation of the same virus-germ. In

---

[1] The above was written in 1896.

other words, the particular rabies of a group of experiments would be reproduced and "restored" with every inoculation, however fragmentary. But a prophylactic germ-disease is not determined by a quantitative micro-organism. True ; all forms of a prophylactic germ-disease have not the same potency of virulence any more than have all forms of rabies. The individual micro-organisms of these varying forms have not the same unvarying capacity for germination any more than all forms of rabies have the same quantity of rabies-microbe in their specific rabies-unit. The special intensity of every prophylactic germ-disease would appear to depend solely upon the special potency or germinating-capacity of the individual micro-organisms, not upon the quantity of such individual micro-organisms introduced in infection, or how these micro-organisms are combined or organised. It is even conceivable that one such individual micro-organism, of highest germinating-capacity, effectually introduced into the circulation, might induce the severest forms of the malady to be met with ; just as one vigorous thistle-seed introduced into a virgin soil will overrun a tropical isle. But one individual or loose microbe of rabies would produce no such result even in an intensifier. If this be so, one form of a disease like smallpox will differ from another, not so much in the special quantity of its virus-germ introduced, or how this is organised as a virus-unit, as in the special life-activity and germinating-power of the individual germ to begin with ; and this in all probability varies with every pronounced form of the malady. One form of rabies differs from another, on the contrary, not so much in the particular potency of the individual rabies-microbes which it happens to contain ; the potency of the rabies-germ being, *per se*, probably tolerably equal in every form of the disease, as in the special quantity of this practically unvarying rabies-microbe forming it into a special rabies-unit. And the quantity of this uniform rabies-germ which goes to form any special virus-unit, or even the quantity of the specialised unit, will not be precisely alike in any two forms of the malady which at all vary. Whilst, therefore, in all but the simplest or amorphous forms, the fundamental morbific unit in any rabies is a collective or multiple one or multiform, it is, on the contrary, in any form of a prophylactic germ-disease, probably as invariably a simple one. In the one case the morbific germ is quantitative ; in the other case it is essentially qualitative. The variability of the prophylactic germ-disease is due to a variability in potency and life-activity of the individual micro-organism which, *per se*, constitutes its virus-germ unit. For this reason, the virus-germ of such a germ-disease, but only of this, is probably always more or less capable of "modification" into a vaccination, the individual virus-germ being, in itself, as variable and modifiable as a seed itself. On the other hand, it is not less warrantable to infer that the variability of such a germ-disease as rabies is due solely to the quantity of rabies-germ of which its special virus-germ as a complex unit is composed; the rabies-microbe being in itself, and individually, of equal and uniform potency and never varying in its intrinsic virulence or capacity of germination, like the individual elementary cells of a mold, a fungoid growth, or a sponge. The special potency of the induced disease is, in the one case, therefore, but a reproduction of the special potency of the particular virus-germ of the inducing disease at the moment of infection, irrespective of the quantity of infection ; it can never, as in rabies, be of a higher virulence or of a higher protective property than the disease from which it was derived, however much the infection. In such a germ-disease as rabies, on the contrary, the special potency of the induced disease is but the accumulated potency of the virus-germ absorbed in infection and sown in the central nervous system ; and this special potency may be altogether irrespective of that of the inducing disease. It may be either the same potency or greater or very much less, according to the quantity of rabies-microbe introduced in infection, and how this quantity is from the outset specialised[1].

[1] Whilst this work was passing through the press Professor Sormani, of the University of Pavia, announced, in January 1903, his discovery of the microbe of rabies. And the authenticity and the valuable significance of this discovery have been placed beyond doubt. From Professor Sormani's investigations, which have lasted for many years, it is certain that the rabies-microbe is most minute. It but begins to be seen when enlarged by " twelve to fifteen hundred diameters"; and to study it adequately is only possible at an enlargement of "two to three thousand diameters." The adequate study of so infinitesimal a micro-organism is obviously enough only possible with the latest and the most powerful microscope. Still more significant, Sormani has clearly revealed that the rabies-microbe is in reality "polymorphous," not simple. It has many appearances and shapes under the most powerful microscope. In one case it appears as a cloud of amorphous particles, in another case like a flake of wool: and in another it possesses "*numberless ramifications.*" Unquestionably this is a significant discovery. But the results, surely, confirm in striking detail the theory propounded above.

CHAPTER VII.

MODE AND ROUTE OF CONVEYANCE OF THE RABIES-GERM TO THE CEREBRO-SPINAL SUBSTANCE.

Is the rabies-microbe, like that of tetanus, planted in the connective-tissue of the periphery, this constituting its specific seat of cultivation? Does the micro-organism ever germinate in the peripheral tissue at all, the virulent product ultimately elaborated by the micro-organism, like that of tetanus, erysipelas, or diphtheria, alone entering the circulation, and invading and irritating the central nervous system? If this be the fact, why should a mere variation in the site of infection, or in the amount of the rabies-microbe in the infection, change the form and the character of the rabies thereby induced? Unlike rabies, tetanus is as severe from an infection occasioned by a rusty nail or by a splinter of rotting wood puncturing the hand or foot, as from an infection due to an extensive frostbitten mortification of either the one or the other. Mortification, extending into bones, is deemed the most favourable of all conditions for the incubation of the tetanus-bacillus, and by many surgeons it is still viewed as the most frequent occasion of the disease.

"It is the fact," says Mr Power, "that tetanus is peculiarly liable to follow wounds in injuries in which foreign bodies or necrosis and gangrene are present[1]."

But tetanus is not confined to these injuries; and the majority of such wounds is very frequently followed by erysipelas, septicaemia, pyæmia, &c., the micro-organisms of which are still more common. Gangrene or necrosis, on the scale characteristic of frost-bite or gunshot-wound, is by no means essential to the causation of the disease. Flügge and his coadjutors, as Mr Power himself has

---

[1] "Bacteriology in its relation to Surgery"; Bradshaw Lecture by Henry Power, M.B. *Brit. Medical Journal*, Dec. 2, 1886.

admirably shown, invariably induced it with the finest of subcutaneous injections. Tetanus is as grave from a mere puncture of the thumb or toe as in the case of a limb crushed and lacerated by machinery. A youth came under my care who incurred tetanus after a fall with his bicycle on a rough country road near a farm-yard. There was only an insignificant wound in the hypothenar eminence of his hand, which in a few days healed[1]. Nay, it is certain that a simple puncture is much the most frequent mode of infection, and that the "idiopathic" tetanus of our fathers is probably due to no other than the slightest possible infection of this kind. A case of a child, four years old, also came under a friend's notice, caused by the onslaught of a barn-fowl, which angrily rushed at the little boy from a dung-heap in a farm-yard. Although but slightly scratched in the face and neck, a severe form of the malady, which was fatal, speedily was induced in the child. Again, tetanus has been recorded to have ensued from the rotten fibres of a whip having been stuck subcu-taneously in the face from an accidental flip. And such cases are probably due to the fact that the bacillus of tetanus is particularly rife in a badly-drained stable or farm-yard, which is pre-eminently its "home."

Here, as in diphtheria, erysipelas, &c., the micro-organism in the site of infection is fixed, and of the most limited amount and area. The peripheral connective-tissue in this site of infection in reality constitutes its specific culture-ground. In this case, likewise, only the virulent product, elaborated by the micro-organism, enters the blood and lymph streams, to do its remote, lethal work in the spinal substance. And this it will do, and to the same extent, whatever the site of infection, and with the most limited quantity of tetanus-bacillus in this site. One site of infection is as effective for producing the disease, and the same form of the disease, as another. Is this true of rabies? Why in the latter should mere proximity to the cerebro-spinal axis determine the amount of infection? Why should a mere *fractional* amount of the virus-germ in the cerebro-spinal substance, on a second transmission through an intensifier such as the rabbit, restore the integral virulence of the initial rabies? Is this true of the virulent product of the tetanus-bacillus? Does it hold good of Koch's tuberculin, or of serpent-venom, or of strychnine, morphia, alcohol, or of any other virulent product? In all these

---

[1] The *Lancet*, Sept. 24, 1898, "A case of Tetanus treated with Tetanus-serum," by David Sime, M.D. The case was successful.

cases a fractional amount can only do a fraction's work, and will never recover the full initial virulence from which it has been obtained. It is certain, therefore, that the rabies-germ, not less than the virulent product of the germ, whether or not it germinates in the peripheral wound, invariably reaches and germinates and elaborates its virus or virulent product in the central nervous system. It is to be found in the cerebro-spinal substance, when completely absent from the connective-tissue of the peripheral wound.

What, then, takes place after the process of infection? How and by what means is the rabies-microbe so invariably conveyed from the periphery? What becomes of it during the so-called incubation-period of the disease, a period ranging from a few days to many weeks, and, in man, to even a space of years? Since the rabies-microbe, sooner or later, finds its way to the central nervous system, through what medium or media is it thus so invariably conveyed? Is there one more than another which may be viewed as its normal track of migration? Being so essentially a virus-germ of nervous substance, it might naturally be assumed, and, in point of fact, it has been inferred by many authorities, that the rabies-germ is conveyed from the peripheral wound to the cerebro-spinal axis through the peripheral nerves themselves. Thus, as we have already seen, Brown-Séquard was so impressed with the fact that the virus-germ was a virus-germ of nervous substance, and of nothing else, that he graphically defined the disease as "*an ascending neuritis.*" In other words, it has been assumed that the rabies-germ introduced into a wound grows from this site of infection and ascends directly through its peripheral nerves to the deepest nerve-centres of the cerebro-spinal axis itself; this process of progressive multiplication and propagation constituting the incubation of the disease. The peripheral nerves of the rabic wound or wounds are in every direction, so to speak, as the very roots of this virulent, steadily-growing upas-tree. Duboué and other able investigators were of the same opinion, and Dr Gamaleia, of Odessa, explains the incubation-latency in a like manner[1].

There can be no question, not only that the rabies-microbe is a virus-germ of nervous substance above all tissues, but that it in all likelihood germinates and elaborates its virus in no other

[1] " Dr Gamaleia concludes that the virus, from the study of the symptoms detailed, *can only spread by the nerves, from the periphery or external surfaces to the centre.*" "Hydrophobia ; M. Pasteur's System," by Renaud Suzor, M.D., quoted from Dr Gamaleia's article in *Annales de l'Institut Pasteur.*

structure. Every part of the nervous system, from the centre to the remotest periphery, has been proved capable of cultivating the microbe and of yielding the infective material. Now, since this is the fact, it cannot be doubted that the virulent product, and, if this, also the rabies-germ—for the one will sooner or later follow in the track of the other—are to be found in the peripheral as in all other nerves. Fragments of the pneumogastric, and of the sciatic and the spinal nerves, and even the remotest peripheral terminations of these, have been, in extreme cases of rabies, found virulent, and have, one and all, rabidised. So also have been the intimate structures of the salivary, parotid, and other glands, but probably exclusively the nervous elements of these structures. In the light of such facts, there can be no question that both the virus and the virus-germ are capable of being transmitted, whether passively or actively, through the substance of the nerves themselves. When the disease has once proclaimed itself, this migration through the nerve-tracks is an invariable fact, the extent of the invasion depending upon the severity of the disease or the amount of virus-germ evolved in the disease. Does it follow, however, that such an invasion takes place from the periphery upward, and from the outset of infection, and all through the so-called incubation-period? As, *after incubation*, the rabies-germ is capable of traversing the nerve-tracks in every direction, does it not, or can it not, likewise traverse the nerve-tracks immediately after the peripheral infection, and all through the incubation-period, till the very advent of the disease itself?

Although the existence of the rabies-germ has been conclusively demonstrated in the nerves, and in every part of the cerebro-spinal system, as a matter of fact this has been *only after the incubation-period was really finished*; it has never been demonstrated in such remote structures before the actual culminating point of the disease itself. There is not a single authenticated or recorded case where a fragment of a peripheral nerve, when removed during the so-called incubation-period, or period of conveyance, has imparted the disease. Even when, after incubation, the existence of the rabies-germ is conclusively demonstrated in the remotest peripheral nerves, it is but in the slightest quantities as compared with the amount of the same rabies-germ in the cerebro-spinal substance, or in any other segment of the same nerve nearer the cerebro-spinal axis. In such a disease as tetanus, or diphtheria, or erysipelas, the virus-germ is not only planted in the peripheral site of infection, but at all stages of the disease, from first to last, it is much more copious and constant here than in any other region of the organism. While this is the fact in respect of every germ-disease, whose specific seat of germination is exclusively confined to the peripheral connective-tissue, in the very rare cases of rabies where the terminal nerves are unquestionably rabic, they are much less copiously supplied with the rabies-germ than any part of the cerebro-spinal axis, and distinctly less rabic than any higher part of the same nerve-trunk ; the amount of the rabies-germ increasing in volume as the nerve-trunk approaches the central nervous axis. If the disease were "an ascending neuritis," and if the rabies-germ constantly began its germination and progressive multiplication in and from the peripheral connective-tissue, and through the peripheral nerves, and immediately after infection, why should a comparative scantiness or absence of the rabies-micro-organism in the peripheral nerves, after the incubation is over, and when the virus-germ is at its maximum amount for the case, be so invariable a fact? If, then, rabies be a "neuritis," and since the rabies-microbe most certainly, with its virus, traverses nerves, it must be a *descending*, not an *ascending, neuritis* ; and this, as we have seen, is precisely the fact. Until the rabies-germ actually reaches and settles in the cerebro-spinal substance itself, there is no reason whatever to believe that it multiplies and migrates through the nervous system. There is cogent reason to show that its invasion through the nerves begins in and from the central nervous system, and *after*, not *before*, the incubation-period ; and that it is, in reality, a *descending* progress from the cerebro-spinal axis, not an *ascending* one from the peripheral nerves ; the migration and extension of the virus-germ and its virus being centrifugal not centripetal.

If rabies were an "ascending neuritis," it would follow that the further the site of peripheral infection from the central nervous system, the more potent would the resulting rabies be ; and, conversely, that the nearer the peripheral site of infection to the central nervous system, the less potent the rabies induced. For since the rabies-germ is a microbe of nervous substance, and capable of cultivation wherever nervous-substance exists, it would likewise follow that, on traversing and propagating its way through the nervous system, it would in this very fact gain in potency. The reverse of this, as we have seen, is the invariable law. The further the rabies-germ has to traverse from the periphery, or, in other words, the longer the period which is occupied in its being conveyed from the periphery to the cerebro-spinal centres, the more it loses of its potency. The longer the so-called incubation-period, the smaller the amount of rabies-germ, and the weaker the micro-organism, which will ultimately settle in the cerebro-spinal substance. The rabies-microbe, therefore, if, in any part of the incubation-period, it traverses the peripheral nerves at all, cannot multiply or increase in its migration thither.

From the constancy of such a fact as that one inoculation in the foot and another of the same "virus" in the face or neck, although of precisely the same quantity of the same "virus," do not necessarily produce the same rabies—in a powerful attenuator, such as the dog, the former inoculation may often enough be blighted—the rabies-germ, all through its conveyance from the peripheral wound, must, for some cogent and constant reason, materially decrease in volume and potency, not increase. The less distance which it has to traverse before its ultimate settlement in the bulb or in the lumbar-swelling, or in both; or the shorter the nerve-tracks between the peripheral wound and the cerebro-spinal centres, the more active and the more potent the resulting rabies. For this reason the length of the incubation-period is so invariably inversely as the potency of the disease. Consequently, whether or not the rabies-germ reaches the central nervous substance through the peripheral nerves, it is certain that it cannot possibly proceed through this path by any process of multiplication or propagation; for it does not at any such stage of the disease propagate or multiply. Traversing the nervous substance of the longest tracts of nerve-fibre, and all through the longest incubation-period, does not aid, but quite the reverse, in the germination of the rabific-microbe, or in the elaboration of its virus. But there can be no question that the rabies-germ is a germ of nerve-fibre, and that it does traverse this structure. Since, therefore, in its assumed migration through the nerves all through the longest incubation-period, it neither multiplies nor propagates at any such stage, but quite the reverse, it follows that it cannot proceed from the peripheral wound to the central nervous axis through a nerve-path, however else or by whatever other means it should be so invariably, if so irregularly, conveyed thither, and however much it may traverse nerves after having been so conveyed.

How else, then, or by what other medium, is it brought thither? If not by the peripheral nerves, is it by the blood-stream, or by the lymphatic stream, or by both? It is certain that direct inoculation into either of these streams will rabidise : and, moreover, more rapidly and effectually than by a subcutaneous inoculation; and often enough, for the reasons already assigned, as rapidly as, and much more effectually than, an intracranial inoculation itself. If this be so, as M. Pasteur has justly pointed out,

" The certainty of inoculation by *intravenous injection* of the virus is in itself sufficient proof that the *nerves* are not the sole channels of propagation of the virus from the periphery or surface to the centre, as one theory would have it ; and proof enough, also, that in the majority of cases, to say the least, the absorption of the virus is effected through the blood-system[1]."

Because it has been proved that the nerves are not the channels by which the rabies-germ is conveyed from the periphery, does it necessarily follow that this conveyance is effected entirely through "the blood system"? What is meant by this term, or how much is involved in it? So far as absorption and circulation are concerned, the blood-system comprises at least two distinct currents ; the liquor sanguinis or blood-current proper, and the corpuscular system, or the living circulating constituents, which may be looked upon as the inhabitants of the stream. The blood-system (including in this term the lymphatic system) thus involves a double circulation ; a circulation within a circulation. Which of these effects alike the absorption of the rabies-germ from an infected wound and its ultimate transference to the central nervous system? It may be the fact that intravenous injection, or the direct introduction of the rabies-germ into the circulation, occasions rabies. But it does not follow that in this transfer from the periphery it is the flowing liquor sanguinis which has borne the rabies-microbe. In any inoculation, particularly if large and massive and directly into a vein, the virulent product which has been thus introduced, but not necessarily the rabies-germ itself, may be straightway conveyed to the cerebro-spinal substance, and in an incredibly brief space of time. For when, even after incubation, the cerebro-spinal substance is disseminated through its entire axis with the rabies-germ, it is found that the blood-stream, often enough, does not rabidise at all. There is no rabies-microbe in the stream. This is probably the invariable rule in respect of the entire attenuating class ; and only occurs on the rarest occasions even in the most potent of intensifiers. The rabies-germ will not

[1] *Comptes Rendus*, Feb. 25, 1884.

necessarily be conveyed from the peripheral wound to the central nervous system by the liquor sanguinis ; unless, indeed, injected into the latter stream in the most massive amounts. But assuming, inasmuch as it is not of peripheral culture, but always centric, that the rabies-germ is, not less than its virus or virulent product, invariably borne from the peripheral wound by the blood-current, and directly to the most fruitful tracts of the cerebro-spinal substance, why should there be any difference in the length of the incubation-period from a mere difference in the site of infection? A hypodermic injection of a solution of strychnine or of morphia or of tuberculin is just as effective in one site as in another ; and reaches the cerebro-spinal axis as truly, and practically as rapidly, from one point of the blood-stream as another, simply because it is borne straightway from the periphery solely by the liquor sanguinis, which, as it so happens, is a regular, uniformly-flowing stream, practically never varying in its rate of movement. If it be the fact that alike the rabies-germ and its virulent product are thus conveyed from the periphery, why, therefore, as in many germ-diseases, should not all forms of rabies have practically the same incubation-period? Why should not the rabies-germ be as prompt and as effective in reaching the cerebro-spinal axis as its own virulent product; or one intravenous inoculation of the rabies-germ be invariably just as rapid in the transit as another? This is by no means the case. And it is not the fact ; because the rabies-microbe which in an infection is associated with the virulent product is not conveyed to the central nervous-system by the blood-current, however much and however constantly and promptly the virulent product itself may be thus conveyed. The very irregularity of the so-called incubation-period demonstrates the fact that it is not by the blood-current or ever-flowing liquor sanguinis that the micro-organism is conveyed from the periphery ; for the blood-stream, as just stated, is as regular and as uniform in its flow as the tides. In this important fact lies the reason why M. Pasteur's course of preventive inoculations should "protect" an organism ; for the virulent product thus inoculated will reach the cerebro-spinal substance, being conveyed directly thither by the flowing plasma, long before the micro-organism, which has been simultaneously introduced. This is not so conveyed, but by a much slower, a much more irregular, and a much more circuitous route. The liquor sanguinis, therefore, does not convey the micro-organism from the peripheral wound.

s.   7

The same line of reasoning disposes of the lymphatic stream, or flowing lymph-plasma, as the medium of conveyance. The liquid part of the lymphatic current, like that of the blood, without doubt conveys the poisonous products of pathogenic micro-organisms directly to centric organs, and, most certainly, to the central nervous system. But here again, from the notoriously extreme variability of the so-called incubation-period of rabies, it is obvious that the flowing lymph-stream does not, apart from its corpuscular system, any more than the flowing liquor sanguinis, convey the rabies-microbe, or "the figured elements of the virus," to its destination in the cerebro-spinal axis ; for, however irregular the incubation-period, in this case, likewise, the lymph-current is anything but an irregular one.

In confirmation of this view of the corpuscular medium of conveyance, it is not without interest to recall M. Nocard's deeply interesting experiments with the *dialysed saliva* of rabid dogs. In these cases, it will be remembered, the liquid element passed through the dialyser, when injected into unprotected animals, proved without one single exception absolutely innocuous ; whereas the solid elements, left on dialysis, were always found to be rabic. From such evidence, if there were no other, the rabies-germ is, clearly enough, a microbe of tissue-elements, not of their liquid secretions. And the rabies-microbe, introduced into a rabic wound, is, therefore, conveyed to the central nervous system exclusively by the corpuscular elements of the site, not (except ·when the infection is of the most massive amounts) by the flowing plasma either of the lymphatic or of the blood-stream. Consequently, if the rabies-germ be conveyed to the central nervous system by the blood-stream at all, as most certainly it is, it must be by the organised constituents of the circulation, and by these exclusively. It is the circulation within the circulation,— the wandering shoals of living corpuscular or cellular organisms, in the ever-flowing plasma,—which must be regarded as the constant vehicle of conveyance. From the fact, then, of the extremely irregular incubation-period, it is certain that the rabies-germ is conveyed to its centric seat of germination in the cerebro-spinal substance, exclusively by the irregularly-wandering corpuscular system. And from the extreme length of the period of conveyance in some of the forms of rabies, it is not less certain that the solitary sluggishly-moving corpuscles of the peripheral connective-tissue itself are much more engaged in the transference than the active mobile leucocytes of the circulation.

CHAPTER VIII.

THE ORDER OF GERM-DISEASES TO WHICH RABIES BELONGS.

To what order of germ-disease, then, does rabies belong?

Broadly viewed, all germ-diseases may be divided into two great orders : those which protect the organism from further attack, and those which do not protect enduringly, but, after and in consequence of the protection, positively unprotect. For this reason, the one great order may be conveniently termed the *prophylactic* or non-recurrent type, the other great order, the *preventive* and recurrent type. Under the first head would be comprised such germ-diseases as smallpox, anthrax, syphilis, scarlatina, measles, whooping-cough, &c. ; under the second head, such germ-diseases as malarial fever, influenza maligna, acute rheumatism, erysipelas, pyæmia, diphtheria, tetanus, &c. The second, or preventive type, is much larger than the first, and, still more significant, of far wider range over the animal kingdom. This important distinction, if there were no other depending upon it, differentiates the entire realm of germ-disease into two highly-characteristic orders, which are not only different from, but, in every fundamental feature, a contrast to each other ; the difference being that of kind more than of degree.

Every disease of the first class, however otherwise differing from all others of the same order, such as whooping-cough and smallpox, is alike in being strictly prophylactic or practically non-recurrent ; whilst every disease of the second, however otherwise unlike any of the order, such as tetanus and diphtheria or erysipelas and ague, is alike in being more or less recurrent, or the protection which it imparts being far from enduring.

A typical example of the change produced from such a germ-disease as smallpox, anthrax, or scarlatina, or any of the prophylactic order, may be likened to the clay figure which a potter puts into his furnace. After due exposure to the heat, on withdrawing it a complete molecular transformation has taken place in the figure. With respect to such heat it is altogether altered, and no amount of exposure to the same furnace will again alter it. Its passage through the furnace has "protected" it from the furnace permanently. A typical example of the change produced by such a germ-disease as ague, influenza maligna, diphtheria, erysipelas, or by any of the recurrent and preventive order, may, on the contrary, be likened to a similar figure, but of marble, thrust into the same furnace; from the first the furnace-heat will erode and deteriorate it. Thrust it without delay into the furnace a second time and it will crack and disintegrate. Thrust it into the furnace a third time, and it will probably crumble into dust, collapsing, even if years should have elapsed, the more surely for its first and second exposure. Its various passages through the heat have positively unprotected it, having progressively prepared it for collapse.

If so radical a distinction exists between germ-diseases, manifestly enough rabies cannot belong to both orders. To which does it belong? If it is really of the prophylactic type, and, therefore, a non-recurrent germ-disease, then, it is probable, if not certain, that it is capable of yielding a modified micro-organism, which, in consequence of its modification, will, like vaccine or the "modified-virus" of anthrax, be capable of stamping out its disease in the animal kingdom. This has been unhesitatingly claimed in respect of M. Pasteur's course of inoculations of rabies-virus. If, however, it should so happen that rabies belongs to the preventive or recurrent type, in spite of the "protection" which its virus unquestionably induces, a somewhat different conclusion must be arrived at. For if the virus-germ of the disease is not, in itself, and to begin with, prophylactic, there is no reason to believe that it is capable of being modified into a "vaccination," or that its micro-organism is, *per se*, modifiable at all. As presumably belonging to the recurrent, preventive type, rabies therefore, unlike smallpox or any strictly prophylactic germ-disease, is not to be extinguished by an inoculation of its own micro-organism. The virus or virulent product of the disease, as apart from the virus-germ, may "protect" for a time, but, like that of probably the entire recurrent and preventive order, it will lead to a condition of unprotection.

Nevertheless, there is strong evidence to show that M. Pasteur,

himself, from the first to the last of his great research, assumed the
disease to be strictly prophylactic. Nor after his triumph over
anthrax was this an unnatural inference ; for this germ-disease is
distinctly prophylactic, the micro-organism, like that of smallpox,
scarlatina, and probably of the entire prophylactic order, being cultivated exclusively in the constituents of the blood-stream. And
this dominating conception of rabies is not less emphasised in the
best English expositions of the disease. The genuinely prophylactic
type of germ-disease is constantly at hand to lighten up every
obscure point of the malady which presents itself. One never finds
any allusion to the analogies presented by erysipelas, ague, diphtheria,
alcoholism, &c., or even to tetanus, itself, although so closely allied,
or to any germ-disease of an unquestionably recurrent and preventive character.

Is the virus-germ of rabies capable of modification into a vaccination, and in the sense that the micro-organism of vaccine is a modification of that of smallpox ? Is it, as an individual microbe,
modifiable at all ? Has this fact been satisfactorily made out ?

What was the achievement attained in respect of anthrax ? In
this case M. Pasteur eliminated the virus-germ of the malady ; and
he not only *attenuated*, but, in doing so, he also *modified* it. He
cultivated the micro-organism in a suitable gelatinous medium ; and,
in virtue of the cultivation, he distinctly modified it into a very
genuine "vaccination"; the capacity of the pathogenic micro-
organism in its original state to impart prophylaxis being completely
retained in the "modified" state, whilst its virulence was attenuated
to a minimum. This was in the strictest sense of the word a modification of the specific micro-organism which was hardly less
efficacious, as a vaccination, than vaccine itself. With this very
genuine modified virus-germ, herd after herd of healthy sheep and
cattle by the million were "protected," and one of the most disastrous
diseases of our domestic animals was practically abolished. Grand
as the treatment has been, it has, however, been, if possible, even
more triumphant in principle than in practice. For if the pathogenic
micro-organism of so deadly a disease can be eliminated and cultivated into the most effective modified virus-germ, so may that of
scarlatina, syphilis, measles, whooping-cough, &c., or of every germ-
disease of the genuinely prophylactic type. M. Pasteur's triumph
over anthrax, therefore, is really a triumph over the entire prophylactic order to which it belongs. But the achievement was possible

because the specific micro-organism of anthrax was really modifiable and "modified" by M. Pasteur. And it was so completely trans- muted into a prophylactic vaccination, and altogether so strictly analogous to vaccine, because anthrax is a prophylactic, not a pre- ventive or recurrent, germ-disease ; and for this reason the micro- organism of the disease is so essentially a modifiable one. The specific micro-organisms of the entire preventive order, whilst capable of being attenuated and intensified, are not modifiable ; their protective power being attenuated with their pathogenic, and strictly in accordance with it.

Now, as a clue to the possibility of a "protective," if not even a genuinely prophylactic treatment, M. Pasteur was the first investi- gator to point out, as a principle of paramount importance, the significance of the special micro-organisms which are at the root of the germ-diseases that are *"common to man and to the lower animals."* Thus, before his investigation of rabies he had already proved, in the case of anthrax, that a germ-disease, which was common to man and to animals, was capable of being stamped out with its own modified virus-germ, and on strictly prophylactic principles. And smallpox, as universally acknowledged, is preeminently such a germ-disease ; this too, like anthrax, being, significantly enough, common to man and to cattle. The vaccinal treatment of this disease, as founded by Jenner, is the beau-ideal of all *prophylaxis.* Since this is the fact, why not apply the same principle of *modifying* the virus-germ— not at all its virus—into a vaccination, in respect of the entire circle of germ-diseases, which are *common to man and to animals?* If this achievement can be accomplished in respect of anthrax and of small- pox, why not of every germ-disease without exception which is common to man and to the lower animals ? If the same prophylactic results could be attained by the same methods of treatment in this particular field of germ-diseases—and the narrower the field, or the more limited their range over the animal kingdom, the more promising for prophylactic purposes—here, to begin with, was a principle which would be a guide, not only to investigation, but to the most promising fields wherein to investigate, and wherein to cultivate with effect "the new microbic-prophylactic viruses." Here, then, one may presume is the fundamental basis of the belief, which has since become the central doctrine of the treatment, that rabies, like anthrax, being a disease, "common to man and to animals," is, *ipso facto*, amenable to "the new methods of prophylaxis." It was mainly because rabies is such a disease that, in spite of "the darkness in which it was veiled," M. Pasteur viewed its investigation with so much promise. In the closeness of the pathological links between man and animal, particularly the domestic animal; in the extreme narrowness of range over the animal kingdom, it is assumed that there is a convenient clue as to the germ-diseases most likely to prove prophylactic, and, if prophylactic, most certain to render on cultivation a modified virus-germ, capable of undoubted vaccination.

Where a genuine prophylactic treatment might be looked for with some assurance, the principle would appear to be, and most probably is, one of paramount importance. Certain it is, that the strictly prophylactic germ-diseases are of the most limited range over the animal kingdom of any order of germ-disease ; and this is a fact of vast significance. The disastrous germ-diseases of the Middle Ages, which have either more or less disappeared, or become but faint reproductions of their original virulent forms, have been, significantly enough, mainly of a prophylactic character. Witness, in this connection, how even the mildest prophylactics of civilized life, such as measles, still decimate a tribe of savages. The specially prophylactic character of such germ-diseases may account for their very limited range over the animal kingdom ; and the narrower and the more strictly limited the range, probably the more profoundly prophylactic the disease. This, as shall be shown in due course, will also account for the final disappearance of the germ-disease in this limited range itself. Since this is so, manifestly enough the prophylactic property, far from being a universal, is a highly specialised one in the animal kingdom.

Is rabies, then, such a limited germ-disease as this? There can be no doubt that, like anthrax, smallpox, syphilis and probably the entire prophylactic order, it "affects animals in common with man," and particularly the domestic animals. Outbreaks of rabies in deer, sheep and cattle have been known from time immemorial. But it does not follow, from even so significant a fact, that "the circle of practical applications," which has resulted in so many "new microbic prophylactic viruses," will do, or has done, anything of the kind for rabies. Accepting the principle as of fundamental importance, that a germ-disease which is common to man and some of the lower animals, affords an unfailing index of its capacity to yield a distinctly prophylactic vaccination, whilst rabies, like anthrax, affects without doubt *man and cattle* ; on the other hand, unlike any strictly prophylactic germ-disease, but marvellously like the preventive and recurrent order, it is *common to man and probably to every verte-brate animal.* The rabies of the dog, man, ape, cat, rabbit, deer, guinea-pig, sheep, cow, horse, even the fowl, may be transmitted to every hot-blooded, or possibly even vertebrate animal. Could this be done with smallpox, scarlatina, measles, or whooping-cough? There is, apparently, no class of hot-blooded animal which may not be rabidised, or in which the rabies-microbe may not germinate. In its destructive virulence through the animal kingdom the virus-germ of rabies is, therefore, too *"common."* The micro-organism is con-fined, in its range of germination, to no special group or groups; but, on the contrary, is probably universal. In its devastating range over the animal kingdom it is as irrespective of class or order as erysipelas, pyæmia, diphtheria, tetanus, serpent-venom, opium or alcohol, which, although certainly likewise "protective," for a time, are not prophylactic, or capable of yielding a prophylactic modified virus-germ. If extreme narrowness of range of attack over the animal kingdom be an indication of a prophylactic character, the virus-germ of such a disease as rabies, which in its morbific results, far from being specialised to man and a single group of domestic animals, is common to the animal kingdom, does not promise very favourably for prophylaxis, or for being modified, either by cultivation or by transmission, into anything like a genuine vaccination. And this wide range of attack, so characteristic of rabies, but which is so unlike a strictly prophylactic germ-disease, or the entire prophy-lactic order, is precisely akin to a strictly preventive and recurrent germ-disease, or to the entire preventive order. Has, then, the micro-organism of rabies been modified into a form capable of imparting the pronounced and enduring protection of the most potent variety of the disease with a minimum of its virulence? This has been alleged.

"It may be deemed *certain* that M. Pasteur has discovered a method of protection from rabies, *comparable with that which vaccination affords against infection from smallpox*[1]."

If the protection imparted by rabies-virus be comparable with that imparted by smallpox or its modified virus-germ, vaccine, it must be due to the fact that rabies, like smallpox, is essentially a prophylactic germ-disease. If so, the protection induced must be

[1] Report for Local Government Board in respect of M. Pasteur's treatment of rabies. The above, here, purposely italicised.

equally permanent, and for the same reasons. This, however, is not the fact. The character and the duration of the protection imparted, and the mode of its production, are very different from that of a prophylactic disease, or of its modified virus-germ. M. Pasteur's group of inoculations "protects" from rabies, not only *before* infection, like vaccine, but, unlike vaccine, also considerably *after* infection ; it would appear to protect as absolutely at the one stage as at the other. This extraordinary property is its most characteristic feature ; but, in itself, distinguishes it from any modified *virus-germ*, and links it to the *virus* of every preventive germ-disease. That M. Pasteur's course of inoculations can both *"protect* against" the disease, *i.e.* before infection, and also *"prevent"* the disease, *i.e.* considerably after infection, there can be no doubt whatever[1]. But does vaccine, or any modified micro-organism, prevent the disease or, which is the same thing, protect considerably after infection or when incubation has fairly set in ? This also has been maintained.

"It is known," says Professor Ray Lankester, "that inoculating with vaccine-virus during the latent period of smallpox has an effect in modifying the disease in a favourable direction[2]."

If vaccine, when very early used after infection, modifies the coming smallpox, which is possible, for vaccine has a shorter incubation, it must be on the same prophylactic, not preventive, lines as the smallpox itself ; for it is but the modified virus-germ of the latter. But the modifying power of vaccine, however pronounced *before*, is, *after* infection, by no means well known. Otherwise it would be the infected, not less than the uninfected, who would be so constantly and so successfully vaccinated. It is far from certain that any genuinely prophylactic virus-germ is ever really preventive ; just as, conversely, it is questionable in the extreme if any strictly preventive virus or virus-germ is ever prophylactic. It has not been demonstrated. So much so that the English Committee, in their Report for the Local Government Board, have unhesitatingly asserted that,

"Some have, indeed, thought it possible to avert smallpox by vaccinating those very recently exposed to its infection. But the

[1] The term *"protective"* is defined by the English Committee in their Report for the Local Government Board as denoting the treatment, "which is designed to *protect* a man or an animal *from the risk of becoming infected"*; the term *"preventive,"* on the other hand, refers exclusively to the treatment "designed to *prevent* the occurrence of the disease *in one already infected."*

[2] *Pasteur and Hydrophobia*, by Prof. Ray Lankester, *Nineteenth Century*, August, 1886.

evidence of this is, at the best, inconclusive. And M. Pasteur's may be justly deemed the first proved method of overtaking and suppressing by inoculation a process of specific infection[1]."

It would appear, therefore, to be perfectly possible for a germ-disease to be powerfully prophylactic without necessarily being preventive; just as, on the other hand, it is certain that a germ-disease may be most potently preventive, without necessarily being prophylactic.

Nevertheless, it is unquestionable that M. Pasteur's course of rabies-virus protects from rabies, and not less obviously than his modified micro-organism of anthrax protects from anthrax, or than vaccine from smallpox. Such as it is, the protection which it imparts, both before and considerably after infection, is of the most pronounced character.

Is, however, "protection" of the kind which characterises rabies so rare a phenomenon? There is not a germ-disease which does not in a measure, and for a time, protect from itself. One sees this phenomenon even in the habitual use of the simplest, not to say of the deadliest, drugs and virulent products. It may be objected that there is a vast difference between mineral and vital properties.

Take, then, a considerable step higher, and directly to vital properties. Consider alcohol and alcoholism. This is very much nearer to rabies, if not on the actual confines of the malady. In this agent we have the virulent product of a germ which is as specific in character as the virus-germ of rabies itself. The alcohol, elaborated by yeast in a saccharine solution, is a typical virus, or virulent product, or soluble ferment induced by a micro-organism. In this light, it may be said that alcoholism, especially acute alcoholism, is in reality a germ-disease, or by far the most important half of a germ-disease. Nor, as a virus, is alcohol unique, in acting *per se* or in producing the specific lesions of the disease, altogether apart from its micro-organism. As it so happens, the virulent product of not a few germ-diseases has, like alcohol, been absolutely separated from the specific micro-organism which alone produces it; and, again like alcohol, these isolated "bacillary products," when inoculated in sufficient quantity into animals, have, one and all, produced the morbid phenomena, *ante-mortem* and *post-mortem*, characteristic of their respective diseases. Thus, the bacillary product of the *bacillus tuberculosis* has been separated with great genius by Koch from the

[1] Report for Local Government Board.

micro-organism which elaborates it.   Unfortunately, although frequently attempted, this feat has not yet been accomplished in respect
of the rabies-microbe.   Consequently, in every inoculation, both
agents—the rabies-microbe and its virus—have to be introduced into
the system together.   But the bacillary products of diphtheria and of
tetanus and of several more germ-diseases have in like manner been
separated ; and these virulent principles have, like alcohol, irrespective of the special micro-organisms producing them, been found
sufficient to induce the phenomena of their respective diseases.   It is
the virus, not the virus-germ, of diphtheria and tetanus, and of all
germ-diseases, which alone kills.   And all these virulent products, or
every virus or bacillary product, elaborated by pathogenic micro-
organisms, are produced, as M. Pasteur conclusively demonstrated, by
a process strictly analogous to, if not identical with, the process of
yeast-fermentation.   Alcohol, then, is a morbific ferment elaborated
by a specific micro-organism, not less so than the virus of rabies
itself.

Moreover it is capable of producing morbid phenomena which are
closely, even startlingly, allied to those induced by rabies-virus.   Not
less than from an excess of alcohol, the morbid explosion arising from
the rabies-virus is essentially an intoxication of the nervous system ;
perhaps the most appalling intoxication known to man.   So far as
the pathogenic properties of the respective virulent products are concerned, the alliance is of the closest.   The diseases produced in their
various forms, modifications and "varieties" are marvellously akin.
Thus, from alcohol, there are a *mad drunkenness* and likewise a
dead drunkenness ; just as, from rabies-virus, there are a *furious
madness*, and likewise a *dumb* or *mortal madness*, or, in other words,
a convulsive-rabies and a paralytic-rabies.

But, so far as the "protective" and the "preventive" properties
of the two viruses are concerned, what does one find ?   A graduated
course of alcoholic drink "protects" from getting drunk ?   So much
is this the case that it is hardly too much to say that an habitual
drunkard of 10 glasses of spirits *per diem*, if one may so express his
capacity to stand alcohol or the intensity-point of his "protection," is
probably one of the soberest of the men who drink.   But, in spite of
the comparative sobriety, one may safely take the amount of such
immunity as a test of the drinking habit, and as a clue to the true
history of the case.   It is not the "incapables," or the "dead drunks,"
or even the violently "mad drunks," who so inevitably find their way

before magistrates, that are the most hopeless drunkards ; their utter incapacity to tolerate ardent spirits is even a healthy feature. It is the daily drinker, and never absolutely "incapable," who is the most serious of all drunkards. Such a "protected" subject detests intoxication, and is quick to detect and resent the insinuation, even more so than the punctiliously temperate. The man who can stand with immunity, *i.e.* without getting intoxicated, 10 glasses of spirit *per diem*, is no recent drinker. He has earned his protection with a vengeance ! Even a drinker of only a 5-glass capacity *per diem* will drink with immunity, and for a long time apparently with impunity, what will make a healthy young man or woman, who has never tasted spirits, as *"furious"* as a rabid dog. In like manner, a thoroughly seasoned drunkard will drink with the same immunity what will stagger or infuriate even the man of a 5-glass capacity. The drinker of a 10 to 12-glass capacity *per diem* is practically as "protected" from intoxication as a dog is protected against rabies, which has been completely inoculated with M. Pasteur's entire course of rabies-virus, from its 1st up to its 10th or 12th or highest intensity-point of virulence. But let a drinker of a 5-glass capacity, or even smaller, increase and strengthen his capacity for alcohol, as at this stage he will unconsciously do, steadily rising from a 5 up through the intermediate capacities even to 10 glasses of spirit *per diem* ; and, by this time, he too will have become as thoroughly seasoned to resist intoxication as the most successfully inoculated dog to resist rabies. What, therefore, is to be observed in the graduated course of the inoculations of rabies-virus, is not only analogous but precisely similar to what, stage for stage, is to be seen in a graduated course of alcohol. Just as a protected dog, which has been inoculated with a course of rabies-virus, ranging from zero up to the highest intensity-point of virulence, will resist the "raving" or "furious," and, at last, even the "dumb," or the most paralytic, form of rabies ; so, in like manner, a man seasoned up to a 10 or 12-glass capacity of spirits *per diem* will resist both the raving mania and the comatose paralysis of alcoholic drunkenness. In each disease, if the virus be methodically graduated in administration, sooner or later it induces absolute protection. In each case the cerebro-spinal system is the prime seat of disturbance ; and in some, of an extremely sensitive nervous-system, far more exclusively so than in others. Still more important, in each case the protection, such as it is, is solely determined *by the amount of the virus in the system.*

Again, in the course of his experimental investigation, M. Pasteur early made the discovery, which may be taken as a fundamental law of all such protection, that a virus of low intensity of virulence, whilst it cannot avert the consequences of a much stronger, nevertheless renders an animal insusceptible to the virus of the next intensity-point of virulence and even lowers to a definite but strictly commensurate extent the virulence of the highest. The first in the protective scale, if it will rabidise a rabbit, is too feeble to rabidise a dog. But, nevertheless, it is found that it is potent enough to "prevent" the second from rabidising the animal ; that is to say, it has practically converted the second into the first virus of the protective scale. For the same reason the first two inoculations will prevent the third, and the first three the fourth, from rabidising, and so on, until the next to the most potent of the group is reached, when a canine-rabies, of a virulence equal to that of the most potent inoculation, will be completely averted. This progressive protection, with its methodical accumulation of virus in the system, is the *sine quâ non* of the inoculative treatment. One inoculation, and of but a mere infinitesimal drop of the rabies-virus, as in the case of vaccine or the modified virus-germ of a prophylactic germ-disease, would neither protect an animal from rabies, nor prevent the disease. But will anyone deny that precisely the same set of phenomena is to be seen, stage for stage, in a graduated course of alcohol? One glass of brandy may, in itself, be too weak to produce intoxication in a man who has never tasted spirits, although, significantly enough, never too weak in a child. This one or initial glass may be, so far, viewed as at the zero-stage of the protective scale. But the daily habit of one glass of brandy will be sufficiently potent to, very soon, prevent a second from having any more intoxicating effect than one. And for the same reason, the daily habit of two glasses will prevent a third, and of three a fourth, and so on until a tenth, or possibly much higher, is reached, from having any more intoxicating effect than in the first instance a glass of brandy possessed. A drinker of a 5-glass capacity *per diem* is in reality not more intoxicated after his sixth or seventh glass of spirits than a man who has never tasted spirits will be after a first or second glass. A confirmed drunkard of a 10-glass capacity *per diem* will drink with immunity what would make the man who has never tasted spirits a paralysed idiot or " *dead drunk*," and even the drinker of a 5-glass capacity a raving maniac or "*mad drunk*." One given amount of alcohol in the system would appear, precisely as one grade or one uniform amount of rabies-virus, to protect up to this grade, and exactly in proportion to it. The protection imparted by each virus is essentially a quantitative protection; and the analogies of the two diseases are so strong that their differences would appear to be those of degree more than of kind, as if the rabies-virus itself were but the deadliest of ferments. How different is this "protection," or its duration, or its mode of production, from that imparted by vaccine or by any modified micro-organism of the prophylactic germ-diseases! On the other hand, how marvellously like it is to the protection imparted by the virus or "bacillary-product" of every preventive germ-disease! A prolonged and carefully-graduated course of Koch's tuberculin will protect for a time an uninfected organism against tubercle, and, employed early, even "prevent" the disease. In like manner, a graduated group of inoculations of the rabies-virus both protects from and prevents rabies. But this is precisely what might have been looked for. After such a mode of inoculation it would have been curious if there had been no *quantitative* protection, strictly determined by the amount of virus inoculated.

Admitting the high preventive property of rabies-virus,—but it is not higher than that of the virus of tetanus, diphtheria, tubercle, &c., or even of alcohol or opium,—what is the character of the protection which it imparts? Is it as enduring as in the first instance it was absolute? Is it in this all-important property to be compared with that imparted by vaccine or by any prophylactic micro-organism, whether modified or not? Is it, in point of fact, to be distinguished *in duration* from the protection imparted by any recurrent but preventive virus? Analogy would appear to indicate that, whilst thorough enough at the end of a course of rabies-inoculations, or still more so after a series of courses, it must be of comparatively short duration. Nay, further, the more virulent the virus at last introduced into the system, or the greater the quantity of virus employed to protect, the sooner will the high protection occasioned thereby begin to fade. Where a virulent product, as opposed to a virus-germ or the modified prophylactic micro-organism, is the factor of the protection, as it is the sole factor of the disease, the evanescent character of such protection, however high to begin with, will not be exceptional. This rapidly-fading character holds good more or less of every preventive and recurrent germ-disease. It is preeminently true of erysipelas, acute rheumatism, influenza maligna, ague, diphtheria, and many more ; all of which are, consequently, recurrent. Probably, the time immediately after an attack of any such germ-disease is the safest during the entire period of protection. But how long does the protection last, however absolute it may be to begin with?

This, again, could not be better illustrated than in the case of alcohol. Take the case of a restored drinker of, at one time, it may be, a 10-glass capacity *per diem,* or even considerably higher. Is this amazing protection against getting drunk enduring, or as permanent as the protection given from a single vaccination or from any modified prophylactic germ? In a short time, if he be a healthy man and of good recuperative power possibly within a year, the pristine protection, far from being absolute, will have so far faded that, should he now relapse, he will find to his cost that he has no longer even a 6- or 5-glass capacity of spirits *per diem.* True; he will be protected up to this point. But on altogether renouncing alcohol, how long will this remaining immunity last? In the absence of the virulent product which has occasioned it, even this latter amount of protection will systematically fail and fade.

Nor, in its duration, is the protection from rabies-virus, any more than in its character and mode of production, in any way different from this. The precise duration of the protection afforded by the course of rabies-virus must in the meantime be somewhat problematical. As yet there has, perhaps, been no adequate time to thoroughly test this important point. But, fortunately, there is not wanting some evidence bearing on the subject, and from which it is certain that even the most pronounced rabies-protection begins to fade in a comparatively short time, much shorter than after vaccination, or than after the inoculation of any modified prophylactic micro-organism. Take, for example, the following invaluable note by M. Pasteur himself ; although it is intended to reveal, curiously enough, the actual durability of the protection :

"I may add a few words on the duration of the immunity conferred on our vaccinated dogs. As you are aware, I have at Villeneuve-l'Étang a large kennel, where I have kept for two years a considerable number of dogs, which I had rendered refractory to rabies.

"At the end of the first year I tried on a group of them the criterion-inoculation, by trephining and injecting the ordinary street-dog virus. Eleven out of fourteen resisted.

"This year, again I tried the same experiment on six more, which had been vaccinated two years previously.   Four out of six came out immune[1]."

Here, apparently, after only one year's duration, more than a fifth succumb to the disease on the reinoculation of a canine-virus.   In other words, of dogs which have been completely "protected" against the most potent canine-madness to be met with, not less than 21 per cent. succumb to reinfection within a twelvemonth ; or actually 33 per cent., or not less than a third of the number, at first so completely protected, succumb after two years, and, moreover, with "the ordinary street-dog virus," which is far from so potent as that against which, but shortly before, they were so thoroughly protected.   Where, in such results, is there any evidence of the continuance of the imparted protection ?   A carefully graduated course of alcohol or of opium itself would protect probably as long and as effectually.   If the protection induced by vaccine were of as evanescent a character, it would be of but little or no avail in stamping out smallpox.   But it is precisely this lasting quality of the prophylactic inoculation, or the enduring and absolutely uninjurious character of the prophylaxis, and, moreover, from an infinitesimal amount of the inoculation, which makes vaccine, and probably the modified micro-organism of every strictly prophylactic germ-disease when it comes to be "modified," so totally different from rabies-virus, or from that of any other strictly preventive germ-disease.   This renders vaccine and the modified micro-organism of anthrax so constant and unfailing in protecting the healthy million, and in thus extinguishing the disease.   In spite of the startling and very massive amount of the protection imparted by rabies-virus, it is precisely its evanescent character which renders it valueless for protecting the race, and which links it to alcohol, and, still more, to the virus of erysipelas, diphtheria, ague, tetanus, and to that of every other recurrent and preventive germ-disease.

But, it may be said, as the virus of rabies unquestionably protects, and, for a time, as profoundly as any known prophylactic inoculation, any given district by a periodic reinoculation might be permanently protected against the disease.   By this means the malady would sooner or later be as practically extinguished as small-pox by vaccination, or anthrax by its modified virus-germ.   A process of systematic and even compulsory reinoculation would possibly not be impracticable in any civilized country.   But it is certain that on account of the rapidly fading character of the protection imparted

---

[1] *Annales de l'Institut Pasteur*, Letter to Prof. Duclaux, Paris, Dec. 27, 1886.

by the preventive group of inoculations, constant and very frequent reinoculation would be absolutely imperative. As this procedure would protect the healthy and abolish the disease, why has it not been established everywhere, where rabies prevails; or, still more important, why has it not been proposed anywhere? Why has the "preventive" property of the inoculation been so exclusively relied on? It has been as wholly employed in this capacity as the protective or strictly prophylactic property has been exclusively employed in respect of vaccine or of any other modified prophylactic micro-organism.

What would be the ultimate effect of enforced reinoculation of the rabies-virus, if carried on thoroughly and systematically even for a few years? Would it be different from the persistent seasoning-process of any other "bacillary product" or preventive virus? Is the virus of rabies, then, so very harmless, even in the most graduated process of inoculation? If so, it is very different from any other pathogenic product, or from the virus of any other germ-disease. Nevertheless, it has been assumed and frequently asserted, that in the longest course of inoculations the virus is practically as bland as the sterilized bouillon which holds it in suspension. The amount of rabies-virus which an animal is capable of tolerating, and apparently with impunity, is startling. Man has been inoculated and reinoculated with the fullest courses of virus, and with no other obvious result than complete protection. In the dog the entire range of M. Pasteur's inoculations has been over and over again administered. They have, likewise, in the most massive form and amount been boldly injected into the circulation, both before and after infection, and within the space of "two hours." Nay, further, so enormous a quantity as from two to ten hypodermic syringefuls, and of the most potent paralytic rabbit-virus to be met with, has been at once inoculated; and when it did not thereafter rabidise the animal it had no other apparent result than complete and absolute protection against the disease in its severest forms, converting the animal into an "immune." Why, then, it may be insisted, should not a frequent and persistent periodic process of reinoculation be feasible enough, and permanent protection be thereby established everywhere?

It is true that the longest or most potent course of rabies-virus has not produced rabies. But even this phenomenon is not unique; it is characteristic of the virus of every preventive germ-disease, nay, even of every virulent product. It is not less true that the

longest and strongest course of alcohol does not necessarily produce
a chronic condition of either *mad* or *dead drunkenness*. The
quantity of alcohol which a thoroughly seasoned drinker will at last
tolerate, and apparently with impunity, is hardly less amazing than
the amount of rabies-virus which a severely inoculated animal may
endure. Long-standing or chronic alcoholism does not necessarily
produce intoxication either of the furious or of the paralytic form,
but, on the contrary, precisely like the rabies-virus, protects from
both conditions. The morbid results which it produces are of a very
different order. In like manner, it is not rabies or hydrophobia
which the most prolonged course of rabies-virus produces, it will
protect profoundly from any such intoxication. The lesions which it
will produce will be of a very different stamp, for there are other
tissues and organs to simultaneously injure beside the nervous
structure, and these morbid results will be none the less insidious for
the protection from rabies which the course of virus affords, and
none the less serious that they are so totally unlike rabies in any of
its forms.

That such results are ever produced has not yet been experimentally determined. Certain it is, however, that if, three or four
times a day, the daily inoculation of hypodermic syringefuls of the
most potent rabbit-virus, and continued for weeks, on a group of
dogs which have already been completely "protected," does not in
the end find out and emphasise every weak organ and system of the
animal, there can be no reason why such courses of inoculations
should not be continued periodically at the shortest intervals, and all
over the world. As already stated, the rapidly fading character of
the protection imparted demands nothing short of this treatment.
But although the course of inoculations never produces rabies, this
is no proof that, if long continued, it will occasion no other injury.
There is not wanting a somewhat suspicious class of cases which, in
spite of so much immunity and apparent impunity, would seem to
indicate this possible danger. In the case of prolonged or repeated
administrations of rabies-virus, or sometimes of one massive injection
of a virus of high power, the sudden death of the animal, and without
rabies being produced, is not unknown. As stated already, such a
case occurred in the group of nineteen control dogs which were
crucially experimented upon by M. Pasteur before the French
Commission. One of the animals prematurely collapsed and very
suddenly died, "*but not of rabies.*" Another such case, strangely

enough, occurred in Sir Victor Horsley's equally crucial experiments on behalf of the British Commission.

"The *protected* dog, No. 6," says Sir Victor Horsley, "was bitten on three different occasions ; by a furiously rabid cat on September 7, 1886 ; by a furiously rabid dog on October 7, 1886 ; and by another furiously rabid dog on November 6, 1886. It died ten weeks after being bitten for the third time, *but not of rabies.* It had been suffering with diffuse eczema during the whole of the time that it was under observation ; and it died of this[1]."

In such a case there most certainly would be, after death, no sign of rabies, any more than, after death from alcoholism, there would necessarily be any sign of *mad* or *dead drunkenness*, or even of *delirium tremens.* But that is no reason why the virus of rabies was absolutely innocuous. What effect had the rabies-virus, so persistently maintained at a high virulence, and for so long a time—the protected animal was bitten by a rabid animal every month for three months—and on the progressive and general degeneration of the tissues? Was it not comparable with the blighting effects of alcoholism, with its fibrous and fatty degenerations and blocked or ruptured capillaries in every organ? Is even diffuse eczema, with the other secondary lesions, never induced by chronic alcoholism? If so, it might well be by rabies-virus, which is so much more virulent. Were the protective group of inoculations to be as periodically employed as the very fading character of the protection would necessitate, the few "accidental" deaths which, even now, mysteriously occur, would not be lessened.

In like manner, it is conceivable that by a very carefully graduated course of alcohol a man might steadily become a drunkard of an 8 or 10 glass-capacity *per diem*, without once having been fairly intoxicated! But even if a complete course of alcohol as severe as this were as successfully undergone, and with as complete an immunity as in the case of the most prolonged course of rabies-virus itself, which is not only perfectly possible but of frequent occurrence, would anybody assert that the alcohol in such a man, because he never happened to be noticeably drunk, or even intoxicated at all, was absolutely innocuous?

It is a notorious fact that, in spite of the protection which a long course of alcohol has imparted, and with such apparent impunity, it is all the more surely and widely doing its lesional work, and much

[1] Report for Local Government Board, Prof. Horsley's Abstract Report A, p. 3.

more thoroughly than if the man were often drunk. In this malady, as in rabies, the cerebro-spinal system is the prime seat of the disease. But if the nervous system be "protected" by the virulent product, although in a large percentage the first to succumb, other tissues and organs are affected by it. The heart, the blood-vessels, the liver, the stomach, the lungs, the skin, but, above all, the kidneys, are all more or less degenerated. And these insidious lesional effects are not any less blighting for the absence of a stormy outburst of intoxication, or because the nervous system, the main seat of the disturbance in a healthy man, is so marvellously "protected." The protection itself, or the absence of any such nerve-storm, is but an indication of a diseased condition ; for no healthy nerve-tissue will tolerate without a nerve-explosion such an amount of the virulent product. The confirmed drunkard's unquestionable "protection" against such an outburst has not saved him, but in every direction has prepared him for an inevitable break-down ; so much so, that at last a slight chill, a slight indigestion, the merest *nomen morbi*, which would injure no healthy man, kills him in an hour or two.

And the same may be said of ague, and of all equally recurrent germ-diseases. So much so that one has at last but to glance at the ague-stricken patient to see that he is dying on his feet ; and, as in the case of alcohol, in the end a trivial illness collapses him in a few hours. The malarial-virus has unprotected him from any trivial illness and all the more effectually for having "protected" him against the "paludal" micro-organism so often and so long. In each of these, and all similar virus-protections, the immunity imparted is far from a healthy sign. Would then a periodic reinoculation of the most potent rabies-virus to be obtained be feasible ? The protection which so distinctly "preventive" a virus invariably occasions is in itself, as shall be shown more fully at a subsequent stage, essentially a pathological condition. And for this reason it is so unenduring, and, in a healthy subject, so rapidly fading even in its highest grades.

Lastly, not only is the protection imparted by a preventive virus more or less fading, but, on its disappearance, the pathological condition involved in the immunity is revealed by an increased sensitiveness or liability to the pathogenic micro-organism, against which for a time the animal has been so wonderfully protected. An indication of this superinduced liability is again to be seen in respect of alcohol. The man who has allowed himself for any length of time to give way to excessive drink, or to be thoroughly "protected," is, on abstaining from alcohol, not really safe to touch a glass of wine for months thereafter, or, if the alcohol-protection be very pronounced, even for years. His organization with respect to the virus is in a very different condition from that of the man who has never tasted spirits; by the protected condition, for a time, having been converted into the most inflammable material. But this liability with positive recurrence is still more obvious in respect of the preventive germ-disease. The specific culture-ground of the micro-organism is but increased and rendered still more favourable as a germinating-ground for the action of the preventive-virus in establishing the morbid condition of protection. When, along with the disappearing preventive-virus which has occasioned it, the protection begins to fade, the lesional after-effects will reveal themselves, if not in positive disorganization, in an increased liability to the virus-germ, against which for a time, and a very definite time, the organism was so strikingly defended. So far as the entire non-prophylactic or strictly preventive class of germ-disease is concerned, this is probably the fundamental reason of their stubborn and occasionally most persistent recurrence. And, possibly, this condition of unprotection may last for a period corresponding to the period of protection itself. If, consequently, there be, as unquestionably there is, a protective scale in respect of every preventive germ-disease, there is probably also, depending upon and determined by it, an unprotective scale, closely following in its wake, and which is in reality at the root of every form of recurrence characteristic of such a disease. Not that the increased liability, even in the most recurrent of such maladies— as erysipelas, acute rheumatism, influenza maligna, ague, &c.—is permanent, any more than the condition or period of protection; for it is due to the same cause, a more or less unenduring preventive-virus.

To what order of germ-disease, then, the prophylactic or the preventive, does rabies belong? From the quantitative form of the protection imparted by the rabies-virus, and from its fading character, if there were no other evidence, it may be safely asserted that its virus-germ is distinctly a preventive, not a prophylactic, micro-organism, and that rabies itself is essentially a preventive germ-disease.

Nevertheless, if M. Pasteur's research had revealed nothing more than the existence of two such radically different orders of germ-disease, it would have been of inestimable value. In the light of his investigation of rabies, alone, it may be unhesitatingly asserted that germ-diseases are either of a preventive or of a prophylactic type ; but that, if of the one, most certainly for that very reason not of the other. Nay, further, as by his creation of the "modified" prophylactic micro-organism of anthrax, which was as godlike as Jenner's discovery of vaccine itself, he has, as already stated, practically triumphed over the entire prophylactic class of germ-disease ; the specific micro-organism of every one of this order, but of this exclusively, being strictly prophylactic and, therefore, modifiable into a vaccination ; so, on the other hand—and it is not a less masterly creation—by his preventive inoculation of rabies-virus he has triumphed, not only over rabies, but over the entire preventive class of germ-disease to which it belongs ; the virus of every one of this vast order, but of this exclusively, being strictly preventive. There is, consequently, apparently no reason why, sooner or later, all germ-diseases may not be overcome by the one method or by the other ; by the preventive virus, if it be a *preventive* germ-disease, or by the "modified" prophylactic micro-organism or virus-germ, if it be a *prophylactic*. Hence, with Lord Lister's most masterly discovery of antiseptic treatment, in time the entire realm of germ-disease may be thus completely mastered.

CHAPTER IX.

PRE-INCUBATION PERIOD, AND INCUBATION PROPER.

THE rabies-microbe of an infected wound, being absorbed by its connective-corpuscles, will be at once conveyed by these to the connective-tissue of the immediate vicinity; and, were this tissue at all favourable for germinating, germination would forthwith supervene. This, however, as we have seen, is not the fact. Rabies would, then, be a germ-disease of as strictly peripheral connective-tissue cultivation as tetanus, diphtheria, erysipelas, &c. The germination of the micro-organism would likewise begin immediately after infection, and, as in these and other germ-diseases, there would be no *preincubation period* whatever. The incubation would invariably be as regular and unvarying as that of the entire class of preventive germ-diseases of strictly peripheral cultivation. Consequently, if at the outset the rabies-microbe is borne to the peripheral connective-tissue by its own "connective-corpuscles," which is extremely probable, for its own fibrous-shell would be the very first resort of the corpuscle, such tissues cannot be the specific germinating-soil, since the micro-organism by no means remains here. In spite of being primarily borne hither, it is, thereafter, sooner or later, conveyed to the cerebro-spinal substance, far enough from the peripheral wound. The connective-corpuscle, still burdened with the micro-organism, will once more be stimulated thereby to its amoebiform wanderings. After leaving its connective-tissue, it will find its way into the adjacent lymphatic channels, and, restlessly migrating from fibrous site to fibrous site, will ultimately bear the micro-organism in its interior to centric structures far enough removed from the periphery.

If the amount of rabies-germ introduced be insignificant and far away from the cerebro-spinal axis, it may take, relatively, a most prolonged and irregular route and a very long time before it will be conveyed to the cerebro-spinal substance; this process of conveyance, or pre-incubation period, lasting for, it may be, many months. If the amount of rabies-microbe be large, or even if small, when introduced in a site most favourable for absorption, such as a lymphatic sac, and in the immediate vicinity of the cerebro-spinal substance itself, such as the arachnoid, it may take but the briefest time before the micro-organism is sown profusely in its specific germinating-ground. In this case the pre-incubation period lasts probably only for a few days, or not much longer than in the case of a preventive germ-disease of strictly peripheral cultivation.

In the prolonged process of conveyance why, however, it may be asked, should not the rabies-microbe be destroyed and devoured by the phagocytic leucocytes of the circulation? This holds true of the specific micro-organism of the preventive germ-diseases of exclusively peripheral cultivation. The freed micro-organism of one and all of this section, on entering the circulation, is immediately devoured by the leucocytes or, if in any amount, stubbornly confined by these very bodies to the peripheral connective-tissue. And if, on infection, the rabies-germs were free and in small numbers in the circulation, there is reason to believe that they would be similarly attacked and destroyed, as possibly not unfrequently occurs in attenuators, such as the dog. Why, then, does not this invariably occur? Simply because the rabies-microbe is, itself, not free in the blood or lymph streams. It is embedded in the interior of the wandering connective-corpuscles. But this very enclosure in a barren vehicle, if it prevents it from germinating, also everywhere effectually defends it from the phagocytic leucocytes of the circulation. And it is probable that this also holds good of the micro-organism of every recurrent germ-disease. One and all of them are defended from the attack of the leucocytes in the very fact of being conveyed so passively within the substance of the wandering connective-corpuscles which have absorbed them. By this means, and in this method, the "spores" of the "paludal parasites" of malarial fever are in all probability so constantly conveyed to the spleen; and the spores of even so essentially a peripheral germ-disease as tetanus are occasionally conveyed to the spinal substance itself.

So far, it has been assumed that in the transit from the peripheral connective-tissue to that of the cerebro-spinal substance the rabies-germ undergoes no multiplication. Does not the micro-organism, immediately after infection, germinate in the peripheral connective-corpuscle which really absorbs it? Were this the fact, it would not be exceptional. It is precisely what takes place in respect of the specific micro-organisms of anthrax, syphilis, scarlatina, smallpox, and probably of every prophylactic germ-disease. One and all of them germinate exclusively in the wandering cells of the circulation which absorb them after infection. But the rabies-microbe germinates in no specialised cell like the leucocyte of the circulation or of the spleen and the marrow of bones. Does then germination occur, if not in the leucocytes, in the much less specialized peripheral connective-corpuscles themselves, and, moreover, all through their wanderings from fibrous site to fibrous site? There is no proof of any such phenomenon, but rather the reverse. The microbe would appear to be merely passively conveyed by the peripheral connective-corpuscle to its ultimate destination in the connective-tissue of the cerebro-spinal substance; all through this process the absorbent corpuscle being neither a phagocyte nor a germinator.

If, however, germination takes place in the interior of the connective-corpuscles then, as just stated, incubation would invariably begin immediately *after* infection. Precisely as in the prophylactic order, the incubation would invariably be of the same duration for every mode or kind of infection. Where the micro-organism germinates solely and exclusively in the leucocytes of the circulation, mere site of infection makes no difference in the incubation-period, for there are leucocytes in every site. For such a micro-organism, the specific seat of cultivation must, consequently, be everywhere where the circulation permeates; and for such a disease the incubation-process must, therefore, be immediate and always of the same duration. Hence, the incubation-period of every prophylactic germ-disease is so regular and normal and can be predicted almost to an hour. And the same holds good of the entire order of the strictly *peripheral* preventive germ-diseases. Here, likewise, the micro-organism on infection at once reaches its specific seat of germination, and germination immediately ensues. Hence, in this class, not less than in the prophylactic order, mere site of infection makes no difference in the character of the malady induced; and the incubation-period is as constant and normal from one site of infection as from another.

But this by no means holds good of such a germ-disease as rabies. The genuine incubation begins only at an indefinite period after infection. The so-called incubation-period, which is so irregular and varying, is in no sense the genuine incubation, but a *pre-incubation period*. And, in every likelihood, the genuine as opposed to the apparent incubation is as normal and regular as that of any other germ-disease, and, probably, of much the same duration as that of tetanus. The apparent difference between the incubation-periods of tetanus and rabies can only arise from the fact that the bacillus of tetanus is strictly of peripheral cultivation, and that its process of germination supervenes immediately after infection ; whereas the rabies-microbe is not peripheral in cultivation, but far removed from such structures ; and hence its true incubation is correspondingly delayed. This pre-incubation period corresponds to the time occupied in the conveyance of the microbe from the peripheral site of infection to the central nervous system. Nor is this phenomenon unique. There is a whole class of preventive germ-diseases of *centric* connective-tissue cultivation, in respect of which this is probably the rule, and where the pre-incubation period is equally indefinite and irregular. The bacillus of tubercle, *e.g.* may float through an animal in one absorbent corpuscle after another, or linger in certain tissues for, it may be, months, without necessarily multi-plying, or before it is actually deposited in a fit "nidus" of germina-tion, such as deteriorated osseous or serous or other connective-tissue. The same is probably true of the micro-organisms of cancer and of leprosy and of not a few more germ-diseases. If, then, the rabies-microbe is conveyed to the central nervous system by the peripheral connective-corpuscle without germinating, it would appear to be the characteristic mode of transference of the entire order of centric preventive germ-diseases.

But if, immediately after infection, as in anthrax and in the entire prophylactic order, or, as in tetanus or diphtheria or the entire preventive order of exclusively peripheral cultivation, the rabies-germ began to multiply in the absorbent corpuscles, the germination being maintained at a multiple rate all through the process of con-veyance, then it would follow for such a micro-organism that the further the peripheral site from the central nervous system, or the longer the incubation-period, the more rabies-germ would be culti-vated in the process of conveyance and, ultimately, sown in the cerebro-spinal substance. Consequently, the more profound would be the rabies thereby induced. Conversely, it would also follow, which is as far from the fact, that the nearer the peripheral site of infection to the central nervous system, or the shorter the incubation period, the less rabies-microbe would be cultivated in the process of conveyance. Consequently, the feebler and the less pronounced would be the rabies thereby induced. If the rabies-germ be really culti- vated in its absorbent connective-corpuscles, and during the entire process of its transference from the periphery, as in the case of micro- organisms of germ-diseases which after infection directly incubate and multiply, why should the mere quantity introduced determine the duration of the pre-incubation period, as likewise the character of the malady induced? It is obvious, then, that the rabies-microbe under- goes in the pre-incubation period, or through the entire process of conveyance from the periphery, no germination whatever. The wandering corpuscular system of the peripheral connective-tissue, however readily and certainly it may absorb the micro-organism, and bear it from one site of connective-tissue to another and a deeper, is in no respect its seat of cultivation. The connective-corpuscle which absorbs it simply conveys it.

All through this pre-incubation period, the rabies-micro-organism, it may safely be inferred, does not multiply. There is ground to show that, at least in attenuators of the disease, rather the reverse is the fact, that is to say that it undergoes, if anything, a process of diminu- tion and positive deterioration. How otherwise should, by a mere difference in site, two inoculations of the same rabies-germ, and of the same amount, produce any difference whatever, not merely in the pre-incubation period, which is comprehensible enough, but in the disease itself? If the rabies-microbe is not more or less diminished in the course of its transference from the periphery, and in proportion to the length of time taken up by the transference, it is certainly not increased. From such facts it is obvious that it is not even main- tained either in its original amount or in its original potency. How different is this from the prophylactic order of germ-disease, or from any of the strictly peripheral preventive group! It holds true, how- ever, of rabies, because by the time the rabies-germ has reached and settled in the cerebro-spinal substance, and has not germinated in the entire course of its transference from the periphery, it may well have diminished in amount and become more or less spent, providing the pre-incubation period be at all prolonged, and providing the micro- organisms at the moment of infection were in anything like an enfeebled, much more a moribund condition, which, probably is no uncommon event.

The rabic bulb or spinal substance of an animal which has just died of the disease, and an emulsion of which constitutes the artificial inoculation, contains rabies-germs in every stage of degeneration and decay, in spite of the fact that in this site they are in a more vigorous and potent condition than in any other in the rabidised animal. As we have seen, even the virulent salivary-secretion of the most profoundly paralytic rabbit-rabies consists of a still larger proportion of such degenerating and degenerated forms, and are analogous to the same "degenerating and degenerated forms" seen in malarial fever, but which in this latter disease crowd the lymphoid corpuscles of the circulation and spleen, not the salivary corpuscles. Now, in both the artificial and the natural infection, there must be many such moribund and, it may be, even dead microbes, blended with the vigorous and healthy. But the dead microbes will, like any other extrinsic organic material, be at once taken up by the absorbent corpuscles of the site and straightway demolished; and the degenerated and moribund microbes in a prolonged pre-incubation period will ultimately die before reaching the cerebro-spinal substance. In an infected animal, a vigorous rabies-microbe may live for months before rabies is actually induced; for it is pre-eminently and even solely a micro-organism of *living,* if of enfeebled, not of *dead* tissue, much less of *plasma sanguinis.* Hence, the 6 or 7 days' rabbit-rabies will, after one day's exposure of the rabic marrow, induce a rabies of 8 or 9 days' incubation; after a few days' exposure, a rabies of 15 or 16 days' incubation; and after only a week's exposure, the bulb will, often enough, fail to rabidise a dog or any attenuator of the disease. Thus, whilst in dead tissues it is found impossible to keep the rabies-microorganism alive for a few days, or to prevent it from speedy death, so different from the micro-organism of many germ-diseases, anthrax, diphtheria, tubercle, &c.; in a living animal, on the contrary, providing this animal be of enfeebled nervous constitution, or suffering from any form of fibrosis in the spinal substance, and, on the other hand, providing that the micro-organism itself is not degenerated, to begin with, or absolutely moribund, it is found impossible to kill it, even, sometimes, in spite of the earliest and the most powerful "preventive" treatment. The microbe, if healthy, maintains for months its vitality in the living organism in a quiescent state, as it is being borne through the system in the interior of the wandering connective corpuscle, like the stoned fruit swallowed and conveyed by a migratory bird to a new and a virgin soil.

If the rabies-microbe does not germinate in the absorbent corpuscles in the process of being transferred from the peripheral to the cerebro-spinal connective-tissue, it follows that the micro-organism will not elaborate its virus during the entire pre-incubation period. When, then, and where, or in what site does it so invariably elaborate and eliminate it? Even assuming that germination begins immediately after infection, and in the connective-corpuscle which absorbs and conveys it, it by no means follows that at any such stage the micro-organism eliminates its virus. Nevertheless, it has been insisted upon that, however little the micro-organism may multiply, it may at least elaborate and secrete into the blood-current its specific virus, all through the transfer from the periphery; and that this steadily-secreted virus, when in sufficient quantity for the purpose, at length in reality causes the disease. All this may happen, it may be pointed out, even with an infinitesimal amount of the micro-organism in the absorbent corpuscles, and without any very active process of germination. Thus, it is certain that the merest infinitesimal quantity of the tetanus-bacillus in the peripheral connective-tissue will secrete into the blood-stream an amount of the specific virus which will never fail to tetanise. It is true that, like tetanus, and probably every germ-disease, the morbid phenomena of rabies are induced solely by the virus of its specific micro-organism, whether the accumulation in the circulation be rapid or slow, continuous or irregular, and whether it takes place through the entire pre-incubation period, or only after the process of conveyance has been completed. As in tetanus, then, it may be said, rabies may actually require but a minimum amount of the micro-organism even in the peripheral tissues to secrete any amount of virus, and, therefore, sooner or later, always enough to induce the disease.

Now, on this assumption, one of two results would necessarily ensue. *Firstly*, in the course of the transference, so much virus would be poured into the ever-flowing liquor sanguinis and all through the organism that the disease would be invariably contracted before the rabies-germ itself would reach the cerebro-spinal substance, just as tetanus is produced by its virus without the specific bacillus necessarily leaving the peripheral connective-tissue, or reaching the central spinal substance. Rabies having been incurred, it would likewise follow that precisely the same form of the malady (as probably in tetanus), and that merely a *convulsive*-rabies, never *paralytic*, would invariably be induced, however massive or potent the rabies-germ introduced in infection. However complex in conformation the micro-organism introduced, and however capable of yielding the most paralysing virulent product to be met with, immediately so much of this virus was eliminated as would be capable of inducing a convulsive-rabies, a convulsive-rabies, pure and simple, would straightway be induced, and this would be the result in an intensifier not less than in an attenuator. Hence, the only difference between one case of rabies and another would be a more or less speedy production of the same convulsive form, proportioned to the potency of the rabific microbe introduced, and of its capacity of eliminating virus. But in all such cases the cerebro-spinal substance would not contain the rabies-microbe, any more than it contains the tetanus-bacillus. Consequently the cerebro-spinal substance would invariably fail to impart infection. This, however, as we have repeatedly seen, is diametrically opposed to the facts. Even a completely convulsive-rabies, where the salivary secretion is unaffected, has the rabies-microbe only in the bulbar substance of the cord.

Or, *secondly*, failing this result, and much more probable in respect of such a germ-disease, or of any equally preventive, there would ensue, even if the rabies-germ should constantly reach the cerebro-spinal substance, precisely what occurs in M. Pasteur's graduated group of inoculations against rabies, a complete " prevention " of the disease; rabies would never occur ! In M. Pasteur's course of inoculations, the gradual increase in the amount of the rabies-virus is the *sine qua non* of its success in treatment. But this steady progressive accumulation of virus is precisely identical to that assumed to take place after infection. Consequently, if the virus be continuously eliminated through the whole of the most prolonged pre-incubation period, either a convulsive-rabies, pure and simple, would be the invariable result, whatever the amount, the site, or the mode of infection ; or by the geometric accumulation of the eliminated virus during this period, "prevention" of the disease would invariably ensue. But neither of these results is in accordance with the facts. It may, therefore, be safely affirmed that the rabies-microbe, with those of the entire division of germ-diseases of centric connective-tissue cultivation, does not germinate in being conveyed from the connective-tissue of the periphery ; and, even if it does, that it yields, nevertheless, no virus whatever at any such stage or during any such process.

Only when the pre-incubation period is over, and when the micro-organism is securely deposited in the cerebro-spinal substance itself, does germination really begin. After being sown in this structure, *the incubation-period*, proper, immediately sets in ; and, as already said, it is probably as regular and normal in duration as that of every other germ-disease. Hereafter, far from being quiescent, having at length been placed in the one fitting germinating-soil in the animal economy, it germinates to its full capacity, this latent process of multiplication of the micro-organism proceeding to the advent of the disease itself.

But there is no evidence that, even in the incubation-period proper, the virus of the multiplying rabies-microbe is elaborated. There is no reason to believe, but quite the reverse, that any pathogenic micro-organism elaborates its peculiar virulent product during any but the final stages of incubation, much less, where such exists, during any stage of the pre-incubation period. If the virus be continuously secreted by the micro-organism in the genuine incubation-stage itself, again, one of the two results, already referred to, in respect of the pre-incubation period, would likewise ensue ; either a completely convulsive-rabies, without any implication of the salivary secretion, would be the result ; or, failing this, by the progressive accumulation of the eliminated virus during incubation, "prevention" of the disease, as absolute as in the case of the preventive inoculative treatment, would be the rule. Therefore it may be unhesitatingly affirmed that not only during the pre-incubation period, but during the greater part of the incubation-period itself, the virus is never eliminated. When it is at last poured forth, germination is practically at an end, and the incubation of the micro-organism is virtually accomplished.

If this be so, it is probable that, so far as the microbe which has elaborated it is concerned, the virus is an essentially pathological, rather than a physiological, product, and an indication, not only of the complete maturation of the micro-organism, but of its incipient decay. On the first outflow of virus into the circulation, all further germination of even vigorous microbes is probably, there and then, and thereby, more or less arrested. Hence a completely convulsive-rabies, a convulso-paralytic-rabies, or a very profound and completely paralytic-rabies, is produced, according to the quantity of virus, which, after germination, is at once eliminated. Thus, it would appear that in the genuine incubation itself, not to say the entire pre-incubation period, the specific virus of the micro-organism is conspicuous for its absence ; the first appearance of the rabies being practically synchronous with the very first appearance of the virus. And for this reason, the incubation period of a germ-disease, not less than the pre-incubation period, where such exists, is invariably so "latent." When the virus is eliminated, all latency is, there and then, at an end. The symptoms and signs of rabies and the whole train of lesions in the cerebro-spinal axis make their appearance ; but they are just as sudden as the appearance of the virus itself, and wholly determined by it.

If this be so, the elimination of virus must be a final rather than an early episode in the history of the micro-organism in the animal economy, and as sudden in its elimination as it is most destructive only to the most specialised tissues. And the particular form or "variety" of the rabies induced will depend upon the particular quantity of virus thus eliminated, and this in its turn by the amount and potency of the rabies-microbe, and how it is constituted, which has rooted in the cerebro-spinal substance. If this be an insignificant quantity, and of the simplest conformation, and deposited exclusively in but one or two slight bulbar centres, the virus at last evolved will only be sufficient to induce a convulsive-rabies, pure and simple. If the micro-organism be in greater quantity, and of more or less complex form, and cover much larger areas of the cerebro-spinal axis, the virus at length evolved will be sufficient to induce a con-vulso-paralytic rabies of more or less severe character. As in such cases the convulsive element is invariably preliminary, and the paralytic the latest, the full amount of virus, necessary to produce all these features, must be elaborated and eliminated even after rabies has proclaimed itself. The onset of the pathogenic product may yet be sudden, but not necessarily complete for the case until a series of onsets have taken place. If, lastly, the micro-organism be in a very large quantity and of the most complex form, and really disseminated through the whole extent of both the sympathetic and the cerebro-spinal substance, the virus eliminated, after germination, however latent this entire process, will be so overwhelming in amount and intense in virulence that a rabies of the profoundest and acutest and of a completely paralytic character will be the result. It is, therefore, improbable that in any germ-diseases the virus is eliminated continuously and progressively, as in the case of the preventive course of inoculations against rabies, or, otherwise, than in a more or less sudden outflow, or series of outflows, and only after the incubation of the micro-organism, which has generated it, is practically at an end. The virulent product of rabies will, consequently, be eliminated virtually simultaneously from every centre of the rabific microbe where the germination of the latter has reached its maturity; for it has, everywhere, been deposited in the cerebro-spinal substance well-nigh simultaneously.

But experimental investigation has shown that a large quantity of rabies-virus, suddenly thrown, *in one inoculation*, into a healthy animal's circulation, if in the vast majority of cases it causes rabies, can also *sometimes* occasion "prevention." A hypodermic syringeful of the most potent rabies-virus to be obtained, suddenly thrown into the blood-stream of a sheep or horse, if it does not rabidise, will, in this percentage, occasion immediate and complete protection. Of this fact, after M. Pasteur's experiments, there can be no question. Take the following, as an example :

"On January 23, 1885, six dogs receive under the skin of the abdomen the half of a syringeful of a broth, holding in suspension the triturated medulla of a rabbit belonging to the 66th passage of the rabbit series. Five of these dogs took *dumb-rabies*.

"The sixth dog resisted the inoculation, and subsequently showed itself refractory[1]."

After such results, it is clear that "prevention," in place of the disease, may sometimes be occasioned by a large amount of rabies-virus suddenly thrown into the circulation. And it would appear that the larger the amount or the more pathogenic the virus thus injected, the more frequently is such prevention induced. It is probable that in this way and by this method the natural "immunes" to be found in the dog-race are occasioned. The "protection," which thus very rarely presents itself in nature, is invariably of the most massive and pronounced character. It must be occasioned, therefore, as invariably, by a maximum quantity of the rabies-virus introduced into the circulation in infection. Suppose a healthy dog, severely bitten and torn deeply in many places, with intravenous infection, by a rabid animal whose salivary secretion is charged with rabies-virus, and in consequence of which a very large quantity of the virus is thereby directly introduced into the circulation, prevention might occasionally be induced. But in the vast majority of such cases, the disease, and not prevention or protection, is the result ; and this is due to the fact that the micro-organism, not less than its virus, is, in

[1] *Annales de l'Institut Pasteur*, Dec. 27, 1886.

large quantity, as suddenly thrown into the circulation, and by the blood-stream quickly deposited in the cerebro-spinal substance. Such cases of spontaneous protection may occur in nature ; but they must be rare in the extreme. So, likewise, are the "immunes" ; although, at least in the dog-race, possibly not quite so rare as is supposed. The very large quantity of rabies-virus, however, which in one injection *occasions* prevention—for, as we shall see, at a subsequent stage, it does not quite *cause* it—it is worth noting, is invariably introduced into the blood-stream immediately *after* the injection, or before the rabies-microbe has reached the cerebro-spinal substance, much more, before the germination of the micro-organism, all over the cerebro-spinal substance, has practically finished. The largest injection, introduced suddenly into the system, at the termination of incubation, or at a late stage of germination, will not occasion prevention, but, on the contrary, accelerate and emphasize the disease.

Why should the virus be so suddenly and so simultaneously elaborated by the micro-organism only at the later stages of in-cubation proper? As the process of eliminating the virus depends probably on the particular age or maturity of the micro-organism itself, or how far its germination has advanced to its full capacity of multiplication, the elaboration and elimination will only require a beginning in one centre to become well-nigh simultaneous over all the centres, ready to supply it. In cases, where the germination has not been quite simultaneous, some centres being possibly slightly more advanced than others, the clusters of germinating microbes through the cerebro-spinal axis not all being exactly at the same stage of growth, the sudden elimination of virus, from every centre ripe, or, it may be, decayed enough, to yield it, would immediately induce the disease, and a form proportioned to this amount. More-over, in so doing, the elimination would in all probability likewise arrest,—in some cases only *temporarily,*—the further germination of the few centres which are as yet unfit to yield virus. This temporary arrest of germination would account for *the intermittent form* of rabies so remarkably characteristic of the hen, and occasion-ally of other animals, even of the rabbit; and also for the intermittent form of every intermittent germ-disease, even malarial fever or pyæmia itself. The same intermittent tendency, and for the same reason, is to be seen to some extent even in diphtheria, erysipelas, and also tetanus, but particularly the latter. In these, as in others, the disease more or less recurs in an intermittent form for a few days, or even a week, before the full amount of virus for the case is eliminated, and the full force of the tetanus or the diphtheria is established. But, at such stages, the serum "anti-toxin" treatment is still of real value; for, even yet, it will be essentially bactericidal, and consequently "preventive." Hence, the form of the resulting rabies will be strictly determined by the amount of virus which at last so directly floods the cerebro-spinal centres, but, above and before all, the bulbar centres where the micro-organism so constantly and so pre-eminently abounds.

Nor is it altogether without proof that the first effusion of the virus from a germinating centre, probably a degenerating one, will, *per se*, in however infinitesimal a quantity secreted into the circulation, immediately induce an elimination of virus from other germinating centres ready to yield it. Consider, in this connection, the bearing of the virus, pure and simple, of the tubercle-bacillus, to the clusters of "latent" but probably germinating bacilli throughout the system, and to the production of the morbid phenomena characteristic of this disease. The extraordinary, widely-spread results obtained from Koch's inoculation of *tuberculin* may be looked upon as an analogue of the virus of rabies and its action on latent clusters of the micro-organism at the time of elimination. In a really tuberculous subject, however unexpected or latent the tubercle-bacillus in the system, what gigantic effects are produced by the slightest inoculation of Koch's tuberculin; effects which are comparable only to the explosion of a whole series of powder-magazines from the paltriest casual spark! The amount employed in the test-inoculation must be infinitesimal in the extreme. But, once in the blood-stream, however infinitesimal in amount, it is capable of producing lesional reactions out of all proportion to the insignificant quantity of the tuberculin employed; reactions not only in the lung-tissue where the *bacillus tuberculosis* may be supposed to abound; not merely in a visible laryngeal infiltration, nor even in a *lupus* of the face; nor exclusively in the joints and bones and serous membranes, but, simultaneously, in one and all of these structures, and wherever the specific micro-organism has a fitting nidus for germination. Is it conceivable that the infinitesimal quantum of tuberculin thus injected in the vast blood-stream should, in itself, produce such pronounced and widely-spread lesional effects? It is more probable that, minute as the tuberculin is, it acts directly and simultaneously upon the bacilli, or clusters of bacilli, which in connective-tissue site after site, are, of themselves, on the point of yielding this same virulent product, exciting them everywhere to secrete their virus. After such an injection, all over the fibrous or connective-tissue structures which have served as a germinating-soil, or wherever there are clusters of bacilli ripe enough to yield the virus, an amount of "tuberculin," purer even than Koch's, which in so infinitesimal a quantity in the blood-stream has started the process, is simultaneously and suddenly evolved by the germinating tissues to produce the reaction. The simultaneous reaction is due to the ever-flowing blood-current. Koch's inoculation of the bacillary product is, therefore, but as a spark which ignites a very vast conflagration, starting a process of virus-elimination from the clusters of bacilli in so many tissues which is as simultaneous as it is widely-spread.

And it is possible that, on the process of germination coming to an end, this is what occurs whenever the virus of a germ-disease is eliminated. Consequently, it is highly probable that the elimination of the virus of rabies is a relatively sudden and final and pathological process in the history of the micro-organism in the animal economy, being an indication that the specific microbe has reached the culmination of its latent, germinating life to the point of decay. It is a process, moreover, which, when once initiated, on account of the virus being secreted into the ever-flowing blood-stream, is virtually as simultaneous as it is universal over the entire field of germination, fit to yield it.

CHAPTER X.

RABIES, A GERM-DISEASE OF CENTRIC, NOT OF PERIPHERAL CONNECTIVE-TISSUE.

IMMEDIATELY after infection, then, the rabies-germ, like that of every other germ-disease, is at once taken up by the absorbent corpuscular system at the site of infection, but, in respect of such a germ-disease, in all probability pre-eminently by the corpuscles of the peripheral connective-tissue. What will ensue thereafter will depend upon what happens to be the specific seat of cultivation of the particular micro-organism absorbed; for various orders of pathogenic micro-organisms have constant sites of cultivation of their own, or special tissues in the body in which they exclusively germinate. If this site be either in the peripheral connective-tissue or in the wandering cellular bodies of the circulation, germination will at once supervene, for the micro-organism on infection will be at once planted in its specific germinating-ground. What will thereafter become of the absorbed micro-organism will depend upon whether the infected animal be, to begin with, susceptible or insusceptible to the disease, or whether its specific tissues of cultivation are or are not capable of cultivating the germ. If the specific germinating ground be reached and fertile, it is of little consequence where infection has taken place; the fact of infection will, sooner or later, involve the tremendous fact of the disease as a fully matured result. If, on the other hand, the animal be insusceptible or an "immune," however "protected," whether by nature or by art, it is of no consequence where the micro-organism has been inoculated, or in what quantity; the "protected" animal will resist the germination of the microbe.

This is well illustrated in the case of the frog with respect to the bacillus of anthrax. In its normal *cold-blooded* condition, the lymphocytes of the animal are powerfully phagocytic in regard to this particular micro-organism. The bacilli which are injected under the skin are rapidly taken up by the wandering cells of the lymphatic meshes, and *in situ* disintegrated and devoured; so much so that in an incredibly short time not one of the micro-organisms injected ·is seen to be free. In a frog, on the contrary, which has been artificially so warmed that it has been practically converted into a *warm-blooded* animal, the lymphocytes, for the time being, are not phagocytic. On their absorbing the bacilli, which under these abnormal conditions they will nevertheless still do, the micro-organisms immediately begin to multiply in the latter. And this process of multiplication continues in lymphocyte after lymphocyte, not only in their movements through the adjacent tissues, but all through the general circulation, even to their ultimate distribution in the spleen itself ; the circulation and spleen being at last so crowded with the swarming bacilli that the process culminates in the outbreak of the disease.

The relation of the absorbent corpuscles of living beings to the pathogenic microbes is, therefore, by no means an unvarying one, even for the same micro-organism. It would appear to be of at least a threefold character. The wandering corpuscle may at once absorb the intrusive micro-organism simply to destroy and devour it ; it may absorb it only to cultivate and germinate it in its own substance ; both of which events we have just seen in the cold-blooded and warm-blooded frog with respect to the *bacillus anthracis.* Lastly, it may absorb the microbe merely passively, neither destroying nor germinating it, only to convey it far from the periphery to remote centric structures which can alone germinate it. Thus M. Metschnikoff introduced certain microscopic fungus-spores into the transparent bodies of a form of *daphne,* and found that

"When small quantities of spores were used, the amœboid leucocytes, collecting around them, took them into their substance, destroyed their power of germination, and, finally, disintegrated them ; while, if many spores were introduced, some of them which were not taken up by the leucocytes germinated and grew through the body[1]."

These facts are not less obvious in the highest animals. Take erysipelas, for example. Although the disease-area in this case is so sharply defined, and the micro-organism itself so strictly localised to

[1] Croonian Lecture for 1891 by Dr Burdon Sanderson, F.R.S.

the peripheral connective-tissue, it gets occasionally into the adjacent lymphatics, and apparently ever struggles for an entrance into such channels; but it struggles in vain. In the inflammatory process which immediately ensues, the intruding micro-organisms are at once surrounded by a massive invasion of the leucocytes of the circulation, with the result that in an incredibly short time the micrococci are found inside the latter in every stage of degeneration, being visible in their interior, transformed into amorphous granules and particles. And the same holds good of diphtheria and tetanus and many more germ-diseases. For a micro-organism of this particular class the leucocytes of the circulation or the wandering lymphoid cells of the spleen, of the interior of bones, and of lymphatic glands, are, manifestly enough, even *normally* highly phagocytic. And this, no doubt, is one reason why the micro-organisms of these germ-diseases are so exclusively located in the peripheral connective-tissues, or why all such diseases are so necessarily peripheral in their cultivation. Were, however, the specific micro-organism of this entire order invariably successful, instead of being invariably defeated, in penetrating into the circulation, as it so happens there is no other connective-tissue in the infected animal which will compare with the peripheral connective-tissue as a germinating-ground. As compared with the active, highly phagocytic gregarious leucocytes of the circulation, and, above all, of the marrow of bones and of the spleen, the solitary, sluggish corpuscles of the fixed, skeletal connective-tissue would appear to show, further than that of mere passive absorption, but little capacity of attacking the bacteria or micro-organisms; and they are not by any means particularly phagocytic with respect to preventive or recurrent micro-organisms. Having absorbed the micro-organism in its own substance, this corpuscle, on returning with it into its own connective-tissue, deposits it there. But, on conveying it straightway to its own tissue, the corpuscle in reality conveys it to the fittest "nidus" for its germination, and in point of fact directly plants it in the richest germinating-ground in the living economy.

A parallel set of phenomena is to be witnessed in pneumonia, a disease which in its most important features—in its sharply defined area, in its dense fibrinous inflammation, in its sudden decline on recovery, and also, thereafter, the rapid and steady disappearance of all inflammatory condensation—so resembles erysipelas that it may be viewed as a pulmonary erysipelas. The micro-organisms, which induce the two diseases, however specific or unlike each other, must be closely allied. In pneumonia, likewise, the germination of the bacterium is strictly limited to the connective-tissue element, but in the mucous, not in the cutaneous periphery. It settles and thrives in such tissue as on no other structure in the lung ; and it is also strictly limited to this primitive connective-tissue element by a perpetual invasion from every side of the leucocytes and lymphocytes of the circulation, which, in this case too, and for this special micro-organism, are powerfully phagocytic. The same more or less holds good of tetanus and diphtheria, also even of tuberculosis, leprosy, cancer, pyæmia, and of many more recurrent germ-diseases. In these, likewise, the connective-tissue of the seat of cultivation, above all tissues, absorbs the specific microbe of the malady simply to cultivate it ; the connective-corpuscles being merely passive vehicles of conveyance to their own special tissue.

This peripheral connective-tissue culture-ground has, perhaps, been the most conclusively demonstrated in respect of such a disease as diphtheria, and by no investigator more lucidly than by the late Mr Ruffer in his valuable observations in regard to the membrane and its surroundings. Here, as already stated, the leucocytes are likewise distinctly phagocytic or germ-destroying with respect to the specific bacilli of the disease, compelling the latter to be exclusively confined to the peripheral connective-tissue, or otherwise in marshalled hosts absorbing them and devouring them outright. Thus, Ruffer found that the leucocytes in and near the diphtheritic membrane invariably contained diphtheritic bacilli in their interior, which showed signs of degeneration varying from a mere difference in the power of retaining gentian-violet to complete disorganization. The bacilli were never found free in the circulation far beyond the membrane, or at all beyond the dense mass of leucocytes, which keep pressing forward, like a life-guard host, on every side of the advancing micro-organisms. The cells of the peripheral connective-tissue, on the contrary, far from preventing the germination of such microbes, would appear, in conveying them to their own tissues, to straightway transmit them into the most favourable nidus ; and, moreover, the phagocytes of the blood and lymph streams, which most unquestionably prevent their germination in these streams, further determine this peripheral connective-tissue as the specific seat of such micro-organisms. Diphtheria, tetanus, erysipelas, pneumonia, &c., cannot fail to be, therefore, pre-eminently fixed and peripheral in cultivation.

In all these, and many more of such preventive germ-diseases, the corpuscles of the skeletal connective-tissue—whether the latter be osseous, serous, areolar, or interstitial, for all are practically the same tissue—as compared with the active leucocytes or lymphoid cells of the blood and lymph streams, would appear to show, not only very little capability of attacking the specific microbes of these diseases, but, on the contrary, a great and dangerous capacity of fostering them in their own peculiar tissue and germinating them.

The connective-corpuscle and its fibre-shell, if one may so term its connective-tissue, which it can leave or take possession of like a hermit-crab, is, for such germs, but only these, the most absorptive, and, on the other hand, the most favourable medium of cultivation of all the tissues of the organism. Clearly enough, there is, then, to begin with, a large and very important class of *preventive* germ-diseases, whose seat of cultivation is strictly external, not centric, this peripheral seat being either cutaneous or mucous.

Not that the preventive order is exclusively peripheral. Even when this is the fact as in diphtheria, erysipelas and tetanus, the specific microbe, as we have just seen, is constantly struggling towards the circulation, or from without inward. The spores of the tetanus-bacillus, for example, as already stated, occasionally find their way to the remote cerebro-spinal substance itself, and are borne hither, probably, mainly in the interior of the peripheral connective-corpuscles and through the lymphatic channels. Again, the micro-organism of such a germ-disease as tubercle (as in the case of lupus) sooner or later penetrates to the deeper or centric structures, and invariably through the lymphatic channels, and in all probability, here too, mainly by the peripheral connective-corpuscles. In respect of tubercle, cancer, leprosy and of this entire order of germ-diseases, the lymphatic channels are probably the normal and most direct route of extended infection. Even such a peripheral germ-disease as pyæmia, sooner or later, always finds its way to centric structures. The pathogenic micro-organism in this case, as in some of the others of the order, is at last so overwhelming in amount, and its virus so exceptionally pernicious to even the leucocytes of the circulation, that the normal phagocytic power of the latter in respect of the micro-organism is thereby paralysed; with the result that, in spite of the seat of germination being in the peripheral connective-tissues, the copiously-multiplying pathogenic micro-organism at length invades the circulation in periodic swarms. All phagocytic power having been overcome by the extreme virulence of the virus, the pathogenic micro-organism is borne passively, not only by wandering connective-corpuscles, but probably even by the leucocytes of the blood-stream or of the marrow of bones, far from the peripheral site, to remote centric structures to germinate afresh, and with the most deadly effect. It is significant, however, as shall be shown presently, that it is still *the elementary connective-tissue* of such centric structures, and these exclusively, where the micro-organism is thus so constantly, if so passively, borne.

Obviously enough, then, there is a class of peripheral preventive germ-diseases capable of germinating in *centric*, not less than in *peripheral* connective-tissue. But, on the other hand, there is a large class of this preventive, recurrent germ-disease, whose specific micro-organism is capable of germinating *only in centric connective-tissue*; in point of fact as exclusively in this tissue as the external or peripheral germ-diseases are cultivated exclusively in the connective-tissue of the periphery.

But the vast order of centric germ-diseases are by no means all preventive; for they do not all germinate in connective-tissue. Of this entire class, there are two important subdivisions; the preventive and recurrent, which are as preventive and recurrent as those of the peripheral connective-tissue cultivation, and, on the other hand, the prophylactic, which, on the contrary, are non-recurrent and not preventive. One feature this entire centric class has in common; unlike that of the strictly peripheral order, the specific micro-organism, either free or absorbed, passes from the periphery directly into the circulation, and is conveyed by its wandering corpuscles, either in the lymph or blood-stream or in both, to the remotest organs. But in the one section, the pro-phylactic germ-disease, the cultivation of the micro-organism begins in the leucocytes immediately after absorption, the germination being exclusively confined to these wandering cells, never in connective-tissue, centric or peripheral. In the other section, or the centric preventive order, germination never takes place in the migratory corpuscles and the leucocytes of the circulation or in any such cells. On the contrary, it begins after its passive conveyance from the periphery, and probably solely by the connective-corpuscles of the periphery and through the lymphatic channels, only in some centric structure which is in no way allied to the leucocytes or lymphoid cells, but very closely allied, as we shall now see, to the peripheral connective-tissue itself.

Of this centric division, take, firstly, the prophylactic section. Most certainly, the specific micro-organisms of such diseases are not settled in the peripheral or external connective-tissues. Even if they, for a time, were, they would not germinate in any such tissue, and they make immediately for the active mobile constituents, the leucocytes, of the blood-stream itself. They find no site of cultivation in any skeletal or fibrous or connective-tissue, whether peripheral or centric. The tissue which forms the special culture-ground or germinating-soil of the one class, the prophylactic, would appear, then, to be of a very much higher and of a more specialised order than that which forms the specific culture-ground of the preventive class. For this reason the preventive or recurrent type of germ-disease is probably so overwhelmingly prevalent over the animal economy, and over the entire animal kingdom, as compared with the strictly prophylactic type, which is invariably limited to only the very highest mammals, in point of fact only to man and his domesticated animals. Thus, in the one order, the *prophylactic*, the wandering lymphoid cells, or inhabitants, of the circulation itself, derived from the spleen, the marrow of bones, and the lymphatic glands, would appear to be the sole medium alike of absorption and germination ; the fixed connective-tissue, whether peripheral or centric, being in no way concerned in the cultivation of the pathogenic micro-organism. In the other order, on the contrary, or the strictly *preventive* type, the connective, skeletal fixed tissue, whether peripheral or centric, would appear to be the sole seat of germination ; the lymphoid cells of the circulation being in no way concerned in the cultivation of the microbe, but rather the reverse. This would appear to be a most important and fundamental distinction between the two orders of germ-disease, and which, perhaps, can hardly be too strongly emphasized. The recurrent and preventive germ-disease germinates in the connective tissue, the prophylactic germ-disease in the corpuscular system.

Of all prophylactic germ-diseases hitherto investigated, these facts have on the whole been most clearly demonstrated in respect of anthrax, which may be taken as a typical example of the order. After infection, the leucocytes of the circulation invariably absorb the bacilli which have been injected within the subcutaneous meshes ; which, however, is so totally different from a preventive germ-disease of exclusively *peripheral cultivation*, where, as already shown, the leucocytes either stubbornly drive them back to their peripheral connective-tissue, or demolish them outright. But after this absorption has taken place, the growth or multiplication of the micro-organism at once commences even in the interior of the absorbing leucocytes ; and this, again, is totally different from a preventive germ-disease of exclusively *centric cultivation*, where, after infection, although corpuscles undoubtedly absorb the specific micro-organisms, and wander sluggishly with them through the tissues and circulations to deeper structures, they in no way aid or induce the germination. And this multiplication of the anthrax-bacillus, with, presumably, that of every prophylactic micro-organism, proceeds all through the process of conveyance from the periphery to the deepest dispersal through the spleen, where the multiplication is still seen to take place even in the minutest structure of this organ. Above all glands or organs, the spleen constitutes not only the ultimate point of distribution of the microbe received in infection, but it is its capital seat of cultivation ; for it is the capital seat of the entire amœboid order of cell. If this be so, the amœboid constituents of the circulation and, above all, of the spleen and of the marrow of bones and of the lymphatic glands, as the main source of the lymphoid system, not only absorb and distribute the prophylactic micro-organisms received in infection, and only these, but constitute their sole and specific seat of germination ; the process of migration, germination, and multiplication up to the advent of the disease itself constituting the incubation of the malady. For this reason, in all probability, the germ-disease is so essentially prophylactic and non-recurrent. The sources of the entire lymphoid or leucocytic system being thus, once and for all, "protected" by such a process of microbe-germination, the entire animal economy will be likewise "protected," and for the same length of time. For, as it so happens, there is no other tissue but these migratory leucocytes capable of cultivating such a micro-organism. The pathogenic micro-organism having once undergone in them the specific process of germination, the lymphoid system will thereafter, and *ipso facto*, for many a year do quite the reverse ; the germination having rendered the leucocytes in respect of such a micro-organism as phagocytic as in the case of that of the most exclusively peripheral preventive germ-disease.

On the other hand, of this centric division, take the distinctly *preventive* section. Not one of this, any more than any of the prophylactic group, takes root and germinates in the connective-tissue of the periphery. The specific micro-organism of this particular section is invariably borne passively from the site of infection to deeper structures, which alone constitute their germinating-ground, not by the active mobile leucocytes of the circulation, but by the connective-corpuscles of the peripheral areolar spaces. And it is conveyed by these, not merely through the blood-stream, but still more copiously, if not exclusively in some, through the lymphatic channels. In this order, the corpuscular system, which really absorbs the pathogenic micro-organism, would appear to be neither phago-cytes nor germinators, but simply passive vehicles. Immediately after infection, the connective-corpuscles, sluggishly moving about in the site, "seeking what they can devour," absorb such microbes, not to destroy them, nor to cultivate and germinate them in their own protoplasmic substance, but, like the seed embedded on the muddy foot of a migratory wader, only to bear them to, and deposit them in, some remote and much more fertile soil, where they can germinate to their full capacity. Although such microbes germinate neither in the peripheral corpuscle and its connective-tissue, nor in the much more mobile, highly specialised lymphoid corpuscles of the circulation, nevertheless, one and all of them induce diseases which are not less recurrent than the micro-organisms which are so exclusively limited to the connective-tissue in the periphery. For in the one preventive order not less than in the other, the specific site of cultivation is still solely in skeletal connective-tissue. Thus, if the micro-organisms of such recurrent diseases as erysipelas or tetanus, diphtheria or pneumonia are strictly peripheral in their site of cultivation,—the former in the cutaneous, the latter in the mucous periphery,—it is not less true that the micro-organisms of such persistently recurrent germ-diseases as influenza maligna, epidemic cerebro-spinal meningitis, probably acute rheumatism, possibly even ague itself, and many more, are by no means of peripheral cultivation, but are borne, often enough very far from the primary point of infection, to a central site which, above all other structures, is alone capable of growing them. Than this centric structure there is no such "nidus" for the micro-organism in the entire body. However far from the point of infection, it is important to note that it is still invariably in connective-tissue structures, and for this reason, if there were no other, such diseases, both peripheral and centric, are so persistently recurrent; for such structures are not only practically inexhaustible, but are really increased and rendered more favourable for germination *for every attack of the disease.*

But there are preventive germ-diseases which, although like the others cultivated strictly in connective-tissue, not in the lymphoid corpuscles nor in any secreting or highly specialised cell, are neither exclusively peripheral nor exclusively centric. Their specific micro-organisms, as already stated, are capable of germinating both in the one site and the other. To this widely-ravaging order, whose micro-organisms are ever ready to settle and germinate in the weakest points of the skeletal or primitive connective-tissues, belong such diseases as tubercle, cancer, leprosy, and in its last development even pyæmia itself. But, here again, even in this most disastrous order, it is the strictly connective-tissue, not the lymphoid cells, nor the muscular, nor the nervous, nor the secreting, nor any other specialised tissue, which constitutes the prime seat of cultivation. So far as the connective-tissue cultivating-ground is concerned, therefore, such pathogenic micro-organisms are in reality of *universal* cultivation.

Now, admitting that connective-tissue of one form or other, and this exclusively, is the specific ground of cultivation for the micro-organisms of the entire preventive or recurrent class, whether peripheral or centric, as opposed to the prophylactic class, is it so certain that the centric structures which cultivate these micro-organisms are also so wholly fibrous or "connective" in form and character, not less so than the coarser areolar tissue of the periphery? What are these centric structures? They are the skeletal, embryonic tissues which form the framework of the deepest and most vital organs; such as the interstitial connective-tissue of the spleen, the lungs, the testicle, the lymphatic glands and of the cerebro-spinal axis, or its delicate fibrous-framework, known as the *neuroglia.* They are such structures as the valves of the heart, the endocardium, the pericardium, the pleura, the peritoneum, the arachnoid, the meninges, and every synovial membrane and serous sac, great and small. In all of these cases how all-important, how integral a constituent, is the connective-tissue element, alone! There is perhaps not to be found in the entire organism, even in bone itself, or in the areolar tissue of the periphery, a purer, simpler form of the primitive connective-tissue. Without this element a serous membrane would be no serous membrane at all. Of what, then, is such a structure composed? There is, firstly, a very thin layer of scaly or tessellated epithelium of the simplest character. There is, secondly, an extremely dense and wholly "fibrous" layer. And, lastly, there is an important "subserous layer of areolar tissue," which loosely connects the dense "fibrous tissue" with the adjacent structures; but this intermediate layer constitutes practically the entire structure.

"The intermediate layer," says Dr Sharpey, "consists of fine but dense areolar connective-tissue, which is in usual made up of bundles of white filaments, mixed with fine elastic fibres ; the former, where there are two or more strata, take a different direction in different planes ; the latter unite into a network, and are principally connected into a reticular layer at the surface beneath the epithelium. The constituent connective-tissue of the serous membrane is, of course, continuous with the usually more lax subserous areolar-tissue, connecting the membrane to the subjacent parts[1]."

Next to the neuroglia of the cerebro-spinal substance itself, the structure is one of the simplest forms of connective-tissue which exists in the adult. Composed of such embryonic skeletal elements, it is not surprising to learn that "breaches of continuity in these membranes are readily repaired ; and that the new formed portion *acquires all the characters of the original tissue[2]."*

This much, however, could not be asserted of a muscle-fibre, of a nerve-fibre, of a nerve-cell, of a secreting-cell, or of any such highly specialised form. The higher the specialisation, the less likely is this specialisation to be restored after a "breach of continuity," or when in any other way destroyed ; the restoration, when it occurs, being on a distinctly lower plane of structure. Is the retinal structure so restored, or are the normal structures of the stomach after gastric ulcer, or even the normal structures of the skin after an extensive burn? But it is strictly true of every form of connective-tissue, and is characteristic not merely of serous sacs and valves and centric interstitial connective-frameworks, but of sinew, ligament, tendon, and even bone ; all of which are in reality likewise but primitive connective-tissue, and therefore so capable of being absolutely restored.

Now, assuming that every micro-organism of the preventive and recurrent order finds its specific site of germination exclusively in this elemental, extremely lowly organised structure, then, provided

---

[1] *Quain's Anatomy*, Vol. III. Serous Membranes (p. cxiii.), by Dr Sharpey.
[2] *Ibidem.*

the micro-organism is conveyed and deposited thither from the point of infection, however long or irregular this process, serous membranes, synovial membranes, valvular structures, the interstitial fibrous-framework of the deepest and most specialised organs, as that of the spleen, or the neuroglia of the cerebro-spinal substance, should constitute a peculiarly favourable and constant germinating-ground, not less favourable or exclusive for special micro-organisms than the areolar tissue of the periphery for the germination of the microbes of strictly peripheral germ-diseases.

The mode of conveyance of this entire order of pathogenic micro-organisms from the site of infection, and the vehicle, and the special channels through which the vehicle traverses, would materially aid in determining these central sites as the germinating-ground ; for, sooner or later, it would invariably bring the micro-organisms precisely to such centric structures. From the prolonged and irregular pre-incubation-period of this entire group, there is reason to believe that the connective-corpuscles of the peripheral areolar spaces are the main bearers of these micro-organisms, not less so than of those of exclusively external or peripheral cultivation. The fact of their being wholly connective-tissue corpuscles would, alone, determine them to absorb at once the pathogenic micro-organisms of the preventive and recurrent type, both peripheral and centric. For it is possible that this same corpuscle might have, permanently adhering to its protoplasmic substance, a very minute film of the connective-tissue substance in which it habitually resides. But this connective-tissue substance is the germinating ground of the entire order of preventive micro-organism. The leucocytes of the circulation, however,—of the spleen, of the marrow of bones, or of the lymphatic glands,—may have no such film. Burdened with the micro-organisms, which they but passively absorb, neither destroying nor germinating them in their interior, these connective-corpuscles convey them, restlessly, to some centric site of connective-tissue which can alone germinate them, and, often enough, by the most circuitous and prolonged of routes, and mainly through the lymphatic channels. What could be more irregular or at times more prolonged than the pre-incubation-period of the tubercle-bacillus ? It may linger in a site, or penetrate through the tissues, for years before finding a sufficiently enfeebled, and, therefore, correspondingly favourable, germinating-ground. As illustrating the part which the corpuscles of the lymphatic current, as compared with the leucocytes of the blood-stream, play on bearing such microbes ; it is significant that, when rabies has proclaimed itself, an inoculation of the blood into a fresh animal hardly ever rabidises, and then only in the case of an intensifier and from the profoundest paralytic rabies of an intensifier. On the other hand, an inoculation of the *lymphatic fluid*, even of so potent an attenuator as the dog, *never once fails to rabidise.* Galtier, confirmed by Bouchard and other investigators, found that, although the blood of a rabid animal was practically never rabic, " the lymphatic fluid was *constantly* virulent," the migrating corpuscles of the stream being loaded with the rabies-germ, and now bearing it in shoals from the swarming cerebro-spinal centres to the periphery, and to well-nigh every secreting organ. It is perfectly possible that the lymphatic fluid might be more or less rabic even in the latter stages of incubation itself; for its corpuscular element will, more than any other, be more or less charged with the ripe micro-organism.

So far, therefore, as the ingathering of these centric micro-organisms is concerned, the more the *connective-corpuscles* abound in the areolar spaces at the point of infection, the more will the intro-duced micro-organisms be taken up and borne, passively, and just as they are, to their germinating-ground in some centric connective-tissue. Small as they are, these subcutaneous areolar spaces con-stitute the outmost limits of the great lymphatic system itself. This is still more true of the areolar spaces surrounding veins, and hence their value for experimental inoculation. These serous spaces, through a prolonged, irregular series of which the deep venous channels pass, are, like the areolar spaces in the subcutaneous layer, "anfractuous cavities, which are limited and defined by a lining of epithelium, agreeing in character with that of the lymphatic vessels; and it may be presumed that their opposite sides are in apposition, or in near proximity, as in *serous membranes*[1]." The various serous cavities of the system, from the farthest areolar spaces in the periphery and around deep veins to the most gigantic serous mem-branes,—the synovial coverings of joints, the pericardium, the arachnoid, the pleura, and, above all, the peritoneum,—are all but lymphatic "lacunæ"; and, as a whole system, constitute, even in the highest animal organism, a most important relic of the irregular, "anfractuous," *invertebrate* circulation. In every direction, and by innumerable outlets and inlets, they are never far removed from clustering lymphatic glands, and in constant communication with the

[1] *Quain's Anatomy*, Part III., p. ccxxxii., by Dr Sharpey.

lymphatic current, like shallow lakes of the current, and with shoals of slowly-moving connective-corpuscles and the more mobile lympho-cytes and leucocytes passing and repassing from hour to hour and from and to every site. A pathogenic micro-organism, then, in the areolar meshes of the periphery is absorbed, passively, by the con-nective-corpuscles of the site, and, providing that the micro-organism does not settle and germinate in its peculiar connective-tissue in the vicinity, cannot fail to be borne in the amœboid wanderings of the corpuscle from fibrous site to fibrous site, to at last centric serous and instertitial structures of most favourable connective-tissue, to be there deposited and to germinate. This holds good occasionally, and, to some extent, even of some of the strictly peripheral preventive germ-diseases. Thus, in tetanus, as we have seen, the "spores" of the micro-organism, which in itself is fixed and exclusively cultivated in the peripheral connective-tissue, are conveyed in the interior of the ab-sorbing connective-corpuscles to such centric structure as the spinal substance. And the same is probably the case in respect of the spores of the "paludal" micro-organisms which induce malarial fever.

Again, pyæmia itself is essentially a peripheral germ-disease, which Lord Lister's great antiseptic treatment has completely sup-pressed. The peripheral wound and its connective-tissues remain to the last its prime nidus of cultivation. Nevertheless, the virulence of its virus is so extreme that at length it converts the very leucocytes of the circulation into passive bearers or vehicles, not merely of the virulent product, nor even of the spores, but of the pathogenic micro-organism itself, and directly into the remotest joints and large serous sacs, or wherever connective-tissue in its simplest elemental forms abounds. And this phenomenon is also to be seen in the case of recurrent germ-diseases which are not peripheral. The centric connective-tissue, in its various forms, is the constant seat of germina-tion. Take acute rheumatism, which is surely recurrent, nearly as much so as ague. If it be a germ-disease, as there is every reason to believe, in every probability its micro-organism, like that of so many other recurrent germ-diseases, is not altogether unrelated to the damp, sour clay-soils where the willows abound. Does it not pre-eminently find its habitat in the connective-tissue of serous and synovial structures? This has been notorious since the days of Hippocrates. It is equally true of tubercle, which, if more chronic in its course than either acute rheumatism or pyæmia, is more widely-ranging over the entire connective-tissue framework. The bacillus of the disease finds a nidus peculiarly fitted for its germination in every form of connective-tissue; in the cutaneous or mucous areolar tissue, as in lupus of the face or of the bowels, in the osseous fibres, in the synovial membranes, in the serous sacs, the pleura, the peritoneum, the arachnoid or meninges, &c., in the fine, connective, interstitial tissue of the lungs, of the testicles, of the lymphatic glands. There is no form of connective-tissue, apparently, if at all weakened or deteriorated, as in the too rapid growth of a structure, as at puberty or even in childhood, which is safe from the invasion of such a micro-organism, or which is not capable of receiving the bacillus and cultivating it, and of constituting a most dangerous starting-point of the disease. How widely-spread over the organism, but also how latent and for how long a time, such isolated nuclei may be, and how invariably in a connective-tissue nidus, have been brilliantly demonstrated by Koch's tuberculin test, which, as a test alone, has made the discovery one of the greatest of our era. The same in all probability holds good of such a disease as leprosy, which in its insidious, sluggish, widely-spread invasion of the connective-tissues, and of these exclusively, would appear to be closely allied to tubercle, but which is still more chronic in its course, and, perhaps, likewise more limited to the *peripheral* connective-tissue. In elephantiasis, both of the leg and scrotum, how overwhelming an element is the connective-tissue and its hypertrophy! The same probably holds good of cancer. The connective-tissues, both peripheral and centric, and probably these exclusively, are invariably the starting-point and nidus of the disease. As in tubercle, there is in this disease no form of connective-tissue which, if at all weakened or deteriorated in structure, as in the premature decay of such an organ as the breast or womb, which is safe from such a micro-organism, or not most capable of cultivating and germinating it. However hypertrophied the connective-tissue which becomes the nidus, the hypertrophy may be taken, not less than the atrophy of the secreting structure, as an index of its degradation. How often does the deteriorated connective-tissue of old scars afford a starting-point for cancer! All these diseases are recurrent, and find their starting-point and germinating-ground in the feeblest or the most withered forms of connective-tissue.

Or, lastly, take ague itself, which of all centric germ-diseases, whether preventive or prophylactic, is surely the most perfect type of a recurrent malady; but, if recurrent, probably likewise really *preventive.* As accounting for the causation of the disease, the

investigations of Laveran, Golgi, Marchiafava, Bignami, and Mannaberg, not to say of Koch, Manson, and Ross, have over and over
again demonstrated that, during the disease, there are in the red
blood-corpuscles, not one, but many "malarial parasites," conveyed
thither or infected by mosquitos. All of these have been graphically
and most lucidly pictured by Manson[1]. It has been assumed that
these "paludal" and "parasitic" micro-organisms have their specific
site of germination in the blood-corpuscles; and that their life-
history in these circulating bodies not only induces but constitutes
the disease. If this be so, ague must be pre-eminently a systemic or
"blood-disease." If this be the fact, why, then, is the malady so
persistently recurrent? Most certainly it is not prophylactic. The
periodic paroxysmal exacerbations of the disease itself are not
like a prophylactic, but marvellously like the most deadly of all the
preventive or recurrent germ-diseases, and pre-eminently, as we have
seen, pyæmia. It is unquestionable that a genuine prophylactic germ-
disease, like smallpox or anthrax, finds its seat of incubation, not in
the connective-tissue, but exclusively in the leucocytes or amœboid
cells of the circulation. It is not less true that, after the disease has
been once incurred, these wandering lymphoid cells, or protoplasmic
beings, so much more highly specialised than any form of the fixed
connective-tissue, have been rendered persistently prophylactic in
respect of the micro-organism; the corpuscles having been converted
by the malady from germinators to the most potent of phagocytes.
Is this, or anything like this, true of malarial fever? One attack of
the disease but predisposes or prepares the germinating-soil for
another. There can be no doubt that the paludal micro-organisms in
the interior of the blood-corpuscles, which have been figured so
perfectly by Manson, are to be found in rich abundance in an ague-
stricken patient; and that in these corpuscles they undergo a complete process of modification. Is this process, however, one of
evolution or of devolution? In spite of the so-called "elaboration"
and "evolution" of the various paludal micro-organisms, or even if
there should prove to be only one multiform micro-organism, the
reverse of anything like true prophylaxis or an enduring protection,
in other words, the most obstinate recurrence, is the invariable result.
It is a recurrence, moreover, precisely like that of the entire preventive
order, which progressively increases for every attack of the malady.

[1] *British Medical Journal,* Dec. 1, 1894, "A Malarial Chart of the Micro-
organisms" by P. Manson, M.D.

It is true that in various "modifications" the paludal micro-organisms exist 'n the blood-corpuscles, and pre-eminently, if not exclusively, in the red blood-corpuscles. But do they germinate in the leucocytes, or the white corpuscles, as in the case of anthrax and the other prophylactic germ-diseases? Do they exist even in the red corpuscles in any noticeable amount during incubation?

What, then, is the red corpuscle, and whence does it come? Huxley thought it the mere nucleus of the leucocyte, specialised for its important work, and derived from the spleen. Other authorities have likewise traced it to the marrow of bones or to the lymph-glands. But, whether merely a naked nucleus or not, is it impossible that it should be a specialised connective-corpuscle, and come originally from the widely-spread connective-tissue? The red corpuscles are far more numerous than all the leucocytes of the circulation, whether of the spleen or of the osseous or lymphatic glands; and they existed in the organism before there was a spleen, and when connective-tissue was still more predominant. If they come originally from connective-tissue, they too might well have to the end a highly specialised infinitesimal film around their proto-plasm of the purest gelatin of connective-tissue, or the so-called stroma. This film, however, would be a fitting medium of conveyance, or even of partial cultivation, of the spores.

Be this as it may, it is undoubted that the micro-organisms appear in the blood-stream in regular periodic swarms. The re-markable periodicity of the disease is its most peculiar characteristic. And this phenomenon is invariably after, not during, incubation. Consequently, their presence in the blood-corpuscles in such sus-piciously periodic shoals is a final, possibly decaying and moribund, not a primary stage in the life-history of the micro-organism in the economy, and is but a disastrous and inevitable effect of the disease, rather than its cause. Nor is this a unique phenomenon in germ-disease. The "various" micro-organisms of the malady, which have been described as so "specific," are possibly but different stages of one and the same form; and these different stages are all in the direction of deterioration and decay rather than of development and healthy maturity. If so, it is a process of devolution and degradation rather than of evolution. It is candidly owned by Manson and other able investigators that the "paludal" micro-organisms are found in the blood-corpuscles, more or less, "degenerating" or in a "degenerated condition," or, often enough, they are "altogether degenerated forms."

But, if the leucocytes absorb them, this process of deterioration may be materially hastened and intensified by their normally phagocytic function. If this be the fact, these wandering bodies in the blood-stream, even the lymphoid tissue of the spleen itself, from which some of these leucocytes are constantly derived, cannot be the main medium of cultivation.

Nevertheless, malarial fever is, *par excellence*, a spleen-disease. It is certain that the spleen itself, and its intimate, highly specialised lymphoid tissue, suffer from the virulent product of the paludal micro-organism far more severely, and much earlier, than any other organ or tissue. Is it possible, then, that this organ is the main, if not specific, centre of cultivation, and the source of all the periodic outbursts of degenerating and degenerated forms into the circulation? It is, surely, an extremely significant fact that spores of the paludal micro-organism are constantly to be found in the ultimate tissue of the spleen, and from the earliest stages of the disease. But, even at the latest stages, they are seldom or never to be seen in the interior of the corpuscles of the circulation. Koch has maintained that, so far as the malarial fever of the tropics is concerned—which, after all, is the prime malarial fever of the world—the spores of the paludal micro-organism are to be found in richest abundance in the ultimate tissue of the spleen. Nor, again, is even this fact unique. As we have already seen, the spores of the tetanus-bacillus are sometimes borne from the peripheral tissues to the cerebro-spinal substance itself. Is it possible, then, that the spores of the malarial micro-organism are conveyed in a similar manner to the remote and deepest tissue of the spleen itself, and by the cor-puscles of the peripheral connective-tissue? At a certain stage of the germination of the spores in the spleen—a stage, in the "elabora-tion," approaching decay and when its virulent product, proper, has been eliminated to do its deadly work—is it inherently improbable that these "degenerating" micro-organisms are periodically flung forth and absorbed by the lymphoid cells of the spleen, and that in the interior of these bodies they find their way, as a swarm, directly into the circulation? Such a fact would be no anomaly. Precisely the same phenomenon is to be seen in pyæmia ; in this case, however, the specific seat of germination being peripheral, not internal or centric. In the case of malarial fever, the eliminated micro-organisms, whether absolutely moribund or not, also find their way into the cells of the circulation, not to be revived in these, or to germinate afresh, but, like micro-organisms of so many other preventive and recurrent germ-diseases, to undergo complete disorganization and removal. And they are borne by these bodies, from within outwards, but not, as in the case of the genuine prophylactic exanthems to the peripheral tissues, to be there completely eliminated from the system, vigorous and capable of infecting, either in an eruption or in a process of ulceration, as in the case of smallpox, anthrax, measles, and scarlatina.

Assuming that the spleen is the specific seat of cultivation of the paludal micro-organism in spore-form, it cannot be in the specialised tissue of this organ, for this is identically the same as the amœboid bodies of the circulation. Although at a certain stage the micro-organisms in a more or less degenerated condition would appear to so plentifully invade the wandering cells of the spleen and the circulation, is it not the fact that the spleen itself is, above all other organs, softened and atrophied in its specialised *lymphoid* structure; yet, on the other hand, hardened and hypertrophied even to monstrosity in its interstitial connective-tissue framework? As a matter of fact, the connective-tissue of the spleen is at length and after much recurrence of the malady as much hardened and hypertrophied, and its peculiar lymphoid tissue as much softened, liquified and atrophied as a tuberculous lymphatic gland, or a tuberculous testicle or lung, or a cancerous breast or pancreas. Which of these elements in the spleen, then, is to be viewed as the germinating-site of the paludal micro-organism or its spores? The specific lymphoid-tissue of the organ, and from which certain leucocytes of the circulation are themselves directly derived, is, for every attack of the disease, progressively degenerated and wasted; as much so as in the case of a cancer of a secreting structure. On the contrary, the interstitial connective-tissue for every attack of the malady is as progressively increased. This, however, and in proportion to the hypertrophy, would only render this tissue a still more favourable soil for germination. Hence, a persistent recurrence would be the inevitable result, for the culture-ground would be an ever-increasing one, and progressively more and more fitting for germination. Is this interstitial connective-tissue of the spleen where the spores of the paludal micro-organisms so early abound, and which is materially increased with every attack of the malady, so small a factor in the persistence of the remarkable recurrence which is so characteristic of the disease? It may, therefore, hardly be too much to assume that the connective-tissue rather than the lymphoid or corpuscular element even of the spleen itself, not less than in the case of other preventive and stubbornly recurrent germ-diseases in respect of other and very special connective-tissue, is the main centre of germination of the paludal micro-organisms or their spores which induce malarial fever.

It would appear then that the connective-tissue, the most primitive and lowly organised in the body—a much less specialised structure than the splenic or lymphoid cells which are the specific culture-ground of every prophylactic germ-disease—is, above all structures or cells, the nidus of cultivation of every microbe of the recurrent or preventive order. Every such micro-organism will not germinate in the same or in every connective-tissue, but only in a form of the fibre, apparently exclusively fitted for its own germination. Not that the pathogenic micro-organism will, *per se*, necessarily seriously impair, however much it may temporarily weaken, the tissue in which it so exclusively germinates. The lymphoid bodies of the circulation in which, for example, the anthrax-bacillus is so invariably borne from the periphery to the spleen, and in the process so continuously culti-vated, are not seriously impaired. On the contrary, they are, in consequence, rendered absolutely phagocytic in respect of the same micro-organism. And this probably holds good of every germ-disease the micro-organism of which is so exclusively cultivated in wandering lymphoid cells, or of the entire prophylactic order. The rule, however, hardly applies to every micro-organism of at least the recurrent order. Some of them, such as the bacillus of tubercle, have been shown by Klein and other investigators to be occasionally phagocytic in respect of the connective-corpuscles which absorb them. And this no doubt likewise at times occurs in respect of cancer or leprosy, and possibly pyæmia, or in the order of germ-disease where the micro-organism is practically *universally* cultivated in connective-tissue. It is the virus or virulent product of all micro-organisms, prophylactic or preventive, not the micro-organisms themselves, which produces the radical change in the cultivating tissues and all deadly effects; and these morbid effects may be remote enough, and on very different tissues and structures, from that in which the virus-producing micro-organism is planted and germinates. In point of fact it would appear to be a general rule, and may be stated and taken as such, that the virus of the pathogenic micro-organism of preventive, recurrent germ-diseases *attacks and deteriorates*, first and foremost, *the most highly specialised tissues of the body*; whilst the micro-organism itself settles and germinates *only in the most lowly organised*, and without impairing them. The simpler and the more lowly in structure a tissue, or the more nearly it approaches in form and character the vegetable-fibre, the fitter nidus will it prove for a micro-organism of the preventive and recurrent order of germ-disease. A pathogenic micro-organism will not germinate in any very highly specialised tissue, however seriously and however soon its virus will impair this tissue.

If simplicity or lowness of structural form, and a corresponding resistance or "refractoriness" to the virulent reaction of a virus, are the essential conditions for the settlement and germination of a pathogenic microbe of the recurrent germ-diseases, this primitive connective-tissue must be the most fitting soil in the entire body, and can only be rendered all the more fitting for its increase in amount from the irritating reaction of the virus of such a microbe. For this reason the connective-tissue, centric and peripheral, is in all probability the peculiar nidus of every micro-organism of a recurrent or preventive order. It is unquestionable that the connective-tissue which is so widely distributed over the animal frame is the most lowly organised in the entire organism, much more so than nerve-cell and nerve-fibre, which are so primarily injured by the virus of tetanus and rabies; much more so than the lymphoid or splenic corpuscles, which are so essential to the cultivation of the strictly prophylactic order of micro-organism. It is the virus, not the micro-organism, itself, which causes this hypertrophy or excessive proliferation of the connective-tissue, just as it is, likewise, the virus, and not the micro-organism, which at the same time causes the atrophy and degeneration and absolute destruction of a specific tissue of an organ, whose connective-tissue has exclusively germinated the micro-organism. Perhaps no better example of the direct, dire effects of a virus, pure and proper, and as altogether apart from its producing micro-organism could be furnished than the case of chronic alcoholism. How common in such circumstances is hepatic cirrhosis or pulmonary or renal fibrosis, or even skin-disease! How often in such cases does tuberculosis or pneumonia of the acutest forms and of the swiftest course ensue!

Once introduced into the interior of a fitting connective-tissue, whether the fibre be of the interstitial framework of the cerebrospinal axis or of the spleen, or of a serous or a synovial membrane, the pathogenic micro-organism would immediately take root, and germinate to its full capacity. The interior of a simple connective-fibre must be all the more favourable soil for cultivation, because it is in reality composed of pure gelatin; and this fact probably renders such structure, above all others, so constantly the specific seat of germination of the entire recurrent and preventive order of micro-organism, both peripheral and centric.   How largely does the gelatinous substance enter into the composition of the various "germ-jellies" and "bouillons" of the bacteriologists or experimental investigators !   All such artificial pabula for the cultivation of the pathogenic micro-organisms are composed almost solely of this substance.   But if gelatinous material of one kind or another, and the purer the better, be essential to germination, once settled in the interior of a connective-fibre, whether the connective-corpuscle be present in or absent from the fibre, the micro-organism could find no fitter soil of cultivation, and germination would thereafter more immediately and more certainly ensue than in the best germ-jelly known.   Consequently, it is no mere accident that each of the micro-organisms of this entire order of germ-disease is so invariably borne to connective-tissue; and that reaching and settling in this structure, in some of its various forms, it should germinate to its full capacity and induce the disease.

Now, to which of these two great classes, prophylactic or preventive, does rabies belong? If to the one order, it will most certainly, and for that reason, not belong to the other.   There is no doubt that the specific micro-organism is cultivated exclusively in nervous substance, and, above all, in that of the cerebro-spinal axis, never in the wandering corpuscles of the circulation; never even in the areolar tissue of the periphery.   Is it possible, then, that it finds its culture-ground, not in the peripheral connective-tissue, nor in the lymphoid cells of the spleen and circulation, nor in the still more highly specialised nerve-cell or even nerve-fibre itself, but in the fine, interstitial connective-tissue framework, or *neuroglia*, of the cerebro-spinal axis, and pre-eminently in that of its higher and bulkier tracts, and in sensory rather than motor roots, or where the neuroglia most abounds? If simplicity or lowness of structure be essential to the settlement and germination of the micro-organism, the delicate connective-tissue of the neuroglia is precisely such a structure.   Most certainly neither the nerve-fibre nor the nerve-cell of the cerebro-spinal substance is so simply or so lowly organised, being in point of fact the most highly specialised tissue, and the latest in its development in the entire economy.   Precisely on this account, both the nerve-fibre and the nerve-cell will be the very first structures to suffer from the presence of the virulent product of the micro-organism, elaborated freshly *in situ* within the neuroglia as its specific nidus.

Accordingly, rabies may be considered a preventive, not pro-phylactic germ-disease, which is cultivated exclusively in centric connective-tissue. Its micro-organism will consequently be conveyed from the peripheral wound or point of infection to the neuroglia or interstitial connective framework of the nervous substance by the peripheral connective-corpuscles, and in all probability through the lymphatic channels, rather than the blood-stream.

CHAPTER XI.

THE PREVENTION AND PROTECTION IMPARTED BY RABIES-VIRUS.

If rabies has been once incurred and recovered from, a state of protection has been thereby induced, the extent of the immunity being determined by the severity of the malady, or by the amount of virus which has been elaborated in the course of the case. And this holds good, not merely of rabies, but of every germ-disease. Even malarial fever, the most recurrent of any, probably protects against malarial fever, *for a time.* The same protective condition may be artificially brought about in one of two ways. It may be induced by a process of vaccination, that is to say by the inoculation of a modified micro-organism of a prophylactic germ-disease ; the micro-organism of this entire order, and not its virus, being alone capable of genuine modification. On the other hand, it may be induced by a quantitative inoculation (or course of inoculations) of the *virus* or virulent product, as opposed to the *virus-germ*, of a preventive germ-disease ; the virus, *and not the micro-organism* of this entire order, being, alone, capable of inducing protection or prevention. But in all such cases the protected condition renders, as long as it lasts, any further germination of the pathogenic micro-organism which has occasioned it abortive. Certain it is, that, so far as rabies is concerned, in an immune animal the rabies-germ never germinates.

What, then, has occurred, after protection has been thus induced, that no such result now ensues? The disease does not supervene, because the pathogenic micro-organism, on its introduction into such an animal, is, for some reason connected with the protective condition, speedily extinguished and demolished. For such an immune animal, whether protected physiologically or pathologically, on prophylactic or preventive conditions, the microbe is not morbific, but inert, even serving as nutriment for the absorbent corpuscles.

How has this extraordinary transformation been brought about? Why should there be so absolute a contrast before and after a germ-disease has been incurred, or between a "protected" and an unprotected animal?   Is this protective condition in all cases of germ-disease alike, and produced in the same way?   Are general immunity, on the one hand, and very special prophylaxis, on the other hand, but synonymous terms, and cover the same protective process and state?   On the contrary, an animal which enjoys even absolute immunity from the pathogenic micro-organism which occasioned it, does not necessarily possess prophylaxis, the protective condition, pronounced though it be at first, being far from enduring.   Wherein, then, do these two all-important, but fundamentally distinct, modes and kinds of protection differ from one another?   What constitutes prophylaxis, on the one hand ; and what immunity, on the other?

What becomes of the rabies-germ on its being introduced into the economy after the disease has been incurred and recovered from— which is very rare—and when a protective condition has been thereby induced?   Nothing could more clearly, if finally, reveal the place which rabies occupies amongst germ-diseases.

According to one theory, protection of every kind has been attributed exclusively to a process of *phagocytosis*, or microbe-devouring; the phagocytic function of the absorbent corpuscles being the essential factor of every form of protection which presents itself. Thus, after such a disease as smallpox or anthrax, and in consequence of the germination of the micro-organism in the lymphoid cells of the spleen and circulation, the leucocytes have, thereafter, become, not merely barren, instead of fertile, soil, but positively phagocytic in respect of the micro-organism.   In like manner, after tetanus or diphtheria, or, which produces the same result, after a graduated course of the virus of their respective micro-organisms, the latter are prevented from again, for a time, germinating, through the phagocytic function of the absorbent corpuscles ; and this function, however previously suppressed, has only been acquired through the stimulation of the virus.   Again, after M. Pasteur's preventive course of rabies-virus, the rabies-germs, thereafter introduced, will likewise be immediately demolished and devoured ; the amœboid organisms having been, in consequence of the preventive course of virus, stimulated into a very positive phagocytic activity, with respect to the special micro-organism. And so in respect of the protection imparted by every germ-disease.

That there is a process of germ-devouring or phagocytosis on the part of the leucocytes there can be no question. Nor is this function peculiar merely to the absorbent corpuscles of the higher and highest animal organisms; it is common to the entire amœboid order of cell throughout the living kingdom, both vegetable and animal. Where such amœboid bodies exist,—and they exist everywhere where there are vital processes,—it is found that they are capable of absorbing and digesting organic substance and of feeding thereon. Nor is this ingestive and digestive function, so characteristic of the entire amœboid order, from the simplest infusorial monad to the most special hosts of leucocytes of the highest animals, by any means confined to merely dead organic material. It likewise holds good of even active, living material. Organised not less than organic substance, and living organised forms not less than dead, constantly constitute the pabulum of the amœboid cell. The discovery that the wandering corpuscles of an organism digested and removed its every effete or decayed structure, led eventually to the not less fruitful discovery that the leucocyte, which is capable of this, is, under certain conditions of stimulation, also capable of taking into its substance certain living micro-organisms and fungoid growths of the lowest forms, and of destroying and feeding on them. But whilst the absorptive corpuscles of the highest animals are observed to take up organic and organised material, such as a clot or fragments of muscle or connective-fibre, or of listerised cat-gut ligature, or of dead bone itself, and to digest them, it is in reality but the revelation of a process which is always going on even in the lowest infusorium ; the function being as primitive as it is permanent over the entire living kingdom, and common to the amœboid order of organism. For the leucocytes, lymphocytes and connective-corpuscles or fibrocytes of the highest animal organization are, there is reason to show, but a persistent and all-important continuation of the primary amœboid form; the function of the latter never being fairly lost even in the highest animals, and always, under stimulation, capable, however suppressed, of being restored. Nature is genuinely conservative and retains in the highest organisms,—even man,—the oldest and most primitive system of the lowest organisms. Phagocytosis is in every probability their chief, as their oldest, physiological function, and has been transmitted serially, from the remotest vegetable itself.

Is it the fact, however, that this phagocytic function is the sole factor of every form of the protective condition? Assuming that phagocytosis is the essential, if not the exclusive factor of prophylaxis, or the protective condition imparted by a prophylactic germ-disease, it by no means follows that every form of the protective condition is due to this cause. Is there any evidence of pathogenic micro-organisms being otherwise destroyed in the economy than by the phagocytic leucocytes? As it so happens, there is absolutely conclusive evidence.

The serum or flowing plasma of the circulation of a protected animal is likewise capable of destroying pathogenic micro-organisms, irrespective of the corpuscular constituents of the blood-stream. The actual germicidal property of the plasma or serum has been established beyond question in respect of many germ-diseases. But it is important to note that this bactericidal property has been ascertained, mainly, if not wholly, in respect of preventive, recurrent germ-diseases, such as diphtheria and tetanus, not of prophylactic germ-diseases, such as smallpox, anthrax, scarlatina. Nowhere has one heard of the serum of a strictly prophylactic germ-disease protecting from the germ-disease, and as a prophylactic. Nowhere has it been alleged that an "anti-toxin serum" is to be obtained from a prophylactic germ-disease, which will protect like vaccine, or any modified micro-organism of a prophylactic. It is true that the "serum" of enteric fever, which may be taken as a prophylactic germ-disease, has been alleged to both "protect" and "prevent." But this fact has not been established.

The prophylaxis established by the prophylactic order of germ-disease is, apparently, the result, not of the condition of the flowing plasma or serum, but rather of that of its corpuscular constituents. Nevertheless it is irrefutable that it is the liquor sanguinis, and not its wandering corpuscular constituents, which is the germicidal agent in the cases of protection imparted by the preventive order of germ-diseases. If there were no other evidence of this fact than the invaluable results obtained by the so-called "anti-toxin" serum-treatment in respect of diphtheria and tetanus, this would be unquestionable. If the "anti-toxin" serum be used *early* after infection, and before the full or maximum quantity of the specific virus of the malady has been elaborated, or, in other words, before profound constitutional disturbance has set in, the diphtheria-bacillus or tetanus-bacillus in the site of infection will be blighted by the serum, and the disease "prevented." The protective serum would appear to be not so much an "anti-toxin" or anti-virus; hence the failures when the remedy is used *too late,* as it is perhaps a germicidal product, or an anti-*virus-germ.* It is probably the bacterium which is destroyed by the preventive serum. Hence its marvellous success when employed *early,* or when little or no virus has been eliminated. And this holds good of every germ-disease which is really capable of yielding a preventive serum ; but this, again, it is important to add, comprises in every probability only the order of strictly preventive and recurrent germ-diseases.

It is unquestionable that, after the protective condition has been induced, the specific microbe of preventive germ-diseases, particularly of peripheral preventive diseases, is destroyed by the liquor sanguinis, and as certainly and quickly as a land-shell or fresh-water fish, which has been dropped into the sea, is destroyed by the sea. But if the liquor sanguinis of an immune animal, whether this animal be protected naturally or artificially, *i.e.* after an attack of the disease, or by a preventive course of inoculations of its virus, is *per se* capable of thus destroying the pathogenic microbe, why, it may be asked, should phagocytosis ever be called in to account for the protective condition imparted? It is true that the leucocytes of the blood-stream, even after a preventive and recurrent, as well as after a pro-phylactic germ-disease, may, and probably invariably do, absorb the destroyed micro-organism like any other dead, organic matter, just as the land-shell or fresh-water fish, which has been killed by the sea, may be thereafter demolished by the wandering star-fish of the sea. But it has been maintained that this absorptive work, highly important as it is, is always subordinate, and in no way induces a protective condition ; in every case of germ-disease the real bactericidal property lying, from first to last, in the liquor sanguinis itself, not in its corpuscular constituents. And the proved germicidal property of the serum of a protected organism has been taken as a fatal objection to the doctrine of phagocytic immunity; or, in other words, to the belief that the condition of protection is ever entirely or even primarily due to a process of phagocytosis, however the latter may be aroused.

For these reasons two opposing schools have arisen, which vividly recall the ancient schools of the solidists and the humoralists. By the former (the solidist) the process of germ-devouring on the part of the wandering corpuscular system accounts for every form of protection, alike prophylaxis and immunity, or whether of long or of short duration. By the other (the humoralists) phagocytosis, *per se*, really accounts for no form of protection; every form without exception being due to the condition of the liquor sanguinis, not of its corpuscular constituents. Consequently, if there be such a phenomenon as *phagocytosis*, which is not denied, whatever its share in the production of prophylaxis, if none whatever in the production of mere general immunity, there is also such a phenomenon as, what it may be permissible to term, *toxicytosis*. To one or the other of these phenomena every protective condition of germ-disease has been exclusively referred. Are these two views contradictory? Because toxicytosis adequately accounts for certain forms of protection, that imparted by all preventive germ-diseases, does it necessarily follow that phagocytosis wholly accounts for none? Neither phagocytosis, or germ-devouring, nor toxicytosis, or germ-poisoning, will, *per se*, account for every protective condition. At the root of each form of protection, and as its prime and essential factor, is a process either of phagocytosis or of toxicytosis. Why should the protective condition be not equally persistent in all protection? why should it be so evanescent after any germ-disease, much more after the entire class of purely preventive and recurrent germ-diseases, both peripheral and centric, since phagocytosis produces *prophylaxis*, or an enduring protection, without reference to the condition of the serum? Nor is it less certain that toxicytosis will not account for every protective condition; for, if so, why should the protection induced be not equally evanescent in all, since toxicytosis, itself, as shall be shown presently, is not lasting? The protective conditions which bring about such wholly different forms of protection must also vary. What, then, are these conditions, and in what does prophylaxis differ from immunity?

As, broadly speaking, there are two orders of germ-disease which are sharply marked off from each other, the preventive, but non-prophylactic, and, on the other hand, the strictly prophylactic, but non-preventive; so, in like manner, there would appear to be two equally great orders of protection, *immunity*, on the one hand, and *prophylaxis*, on the other. The former is characteristic of the entire preventive order, peripheral and centric; the latter of the entire prophylactic order. This fundamental distinction is, again, determined by the fact that in the strictly prophylactic order the pathogenic micro-organism is germinated exclusively in the leucocytes or migratory corpuscular cells of the circulation, the malady being

extremely limited and a very special germ-disease in the animal
kingdom; whereas in the preventive and recurrent order, the pathogenic micro-organism is never germinated in the leucocytes or
migratory corpuscular cells, but exclusively in the fixed connective-
tissue, centric as well as peripheral, the germ-disease in consequence
being by no means limited in its range over the animal kingdom,
but quite the reverse.

As we have seen, the leucocytes of the circulation are, normally,
phagocytic with respect to the micro-organisms of probably the entire
preventive order; that is to say of every germ-disease whose seat of
cultivation is exclusively in the fixed connective-tissue, but, above all,
in the peripheral connective-tissue. These leucocytes are the main
phagocytes of the higher animal forms; but with respect to the
peripheral preventive order of pathogenic micro-organisms, they are
as persistently phagocytic as the lowliest protoplasmic cells. The
lower in the scale of life, whether of vegetable or animal, or the more
it comes in contact and competition with microbic life and approaches
the microbic mode of existence, the more phagocytic in all probability
is the amœboid order of cells, as this fundamental function will be
more frequently called upon as an offensive and defensive weapon in
the life of the cell. For this reason, probably, the vegetable amœboids, and those of the lowest animal forms, such as the sponge, are
so constantly and so highly phagocytic, to maintain their place in
a nether world of micro-organisms.

But so far as even the most active, gregarious, germ-devouring
leucocytes of the circulation in the animal realm are concerned, it is
certain that they are not phagocytic, normally, with respect to a
distinct class of pathogenic micro-organisms. In the entire order
of prophylactic germ-diseases, they in reality prove the seat of cultivation of their specific micro-organisms. Only in these migratory
protoplasmic corpuscles does the micro-organism of a prophylactic
germ-disease really incubate and multiply. And for this reason, if
there were no other, the germ-disease is prophylactic; for in the
process of germination the whole corpuscular system is involved, and
the entire germinating-ground of the very specific micro-organism
will be covered and modified. After an attack of any germ-disease
whose seat of cultivation is exclusively in the leucocytic constituents
of the circulation, the amœboid cells which have absorbed and
germinated the microbe, and through this produced the disease, have
in this fact become phagocytic, and have rendered any further germi-

nation of such a micro-organism all but impossible. How is this latent function called into activity? How is the non-phagocytic leucocyte rendered phagocytic? So much so that the pathogenic micro-organism which, before this process, never fails to germinate in it is now, after this process, as instantly absorbed and devoured as is the micro-organism of diphtheria or erysipelas, or of any other peripheral germ-disease of as strictly connective-tissue cultivation.

Even vegetable-cells and those of the lowest forms of animal life are capable of being repelled or attracted by irritant or non-irritant bodies, such as micro-organisms and their products. However much they may recoil, to begin with, sooner or later, in virtue of the repulsion and the stimulation involved by it, they become proportionally attracted and, thereafter, attack and devour the substance, whether living or dead, or however irritant, with the same efficiency that they devour the most non-irritant and nutritious. And this vital power is characteristic of the amœboid-cells of the highest animal organisation and all through the animal kingdom. Substances of the most irritating character, in the neighbourhood of which leucocytes will everywhere recoil, the same leucocytes will eventually face in shoals and promptly absorb and demolish. Nor is this recoil with subsequent attraction a mere mechanical force, like the drawing of a bow-string with its subsequent discharge of the arrow. Much less is it chemical. The phagocytic function which has thus been exerted is distinctly a vital, not a chemical or mechanical function, and is essentially a physiological, not a pathological process. It has been objected that this is based upon phenomena merely of the vegetable kingdom, and that there is no evidence that even in the vegetable-cells such repulsion and subsequent attraction are really vital, but probably chemical. But if *chemiotaxis*, both negative and positive, like an electric discharge rather than a chemical force, is characteristic of vegetable-cells, for the same reason it will be more or less characteristic of the amœboid system of cells even of the highest animals. The latter cells are much the nearest approach to the former in the animal organisation, being practically but their lineal, if not, in some classes, unaltered descendants, and, with respect to the majority of pathogenic micro-organisms, retaining the same fundamental function.

The phenomenon of repulsion with subsequent attraction is by no means uncommon even in the highest and most specialised animal forms; and in these the process is most certainly vital, not mechanical.

11—2

Take, as an example, the use of tobacco or of any potent vegetable-virus. The habitual use of tobacco for but a relatively short period will produce less and less sickly effects, at last precluding all possibility of nausea and vertigo; and eventually it induces even a positive appetite or hunger for the "alkaloid," deleterious as it sometimes is. So much so that after the longest interval, on a return to the use of tobacco, nausea will not necessarily occur. Is this persistent toleration of so potent a vegetable virulent product, not to say the positive relish and appetite for it, mechanical or chemical? Is it, at last, whatever it may have been at first, even pathological? However pathological in the first instance, it is, ultimately, strictly physiological; and this, as we shall see presently, is probably no uncommon sequence in either the vegetable or animal kingdom. In such a case, the nervous system, in specific and all-important centres, has been very profoundly and likewise permanently affected in the toleration of and positive appetite for the alkaloidal principle. These nervous centres have been affected to the acquirement of an altogether new taste; the pristine irritability having been converted into positive relish. The general acute sensibility has been changed by the virus, not merely into bluntness or toleration, but into a lasting and very special form of sensitiveness, or into what one may term an almost new sense. And it is just possible that in some such way some of the special senses may have taken their rise. Sensitiveness to virulent products, or to their specific microbes, whether this take the form of repulsion or attraction, or of both conditions, consecutively, is, therefore, essentially a vital function, not mechanical or chemical; and is probably of a strictly nerve-character, even in the simplest infusorial organism; the intrinsic vital irritability of the protoplasmic organism being due to its specialised but possibly widely-diffused nervous elements. The conversion of repulsion into attraction, or of shuddering nausea into positive relish and appetite, constitutes a specialisation of the nervous irritability into a distinct sense-centre. How much of the simple, translucent substance of the lowliest protoplasmic being is composed of such undifferentiated nervous elements, who can say?

When, however, an entire system of such cells, as in the case of the leucocytes of animal forms, is under the constant and the complete sway of the most complicated and the most specialised nervous system, this intrinsic sensitiveness will not be lessened, but, on the contrary, intensified and, sooner or later, extremely specialised.

Hence, the system of leucocytes of even the highest animal organisation, where their normal phagocytic function is, in respect of a certain order of pathogenic micro-organisms, in relative abeyance, may yet be rendered positively phagocytic, in direct consequence of the germination of the micro-organisms in these migratory cells. A prophylactic germ-disease having been incurred, there is involved thereby a specific stimulation, not only of the intrinsic sensitiveness of the individual leucocytes which have germinated the pathogenic micro-organism, but, still more lasting factor of the phagocytic function excited, of the all-important nervous supply, both cerebro-spinal and sympathetic, particularly the latter, which is so intimately blended with this lymphoid system in its deepest origin in the spleen, in the marrow of bones, and in lymphatic glands. Phagocytosis, once having been aroused and induced by the germination of a pathogenic micro-organism in the leucocytes, will become habitual against the particular micro-organism occasioning it; as habitual and normal as against a micro-organism of exclusively connective-tissue cultivation.

The prophylaxis established will, therefore, be a more or less permanent protection; for it is due to a vital, not to a chemical or mechanical process. The entire function, when once established, is a physiological rather than a pathological one. The germinating microbe in stimulating with its virus the nervous system but doubly stimulates the latent physiological function of the leucocytic system to phagocytosis, and, if so, to genuine prophylaxis.

But granting the possibility of phagocytosis, and of its being completely restored, if ever suppressed, and also its vast importance in the production of prophylaxis, why, it may be objected, should the system of leucocytes, thus so successfully stimulated, be phagocytic only against the respective microbe which has occasioned it? Why should not the leucocytic-cells, when once rendered phagocytic, therefore be *ipso facto* microbe-destroying against every microbe capable of germinating in leucocytes? This most certainly is not the fact. Otherwise, an attack of smallpox might well protect from scarlatina or measles, or an attack of scarlatina from anthrax or from any other prophylactic germ-disease. Clearly enough, the phagocytic function which has been excited by the germination of a prophylactic micro-organism is a very specific one, and far from being general; and for this reason it is so specifically and so persistently prophylactic. Hence, the more limited the seat of the germination of such a micro-organism, even in the lymphoid system itself, probably the more pronounced and the more specific will be the phagocytosis induced, and the more lasting the physiological protection against such a micro-organism which will be acquired. This is well seen in such a germ-disease as mumps, perhaps one of the most distinctly prophylactic of the entire group. And the same phenomenon is probably characteristic of whooping-cough. In spite of, nay in consequence of, the very limitation and special character of the field of cultivation, both of these germ-diseases are stubbornly and persistently prophylactic, the protection imparted by the maladies lasting for many a year, and often enough for a long life-time. When once the micro-organism has germinated to its full possibility of multiplication there is no other soil of cultivation left. In consequence of the cultivation this limited germinating-ground is rendered for a very long time prophylactic against the particular micro-organism, and mainly through the nervous-system in the very special centres which govern the special life-activity of such organs. After all, even the entire leucocytic system, far-ranging as it is, is strictly limited; confined to the intrinsic tissue of the spleen, the lymphatic glands, and the marrow of bones : the "marrow of bones" being probably but lymphatic cells, or glands of these cells, in an osseous framework. Most certainly, the wandering corpuscular system of the circulation and spleen, in which the prophylactic micro-organisms are, apparently, exclusively cultivated, is not anything like so extensive as the areolar or fixed connective-tissue which is practically unlimited, and which depends upon no capital site of cultivation and no special central nervous system. But the very limitation of the leucocytic system in which the prophylactic micro-organisms alone germinate renders prophylaxis alike specific and constant. If this system be rendered prophylactic, whether through its special nervous centres or through an intrinsic alteration in the irritability of the leucocytes themselves, or through both factors, the entire organism is rendered prophylactic.

Is it so very remarkable, then, that the system of leucocytes which has once been rendered phagocytic against a particular microbe, should remain permanently phagocytic only against the specific microbe which has excited and established, but not created, the phagocytic activity? In this connection, again, consider the case of tobacco, or other virulent product. There is no more reason for the system of leucocytes, if once rendered phagocytic for one micro-organism, being therefore phagocytic for all micro-organisms generating in the same leucocytes, than there is for the protection against tobacco necessarily involving a protection against alcohol, morphia, strychnine, or any other virulent product. The protection imparted by a prophylactic germ-disease is, therefore, very special. Specific phagocytosis having been excited and physiologically maintained in the leucocytes, prophylaxis necessarily ensues. It is not the entire nervous system which has been thus acted upon, but solely the specific centres which regulate the relatively limited leucocytic system. The effect produced is exclusively confined to this system, and has been ulti- mately a distinctly physiological one; and, consequently, it is as enduring over the leucocytic system as in the specific nerve-centres themselves.

If this be so, phagocytosis, as a prime and very special factor of protection, is characteristic of a prophylactic, rather than a pre- ventive germ-disease; that is to say, of a germ-disease whose micro- organism is cultivated exclusively in the leucocytic-cells of the circulation, the phagocytic function being normal to the amœboid- cells of the entire living kingdom. Hence, the protective condition induced is physiological. It is a latent function aroused and specialized by germination, and therefore so enduring. It is not pathological, and therefore not transient; for it is due to the phagocytic habit, with respect to such micro-organisms, which has been revived and established by the malady. But this is distinctly a vital and physio- logical function which is as old as the amœboid system of cells, and by far the oldest and most elementary function in the highest animal forms.

One can, consequently, understand not only how the micro- organism of a prophylactic germ-disease may give rise to phagocytic prophylaxis or the most enduring protective condition, but how even a modified form of this micro-organism, such as vaccine, may likewise give rise to the same protection. However modified the micro- organism, its germination in the leucocytes will still excite the phagocytic function, and induce, thereafter, the same phagocytic prophylaxis as that of the micro-organism of which it is a modification. And, as we have already seen, there is reason to show that only the micro-organism of a distinctly prophylactic germ disease is capable, not merely of attenuation, but of this genuine modification; or, in other words, however attenuated, yet in this attenuated form of retaining the full prophylactic force of the micro-organism of which it is a modification. This by no means applies to the micro-organism of a strictly preventive germ-disease, which may be attenuated or intensified to extreme degrees by culture or transmission, but never can be modified, as a prophylactic micro-organism is modified.

How, then, if not by phagocytosis, is the immunity of the preventive order of germ-disease occasioned? One fact of prime distinction between the two classes of germ-disease is clear, that the immunity characteristic of the preventive order may be induced alike *before* infection and *after* infection. There is, however, as we have seen, no conclusive evidence of a prophylactic vaccination protecting after infection, or when germination in the leucocytes has begun, and thus "preventing" the disease. But protection or prevention takes place, in respect of the preventive class, either before or long after infection and to the same amount in each case, because the leucocyte with its phagocytic function is not concerned, except subordinately, in the production of the immunity. Here, it is not the condition of the leucocytes or of the constituents of the blood-stream, but of the blood-stream itself, or of the ever-flowing liquor sanguinis, which constitutes the essential factor of the immunity. And given this condition of the serum, protection, even *after* infection has taken place and germination has begun, will be as assured as with the same condition of the blood-stream *before* infection. It is the altered condition of the serum which is the prime factor of the protective condition imparted; the entire fluid having been rendered distinctly germicidal. The pathogenic micro-organism introduced in infection is instantly destroyed by the blood-current itself, and the prevention or protection thereby occasioned is not from phagocytosis but from what has been termed above, a genuine toxicytosis. And this process is essentially chemical, not vital, and due to a pathological, not to a physiological, series of events.

What, then, has rendered the serum germicidal? Does the virus itself, which has been elaborated in the course of a preventive germ-disease, or which has been introduced into the blood-stream in a course of inoculations, constitute, in virtue of its very virulence, the germicidal material? This has been asserted. But it by no means follows. There is no proof that any micro-organism is directly or wholly destroyed by its own secretion, however copious and virulent the product. If, therefore, after a preventive germ-disease the liquor sanguinis instantly destroys the specific microbe of the malady on reinfection, it cannot be directly due to the existence in the blood-stream of the virus of the micro-organism, however certain it is that this virus is present in the fluid, even in the largest quantity. Nevertheless, it is certain that the protection from and by a preventive germ-disease is both in amount and in duration strictly commensurate with the amount, not of the specific micro-organism, but of its virus which has been elaborated in the case. As we have already seen in respect of rabies the amount and the duration of the immunity imparted may be mathematically measured by the amount of virus introduced into the system. If, consequently, the virus elaborated in a germ-disease, or artificially introduced in a course of inoculations, does not *cause* the blood-stream to be germicidal, it must, nevertheless, invariably *occasion* this important change.

Since the virus is, *per se*, incapable of destroying its own micro-organism, is the immunity, after all, due to the actual presence of the moribund and dead micro-organisms, which have been left in the system after a preventive germ-disease, or which have been introduced in a course of preventive inoculations?

"Let us not lose sight," says M. Pasteur, "of the very original and very fruitful theory put forward by M. Metschnikoff. Does the vaccinal matter, supposing it to exist, reside in the *dead* micro-organisms[1]?"

But why, even in the largest quantities, should moribund or dead micro-organisms produce any morbid disturbance whatever, much less cause protection and prevention? Effete fibrous and muscular tissue, suddenly thrown on the system, as in the subinvolution of the pregnant uterus, or of the fœtal liver at birth, or in the absorption of pneumonic condensation, causes no such disturbance, but is steadily devoured by the wandering, absorbent corpuscles. Why should not the same result follow in respect of dead micro-organisms? There is every reason to believe that this result does invariably follow. Assuming, however, that in respect of rabies, such absorption, exceptionally enough, does not take place, or at all events with the thoroughness and promptness in respect of ordinary effete tissue; is it possible that the presence of these dead microbes in the circulation, especially in large quantities, if it does not produce the disease, nevertheless prevents the germination of living microbes introduced in their midst, rendering the blood essentially germicidal? We know that the rabies-germ is a micro-organism of *living*, not of *dead*, tissue. In a week or ten days the spinal marrow of the most extreme

---

[1] See *Annales de l'Institut Pasteur*; a letter from M. Pasteur to Prof. Duclaux, Dec. 27, 1886.

paralytic rabbit-rabies, and where the spinal substance has been thoroughly disseminated with the living micro-organism, ceases to rabidise. It is certain that the rabies-germ immediately begins to die on the death of its infected victim. In the dead tissues the rabies-germ apparently cannot survive. Hence the hitherto absolute impossibility of cultivating it artificially, in germ-jellies or in any, even fresh, nervous-structure. Failing to maintain its vitality in dead tissue, is it possible that the dead micro-organisms introduced in a graduated course of preventive inoculations, or left in the system after the development of the disease, prevent the germination of the living micro-organisms introduced thereafter in infection? If this were the fact it would follow that a rabic marrow, 6 or 7 days old, would invariably protect very much better than a rabic marrow only *one* day old; for in the six days' marrow there would necessarily be an immensely larger number of dead microbes—they would practically be all extinct. The six days' marrow, however, if it protects at all, in spite of its many extinct microbes, does not protect anything like the one day's marrow. Consequently, the preventive material in the liquor sanguinis does not consist of the moribund or dead micro-organisms, any more than of the virus or virulent product of the living micro-organism.

Again, it has been suggested that a preventive material may have been secreted into the blood-stream, possibly by the pathogenic micro-organism itself along with its specific virus; a micro-organism within the living organism eliminating more than one product: not only a pathogenic secretion, but, at a still later stage, possibly also a germicidal or preventive material. . Thus, in accounting for the immunity in respect of rabies, M. Pasteur has stated that,

"The facts (of experimentation) agree better with the notion of a *vaccinal matter*, which we may suppose associated with the rabies-microbe, the latter preserving its own virulence intact in all the drying marrows. But the process of desiccation destroys the microbe itself progressively and more rapidly than it destroys the *vaccinal matter*[1]."

M. Pasteur does not here state that "the vaccinal matter" is the intrinsic product of the microbe, and as much so as the virus itself, however incompatible the agents. But it has been suggested. It is surely, however, hardly possible that a micro-organism, which will

[1] *Annales de l'Institut Pasteur.* M. Pasteur's letter to Prof. Duclaux, Dec. 27 1886.

elaborate and secrete a virus, capable of destroying the most delicate, highly specialised of the living tissues (nerve-fibre) yet incapable of impairing itself, or its germinating-tissue, will, nevertheless, secrete another product which will not only be innocuous to the most highly specialised of the living tissues, but protect them from the virus, and at the same time actually destroy the pathogenic micro-organism itself. One might as well expect the serpent to simultaneously secrete with its venom, and from the same secreting-organ, a ferment or protective material, not only which will protect the animal against its own venom—which is conceivable enough—but which at the same time will destroy the venom-secreting organ !

"There are some," says Dr Sydney Martin, "who have considered that the chemical products formed by the primary infective agent, outside the body, or in the natural disease, may consist of a 'vaccine' and a 'toxine'; there is not the slightest evidence of this." "There is also," he states, "no evidence that there is any particular chemical substance which stops the growth of a pathogenous micro-organism. When grown in a flask, it will not develop indefinitely, and it stops, not because there is an antitoxine formed, but because it is choked by its own chemical products, in the same manner as peptic or triptic digestion may be inhibited by the accumulation of the digestive products[1]."

The micro-organism in a flask of gelatinous material at last stops germinating, surely not so much because it is "choked" by an accumulation of its own products—if this ever occurs—as because the culture-ground is exhausted. Want of germinating-soil—inanition —quite as much as a plethora of its own products, kills the microbe. Increase the gelatinous substance "indefinitely," and the germination of the micro-organism will develop indefinitely, as it does in the natural course of the disease. There may be no evidence that a pathogenic microbe produces a virus and at the same time its antidote, or preventive material with respect to the germ itself. But it does not follow because an antitoxin material has never been isolated from the liquor sanguinis, that it does not exist in this fluid. Until comparatively recently, not even a virus, nor a specific micro-organism itself, was isolated. But the hypothetical assumption of the existence of both agents has been very amply justified. Much less does it follow, because a preventive material has never been isolated

[1] *Goulstonian Lectures*, "The chemical pathology of diphtheria," by Sidney Martin, M.D.

from an artificial germinating-ground, that after the disease it does
not exist in the animal system, or even in the blood-stream.   No
such material may have been isolated from a gelatinous medium in
respect of the entire preventive order of germ-disease.   But this
holds good only of these.   A modified virus-germ has been brilliantly
isolated by M. Pasteur himself, in respect of anthrax.   The pathogenic micro-organism of the disease has been cultured and modified
into a genuine "vaccine" in a gelatinous medium, and in this only;
and possibly the same result may follow with the micro-organism of
the entire prophylactic order, the micro-organism of this order
being alone capable of true modification, whether artificially or
naturally.   If there be no evidence that there is any particular preventive material in the liquor sanguinis which "stops the growth"
of the particular micro-organism, why should the growth be ever
stopped at all by the serum of such a case?   Certain it is that
ordinary normal serum will not do so.   Why, after tetanus or diphtheria, should the serum, if inoculated at an early stage, so effectually
prevent the germination of the pathogenic bacillus?   It will not be
denied that after such preventive germ-diseases the serum is distinctly
germicidal.   Why, then, is it germicidal?

The absence of any protective principle in a flask of gelatinous
substance—if such be really the fact, and it is characteristic only of
the preventive germ-diseases—is surely proof positive that the
pathogenic micro-organism itself, however much virus it may secrete,
secretes no germicidal material whatever.   It is also a fairly strong
proof that dead, inert gelatinous substance yields no such principle,
however acted upon by the virus.   The antitoxines which have proved
so successful and so truly germicidal have been obtained from the
serum of animals which have received the preventive inoculations, or
passed through the preventive germ-disease.   There will always be
an absence of the protective material in gelatinous germ-jellies,
however extensive the culture-ground, and however much virulent
product there may be elaborated in it : because, whilst the virus or
pathogenic product is the direct secretion of the micro-organism
itself in even a dead organic medium, the germicidal product, which
induces immunity, is not the secretion of the micro-organism, but in
every likelihood a product of the living and not of dead tissue.   This
is probably the reason why it is absent in artificial cultures, as likewise
it is a reason why it should be present in the liquor sanguinis, after
a preventive germ-disease, or after a course of preventive inoculations

of virus. If, then, there be a preventive material eliminated at all, as from the distinctly germicidal property of the serum after so many of the preventive germ-diseases there is every reason to believe, it is eliminated, not by the pathogenic micro-organism itself, but by the living tissues of the infected animal which have been acted upon by the virulent product of the micro-organism. It is a germicidal product at last eliminated by the living tissues, and in reaction to the deadly virulence of the virus.

It is worth remembering that an amount of the preventive principle in the blood-stream, slight enough to entirely escape detection, might yet prove, all over the circulation, absolutely bactericidal. Who could detect in the blood-stream the infinitesimal quantity of tuberculin employed by Koch to reveal the existence of tuberculous sites, and to test with such brilliant success? Who could detect in the blood-stream, or any part of the system, the small amount of antitoxin-serum used for the prevention of diphtheria? Yet the smallest amount injected, if before the pathogenic micro-organism has eliminated its own virus, or a part of its virus, will prove distinctly bactericidal. It might escape detection, and yet completely alter the properties and character of the liquor sanguinis, rendering it, over the entire circulation, uniformly preventive in respect of the micro-organism which has occasioned it. Hence, it is perfectly possible that the serum of an animal profoundly protected against rabies will also prevent or protect against the disease. This, however, has never as yet been adequately tested.

Assuming, then, that after a preventive germ-disease or a prolonged course of preventive inoculations, a germicidal principle is at last eliminated from the *living* tissues themselves, in however minute quantities, the principle must be a pathological one, and the whole process of elimination strictly morbid. Nor is this unique or surprising. The process is characteristic of the great preventive order, both peripheral and centric, as opposed to the prophylactic class, and is caused by the presence and continued pathogenic action of the virus which has been elaborated in the course of the malady, or introduced in a series of inoculations. We have already seen in respect of rabies, that the immunity induced is strictly proportioned to the amount of virus introduced in the inoculations. Such as the amount and the virulence of the virus, so are the character and the duration of the immunity imparted. But we know that the virus does not, in itself, cause the immunity; it is not bactericidal; at all events, it does not destroy its own micro-organism. Consequently, if the living tissues yield a germicidal product or become themselves germicidal which induces immunity, it is a prevention or protection which is strictly commensurate with the amount of virus in the system. Acting on such tissues for days and with intense virulence, the virus must, therefore, be the cause of the product and of its elimination, or of the germicidal condition, and both must be essentially pathological; for the virus which has caused the elimination or the condition is the most virulent and deadly of agents. Consider in this connection the morbid results of which a germ-disease is capable. Its destructive influence is to be seen, not only in the most vital nerve-centres, although, probably, always primarily in such highly specialised structures, but likewise in well-nigh every tissue of the body. In addition to the nerve-centres and the nervous tissues, there is a simultaneous and a collateral degeneration of well-nigh every secreting-organ. But long before this extreme disorganisation takes place the tissues acted upon must be in a condition of the intensest irritability, the character of their secretions into the blood-stream being morbidly altered. Is it unreasonable to infer that whilst in this irritated condition, and before actual degeneration has occurred, the tissues, in continued reaction to the virus, should themselves become bactericidal, or eliminate a morbid material which will render the blood-stream bactericidal? But if special tissues become preventive or at last elaborate, however slightly, a principle which is, it is precisely because they are not healthy or in their normal condition, nothing like so healthy as they are in a case of prophylaxis, or as are the leucocytes after a prophylactic germ-disease. The prevention induced by the existence of the germicidal material of the blood-stream from the degenerating tissue which affords it, in however small a quantity, must be essentially pathological. Hence the protective condition, such as it is, is more or less transient; and this unenduring character is peculiar to the entire preventive order. In such a germ-disease it will last only so long as there is a bactericidal condition of the special tissues and liquor sanguinis; and the length of its duration in the system will be determined by the amount of virus elaborated in the malady.

So long as there is virus in the circulating fluids to act deleteriously on these tissues there will be a germicidal principle; and in accordance with the extent or amount of both will be the amount of immunity imparted. The protection of the preventive order is

therefore essentially pathological, not physiological; and, consequently, however absolute to begin with, it is fading and evanescent.
The protection of the prophylactic order, on the contrary, is essentially
physiological; and, therefore, however slight, it is enduring, lasting
for years, sometimes for a long lifetime, or as long as the phagocytic
function itself. Is the protection imparted by an attack of erysipelas
or diphtheria or ague permanent? Is the protection imparted by the
longest course of inoculations of the rabies-virus enduring? Will it
compare with that of vaccine against smallpox?

The protective condition imparted by the preventive order is, not
only from its pathological mode of production, more or less transient,
but after the immunity has faded—or, possibly, begun to fade—it is
followed by recurrence of the disease. On fading, the protection has
given place to a pathological condition of unprotection which has really
underlain it. The tissues which have served as a specific culture-ground
for the micro-organism, have, *de facto*, been rendered a fitter nidus than
before the germination. The virus of the disease will have somewhat
impaired or deteriorated the special connective-tissue in which the
pathogenic micro-organism of this entire order is so exclusively cultivated; but it will, at the same time, have materially increased the
amount of this tissue, rendering it a more fitting germinating-ground
than it found it. Moreover, the germicidal condition of the tissues
and blood-stream, entirely through the action of the virus, would be
evolved at the expense of the tissues. Does this not hold good of
malarial fever? Not only does it protect for a time, like all germ-
diseases, but, such as it is, the protection is followed by positive
unprotection, or increased liability for a corresponding time. There
is no more persistently recurrent germ-disease than ague. This
transient and fading protection, however, with recurrence of the
germ-disease, is the fundamental characteristic of the entire preventive order, and marks it sharply off from the strictly prophylactic
order. But the subsequent state of unprotection will, likewise, be
transient, and, like that of the immunity experienced before it, will
be strictly proportioned to the amount of virus which has been
elaborated in the course of the malady, and which has been necessary
to produce it.

But if the virus of a preventive germ-disease causes the morbid
phenomena and occasions the germicidal condition of the blood-
stream and special tissues which results in prevention; and if, therefore, the process of prevention and protection is strictly pathological,

it may not always be so. In an extremely recurrent germ-disease, occurring month after month, and which has been thus transmitted through the suffering race of animals for very many generations without cessation, the virus of the malady, instead of occasioning a bactericidal and preventive condition may, ultimately, have aroused the phagocytic function of the entire amœboid order of cell in the economy. In this way a positive phagocytic function may, in the long run, have been excited and established, not merely in the very active leucocytes of the circulation, of the spleen and the marrow of bones, or of the osseous and lymphatic glands, but finally, in even the corpuscles of the connective-tissue. In such a case there would be attained complete protection from prophylaxis, not immunity or prevention; and the process would likewise be physiological. There would be no pathological germicidal product in the serum; for the pathogenic micro-organism on infection would always be promptly destroyed and devoured by the phagocytes. In this case the preventive germ-disease, however disastrous, would steadily lessen in virulence; and, as the phagocytic function in the leucocytes increased and became established, the germ-disease would, ultimately, become a *nomen morbi*, and then altogether cease. Nor is wanting some evidence to support this view. This final process may have occurred in some of the severest of even the preventive germ-diseases. Acute rheumatism is probably more fatal in the dog than in man; and tuberculosis is more acute and deadly in man than in the cow. But, still more significant, amongst the natives of tropical countries, especially the negro, ague or malarial fever is not anything like so severe, nor by any means so common or persistent, as in the natives of the temperate regions of Europe or North America, who temporarily inhabit the tropics. Why is this? A European or an American will tolerate either the heat of the tropics or the cold of the Arctic regions as well as a negro. It has been suggested that in consequence of the scarcity and the feebleness of the ague which occasionally appears in the natives of the tropical jungles the serum of the negro might be serviceable for preventive purposes.

But the protection, now experienced by the negro, although not yet absolute or superlative, does not wholly consist in a pathological condition of the serum or flowing blood-stream, or of certain tissues. It probably lies solely in the phagocytic function of the leucocytes which has been excited and established by the virus and through very many ages of transmission of the malady through the race.

Thus, ultimately, in both the prophylactic and the preventive order phagocytosis is a most important factor of protection. But in even a persistently recurrent, preventive germ-disease, such as ague, the phagocytic function, with its prophylaxis, can occur and be established only after a constant and incessant transmission of the disease through a race for very many generations, and for centuries upon centuries. Ultimately, the protection in such a case is as physiological or phagocytic as that imparted by a prophylactic germ-disease, and with the serum or blood-stream or special connective-tissues as devoid of a pathological germicidal condition. These, however, may not be altogether without germicidal properties; but this condition will now, as we shall see more fully presently, no longer be pathological, but essentially physiological and absolutely indispensable to the race.

Turning, now, to rabies, what is the nature of the protective condition which is imparted by the malady, or after a course of M. Pasteur's preventive inoculations? On reinfection, how is the rabies-microbe blighted? M. Pasteur, himself, viewed his course of inoculations as strictly analogous to a "vaccination," and the protection which they imparted as a genuine prophylaxis, similar to that imparted by vaccine against smallpox, or the modified-virus of anthrax against anthrax. And this view, as we have seen, is likewise held by some of the highest exponents of the disease, and particularly by the great commission of experts who reported in respect of M. Pasteur's inoculative treatment, for the Local Government Board. If this be so, it must be due to the fact, as already stated, that rabies is, in itself, a strictly prophylactic germ-disease, not preventive. On reinoculation or reinfection, the rabies-microbe will consequently be, after M. Pasteur's graduated course of inoculations, immediately devoured by the phagocytes of the circulation; phagocytosis being the fundamental factor of the protection. Is rabies, then, a prophylactic germ-disease like smallpox? It is certain that the character and the amount of the protection imparted are strictly commensurate with the amount of virus in the inoculations. It is, therefore, a quantitative and virulent protection, the amount of immunity being determined by the amount of virulence. If this is so, as in the strictly preventive order of germ-disease, the whole process is distinctly pathological. Consequently the protection, such as it is, will not be enduring, and this is precisely what one finds to be the fact. The protection is fading and transient, and in no way different from that of any other preventive virus. It is, therefore, as in such cases, probably due to the existence in the system of some germicidal morbid product, which has been eliminated by the living, but deteriorated, tissues, not by the pathogenic micro-organism itself, but in response to its deadly virus. After such "protection" or "prevention" has been acquired, the rabies-microbe, which is there-after introduced in infection, is at once destroyed by the serum or liquor sanguinis to be immediately absorbed and devoured by the wandering absorbents of the blood-stream.

CHAPTER XII.

THE RELATION OF BACTERIAL AGENCY TO SECRETING ORGANS, AND TO THE EVOLUTION OF THE ANIMAL ORGANISM.

Is prevention, then, or prophylaxis the last result of germ-disease? Does the phagocytic function of the wandering cellular system in the long run end bacterial life in the animal kingdom? Is a pathogenic micro-organism, like the rabies-germ, always to be pathogenic? Or is the merely convulsive form of the disease characteristic of the dog, and of the entire attenuating division of the animal kingdom, only to be compared with the slight malarial fever of the natives of tropical regions, being in reality but a fading, final form? Is the micro-organism always to be cultivated in the same centric connective-tissue ; or does this tissue, with the micro-organism itself, never undergo any modification?

That, in the course of time, and in the course of many ages of transmission, there is much specialisation, there can be no question. Certain it is that the strictly prophylactic germ-diseases have, one and all, a tendency to deteriorate and to become less severe, and finally even to disappear. Where, nowadays, are "the plague" and any of the "pestilences" of the Middle Ages, or probably not a few equally disastrous but unknown maladies of pre-historic times? Is syphilis so malignant? Is measles, whooping-cough, or even mumps so severe? But all these germ-diseases are essentially and powerfully prophylactic. Relatively mild or slight as they now are, probably they are not less potently prophylactic than when they were severe. Hence, the value of vaccination. Nevertheless, they are still as deadly as ever in an aboriginal race. It is preeminently the prophylactic germ-diseases which thus deteriorate through transmission,

and ultimately disappear. Erysipelas, pyæmia, diphtheria, tuberculosis, pneumonia, acute rheumatism, tetanus, rabies are still as
malignant and deadly as in the Middle Ages, or in civilised as
in savage life. It is significant that, even now, the distinctly recurrent or preventive order is of the widest range, not merely
through the animal economy itself, but also over the entire animal
kingdom. The lower down the scale of animal life one goes the
more does the exclusively recurrent order prevail, or the more
wholly does the pathogenic micro-organism find its seat of cultivation
in the elementary, skeletal connective-tissue. If the recurrent order
of germ-disease is the easiest to "prevent," with its own virus or
germicidal serum, it is the most difficult to eradicate out of the
animal kingdom; and it is all the more stubborn in its recurrence
the more lowly and embryonic the connective-tissue in which its
micro-organism germinates. The nearer in character this seat of
germination to vegetable or woody fibre, the wider and the more
persistent its hold upon the animal kingdom. In spite, however, of
the specialisation or modification which must take place in the
transmission of a pathogenic micro-organism through the animal
kingdom for thousands and even millions of generations, nay, in
consequence of this fact, there will still be as much difference
between the prophylactic micro-organism of leucocytic cultivation,
and the preventive and recurrent micro-organism of connective-
tissue cultivation, whether centric or peripheral, as there is between
wheat and the wild grass from which it has been derived. And there
will be as much difference between a preventive micro-organism of
centric, and that of peripheral, connective-tissue cultivation, as there
is between one grass and another. The difference will be in reality
as radical and as persistent in the one case as in the other; the
respective micro-organisms being no more "mutually transmutable,"
and, above all, directly and immediately so, than are the wheat and
the wild grass.

Nevertheless, even the most stubbornly recurrent of the preventive germ-diseases, after very many ages of transmission, must
undergo some process of modification and deterioration, and
probably, likewise, solely due to the phagocytic function of the
leucocytes which they ultimately establish. As we have already
seen, this is likely enough in respect of the malarial fever of the
natives of the tropics, as compared with that of the natives of
Europe or North America living temporarily in the tropics. Is

canine-rabies, then, or the merely convulsive rabies of the entire attenuating division of the animal kingdom, such a fading form, and due to the many ages of transmission of the disease through the dog? This does not necessarily follow. A preventive recurrent germ-disease, to be transmuted to a fading, final form, not only must be transmitted through many generations, but must be very frequently and even incessantly transmitted, the disease being constantly and excessively recurrent. Such a germ-disease has been the ague of the tropical regions. Is this true of canine-rabies? Years may elapse without any epidemic arising. The disease has not continuously and incessantly prevailed in the animal. The attenuating property of the dog, as that of the entire attenuating class, may be due to an exceptionally high phagocytic power. But this phagocytic power has not been acquired and established by a transmission of rabies for very many ages through attenuators. There are very different grounds for their stubborn refractoriness to the disease, and for their marvellous power of attenuating its pathogenic micro-organism. The monkey, for example, is even a more potent attenuator than the dog. Yet, in tropical Africa, where the monkey abounds, rabies has never been heard of. How has this animal come to be such an attenuator of the rabies-germ? Most certainly not because the disease has been transmitted through the race.

Is, then, the establishment of prevention or of prophylaxis the only end of germ-disease or of the pathogenic micro-organism? On the contrary, there is probably a very large class of micro-organisms, which, once pathogenic, phagocytes do not attack nor germicidal serum deteriorate, and the virus of which, ultimately, becomes even physiological, and indispensable to the animal in which it is at last incessantly elaborated. And this indispensable bacterial agency is characteristic both of the vegetable and of the animal kingdom, or of every living organism.

In the vegetable, not less than in the animal, kingdom there is constant bacterial agency which is not only harmless to the plant-organisation, but ultimately indispensable ; there is habitual fermentation, and the elaboration of virulent not less than of innocuous products. How do these originate? Have micro-organisms no influence whatever in their production? Why should such virulent poisons as morphia, atropia, aconitin, conium, nicotin, curare, jaborandi, strychnine, croton-oil, be at all stored in a plant, and not destroy it? Most certainly they would not be so stored in any

animal, and with the more injury the higher the animal in the scale
of organisation. But all these products, even the least irritating,
such as that of tea or coffee, are more or less neurotic poisons. For
this reason they may well be stored in plants ; for here there is
no nervous system and no such highly specialised structure to injure.
But the virulent product of every micro-organism which pathologically affects the animal organisation is, likewise, it is worthy of
note, primarily, a neurotic poison. It is the nervous system in its
highest and most specialised centres, both cerebro-spinal and
sympathetic, which is the first system to succumb to a deadly virus
in the circulating fluids. Are these plant-principles, then, the
products of the plant itself, or of a special organ differentiated for
this end? Are the turpentines of the pines, the alcohol of the
palms, the active "essences" of the juniper or of the Indian hemp,
or even the various "perfumes" of flowers and leaves, the direct
and exclusive products of the plant itself? If so, they are in reality
specific "secretions" on the part of the plant-tissues in which they
are so stored, and comparable to bile, urea, pepsin, &c., in the
animal organisation.

    If the active principles of plants are thus specifically elaborated
by special plant-cells it is surely not without significance that, in the
great majority, the so-called "secretion" is eliminated to the bark or
the leaves, or, in other words, to the most deciduous of its organs.
And in this way the virulent product is as effectually got rid of at
the fall of the leaf or the exfoliation of the bark as the virus-germ
of scarlatina is got rid of through the exfoliating skin or mucous
membrane. If, however, these principles are not in any sense of the
term "secretions," are they really the products, direct or indirect,
and extrinsic much more than intrinsic to the plant, of a specific
bacterial action which is constantly going on at the roots? They
may be the products of certain of the plant-cells which have been
acted upon by certain bacterial eliminations brewed amidst the
roots, and thereafter conveyed to the leaves, bark, fruit, seed, and
other such structures. Again, some of these products, and the most
indispensable of any, may be elaborated by specific micro-organisms,
not necessarily in the soil, but occasionally, if very rarely, *in the
plant itself*, in specific plant-cells, specialised with and for this
result. And the micro-organism may be transmitted to these
structures through and by either the flowing sap, or Gardner's
radiating connecting-cells, or both.

If the poisonous extracts in the youngest and loftiest twigs, or even in the seed, are elaborated *ab extra*, it is certain that such principles might be conveyed to any of these structures. A strong solution of morphia, poured over the roots of a camellia or rose in a flower-pot, will completely narcotise it. The alkaloid will be absorbed by the rootlets, and from these conveyed through the plant to the remotest twig or blossom. The leaves will at length curl, and the flowers, one and all, close their petal-lids, and the plant go to sleep for hours. If, therefore, either toxic or innocuous and nutritious products are elaborated through bacterial activity at or in the roots of plants, these principles might well be absorbed by the root-cells and specially relegated to the remotest structures which are capable of tolerating and storing them, and which have been specialised for this end. But the micro-organism which induces such products will not necessarily likewise be absorbed. And this in reality would be but similar to, if not the prototype of, the preventive germ-disease in the animal kingdom of strictly peripheral cultivation.

It is most certain that the immediate environment of the roots of plants is the natural habitat of well-nigh every kind of micro-organism, and that under favourable conditions they are for ever crowding up from this nether region, "seeking what they can devour." One can, therefore, understand why "even light from the sky," as Sir Douglas Galton demonstrated, should prove so fatal to most of them ; for the soil is their habitual home ; and in the soil no light disturbs their dark and weird activities. Nor is the existence of this teeming underground-world altogether inexplicable. According to Lord Kelvin's brilliant hypothesis, the living forms which first made their appearance on earth, far from originating spontaneously and *de novo* in the earth, were brought hither from other worlds, or from the interstellar spaces of ether itself, and mainly through cosmic dust[1]. Startling as this suggestion was when first announced, it has gained wider assent every year. Not that the hypothesis accounts, or was for one moment meant to account, for the origin of life. The origin of life, or even of consciousness itself, is wrapped apparently in deeper mystery the further scientific investigation penetrates into the arcana of Nature. But in the light of this suggestion it is perfectly conceivable why

---

[1] Presidential Address by Sir William Thompson to the British Association at Edinburgh, 1872.

micro-organisms so perpetually overcrowd the superficial soil of the globe and, as still, its simplest primordial living forms; for, with its teeming hosts of micro-organisms, it is as a very celestial mantle for the planet.

It is not merely in extremely populous towns and cities where micro-organisms, pathogenic or otherwise, swarm. Wherever there is overcrowded life, whether of the vegetable or animal kingdom, but particularly the former, micro-organisms exist in the soil in seething shoals, and in the steamy exhalations perpetually float through the adjoining ever-moving air and water. Where there is little or no vegetation or no animal life, as on barren mountain-tops, barren ice-fields, or arid deserts, micro-organisms are conspicuous for their absence.

"Where any such a series of (M. Pasteur's) flasks (of sterilised liquid) were opened, and resealed, in an inhabited room, *or under the trees of a forest*, multitudes of minute living forms made their appearance in them[1]."

It is by means of certain classes of these micro-organisms that all decayed or dead vegetable or animal matter in the soil is sooner or later transmuted and removed. But for this unceasing bacterial agency, and its beneficent underground-work, our planet would, as M. Pasteur has said, speedily become "encombré des cadavres." Through the action of such micro-organisms, dead vegetable or animal matter literally melts and is absorbed by plants to become alive once more. Elements are prepared from the dead matter, and specially *predigested*, by the micro-organisms, for the use and benefit of the vegetable world, which the vegetable kingdom could never prepare for itself. Without this invisible under-world of incessant bacterial agency, the upper-world of life and beauty, and in the vegetable not less than in the animal kingdom, would soon be at a stand-still and cease. Their transmuting activity extends, not only to decayed and dead organised matter,—for, here, the substance is of the loosest conformation,—but to certain mineral or inorganic, not less than to all organic substances; nay, even to gases and to the elements of the atmosphere itself. They are capable of analysing the most complex compounds into their ultimate elements; and, under favouring circumstances, of synthesising the simplest elements into complex compounds. They are capable of modifying the ultimate chemical elements themselves

[1] Presidential Address by Lord Lister to the British Association at Liverpool, 1896

into their various "allotropic" forms or conditions. Vitriol, *e.g.* has been demonstrated by French and American chemists as the product of certain micro-organisms in india-rubber tubing. This is, surely, a marvellously virulent compound to be elaborated in any medium by so simple, so infinitesimal a protoplasmic being! But if so potent an inorganic compound may be thus synthesised by bacterial agency, so may be even the hydrochloric acid of peptic fluids. And if complex organic compounds may be split up into their simplest elements, as in the case of urea and ammonia, so, in like manner, may be even inorganic compounds. It is not merely in the animal and vegetable kingdoms that bacterial agency exists, but probably, hardly less so, in the still vaster mineral kingdom. Whether this be so or not, unquestionably it is solely due to the bacterial agency around the roots that plant-life owes the most important of its food or predigested pabulum. As this is the fact, it is probably likewise directly or indirectly due to specific bacterial agency that even the most toxic plant-principles, if not every "alkaloidal" product whatever, are elaborated, down to the very perfumes of flowers and leaves.

It is not without significance that the plants which most abound in toxic principles are preeminently the plants which grow in a soil teeming with micro-organisms, and particularly with pathogenic micro-organisms. The plant whose habitat is likewise the favourite haunt of pathogenic microbes may be relied on to yield an "alkaloidal" product of some kind, which is certain to be one of the most potent of virulent principles, and like the virus of germ-disease a genuine neurotic poison. Conversely, the plant whose habitat is constantly devoid of such micro-organisms may be relied on to yield no virulent principle. Thus, even the nettle has its poison-sting, killing outright the hardiest caterpillar. The hemlock and the henbane, the belladonna and the aconite, and many more natural grave-yard growths, may be taken as other examples. All these plants grow luxuriantly in a soil teeming with pathogenic microbes. Consequently, every such plant is well-nigh saturated in every structure with the virulent principle characteristic of the plant ; the extent of the saturation depending upon the amount of the micro-organisms in the soil. One and all of our cultivated plants, on the contrary, and our domestic vegetables, carrots, cabbage, turnips, have no such virulent principle. Whilst many of the umbelliferous plants, such as hemlock, are extremely deadly, and never eaten by cattle, some of them, such as the carrot and parsley, which do not grow on fœtid soils, teeming with micro-organisms, have no toxic principle at all, but are harmless and extremely nutritious. Again, the European corn-poppy, which so blazes in waving fields of wheat and oats, yields no opium; nor does the white Indian poppy itself, when cultivated in a well-drained soil, frequently upturned, and freely exposed to the air and light. In like manner the wild belladonna, growing in a densely shaded, stagnant ditch, is much richer in the toxic principle characteristic of the plant, and this principle more concentrated, than the belladonna which grows in a well-drained garden. In all these and many more the virulent product is uniformly diffused through all structures. However otherwise differing from each other in structure and form, and whatever their natural order, only the plants which live exclusively amidst pathogenic micro-organisms are poisonous through and through. And it is important to note that the penetrating, spreading rootlets must be neither too deep in the ground nor too shallow and superficial, or no such principle will be elaborated; in other words, they must be neither below the sphere of the agency of the micro-organisms, nor too exposed to the breezy air and sunshine. The plant must be neither a giant oak nor beech, on the one hand, nor a sand-rush, a grass nor a saxifrage, on the other. It must be habitually located in, what one may term, *the bacterial zone* of the soil.

Now, if virulent products are elaborated in the soil or amidst the tissues of roots, it is certain that they could be absorbed by the plant and relegated to special structures. They might be conveyed by the flowing sap, but without their micro-organisms, to the remotest structures, as the blood-stream conveys the virus of every strictly peripheral preventive germ-disease, without its specific micro-organism. Or, more likely, they might be transferred from the root-tissues to their ultimate destination by and from one to another of Gardner's very remarkable radiating cells, and through a definite specialised train of such connecting-cells. In this connection the recent researches of Gardner on "The Histology of the Cell-wall" are of profound significance. "There can be little doubt," as he justly concludes, "that such connecting-threads occur universally in the cells of *all the tissues* of all plants[1]." But what a united, vital, complex totality does this show even the commonest plant or weed to be! "From this," says Lord Lister, in summarising the masterly

[1] *Proceedings Royal Society*, 1897.

research to the Royal Society, "arises the fundamental conception that the plant-body must be regarded as a connected whole. And the transmission of impulses and of nutrient material from one part of the vegetable organism to another, quite unintelligible as long as the protoplasm of each cell was believed to be shut off from that of its neighbours by a wall of cellulose, receives a ready explanation[1]."

But if "nutrient material" is prepared *ab extra*, or predigested by micro-organisms from dead animal and vegetable substance, and if, likewise, it should be thus absorbed by the vegetable-cells of the roots, and transmitted by and through a train of the latter to every part of the plant; so, in the same way, may other products, toxic not less than "nutrient," which are thus elaborated. This may be habitually accomplished by a very special train of the Gardner connecting-cells, the train, in the course of ages, having been specialised for this very result.

Is it, then, probable that the virulent principles of a plant are elaborated solely in and by the organs where they are so exclusively stored, and as "secretions" of these organs? Is the quinine of the cinchona, or the salicin of the willow, or the croton-oil of the seed, or the atropia of the fruit, or the rhubarb of the root, a secretion proper of the inner tissues of the bark, or of the special tissue of these structures? One might as well assert that urea and uric acid are elaborated exclusively in the urinary bladder, because they are found so invariably in this organ.

By this ceaseless process of fermentation in the immediate environment of the root-tissues—and all fermentation is bacterial—it is even conceivable why the nux vomica tree should yield so concentrated and so potently virulent a principle as strychnine; a principle which, in its pathogenic results, is hardly to be distinguished from the virus or the extremely virulent product of the tetanus-bacillus itself. But if the strychnine of the vegetable kingdom be thus induced through bacterial agency, the virulent product would be elaborated in a mode really analogous to that of tetanus in the animal kingdom. In both cases, the specific micro-organism, directly or indirectly elaborating the toxic product, would be strictly fixed and peripheral in its cultivation. And in both cases the virus elaborated produces in the entire animal kingdom identically the same spinal disease, and amidst the motor, not the sensory, roots

[1] Lord Lister's Presidential Statement to the Royal Society for the year 1897 See *Nature*, Dec. 2, 1897.

of the spinal cord. If, then, there be a specific micro-organism as the main factor of the strychnine of the nux vomica, from its pathogenic results in the animal kingdom it must be closely allied to, if not a member of, the same family as the bacillus of tetanus itself. And, as connected with this possibility, the exceptionally high mortality from tetanus in India is not without interest. Tetanus is much more prevalent in India than in Europe or America; in ancient decayed villages of the country districts and in forests it is more or less a constant and extremely common disease. But India constitutes the exclusive home of the nux vomica; and from this plant-organism strychnine is alone derived. Consequently, if the strychnine elaborated in the plant be the result of bacterial action, manifestly enough the particular microbe and the bacillus of tetanus, whether allied or not, thrive and crowd in the Indian soil as in no other. But it may be said, and with truth, that a bacillus of the tetanus order, or any other micro-organism whatever, has never been detected, much less isolated, from the root-tissues or root-environment of the nux vomica. Has it, however, been really searched for in such a medium?

But such virulent product, whether or not of bacterial agency, or whenever and however elaborated, in becoming specialised to one particular plant, or even to one particular organ, such as the ovary and the seed—the most sensitive and the most modifiable of all its structures—becomes in this fact a physiological in place of a pathological product, constituting an indispensable factor in the plant's "struggle for existence." Now if it be a stable, unaltering product, and of fixed amount and strength, or in any way serving for physiological ends, is it not in reality the "secretion" of the particular organ in which it is so exclusively found, and wholly the product of this organ? Not necessarily so. Secretions are not of fixed amount, or even of a fixed strength or standard. The organ in a plant, or in an animal, which constantly and exclusively stores a specific virulent product, may be specialised simply for tolerating and storing, not for elaborating it, as in the case of the urinary or the gall-bladder in the animal kingdom. Marvellous as is the differentiation which has been involved in the fact of such an extreme irritant as croton-oil being stored with impunity and, it may be, with the utmost benefit, in the seed-cells of a plant, it is not to be compared with the specialisation which has resulted in a hepatic, a thyroid, a peptic, a renal or a salivary cell, which are capable of elaborating out of flowing plasma of a uniform composition such various secretions as bile, thyroid extract, peptic-fluid, urine, and saliva. Specialisation of the tissues of particular organs up to the capacity-point of not merely tolerating but storing the most potent of toxic products undoubtedly frequently occurs in the vegetable kingdom. And than such toleration and accumulation nothing could more effectually ensure the distribution and preservation of the species. Where could its seed be more favourably planted, or how more favourably dispersed, than in the stomach of the wandering, hungry victim which it has poisoned! In so genuine a germinating-soil for sprouting, every micro-organism in the immediate neighbourhood, capable of analysing and transmuting dead matter, and of preparing or predigesting it into a fit pabulum for the young plant, would but aid in the process of its establishment and growth. All the virulent principles, therefore, which are stored in special structures, however deadly the principles over the entire living kingdom, are tolerated and stored, because they are, *ultimately*, whatever they were *primarily*, preeminently serviceable in the plant's struggle for existence, and may be looked upon as at length distinctly physiological accumulations. Nor is the toleration, much less the storing, of the most deadly poisons, and in the most delicate and sensitive structures of the plant, the result of only a few generations of exposure to such toxic products. Have they always been so inert and harmless?

On the contrary, it is not improbable that every such principle was in the first instance, and possibly for many generations thereafter, distinctly an injurious product, inducing more or less pathogenic results even in the plant itself. Take, for example, croton-oil. Before this most virulent irritant, living protoplasmic substance, all over the animal and the vegetable kingdoms, instantly recoils. In the animal kingdom it gives rise to positive necrosis of the amœboid cells. Is it conceivable that so potent and so universal an irritant was tolerated, as it is now tolerated, by the plant in which it was first elaborated? And is it at all probable that the seed, which now solely stores it, and which, as already stated, is without exception the most delicate and vulnerable structure of the entire plant, was originally as capable of tolerating and storing it? It took in every likelihood very many generations of differentiation of certain of the plant's cells, and at great sacrifice to the order of the plant, before so toxic a product ceased to be toxic, or could be stored by its seed. In like manner, it is possible that the strychnine of nux vomica, far from being in the first instance, as it now is, exclusively stored in the seed, was eliminated through the deciduous structures, such as the bark and leaves, and thus effectually and periodically got rid of as, at first, an injurious and, then, a useless product. Only by a prolonged process of differentiation on the part of the plant-tissues, and, at last, of the special cells of the seed itself, has the toxic product been converted into a physiological product of the first importance in the welfare of the plant.

And it is not merely in the welfare of the individual plant, as when the virulent principle is confined to the leaves, as in senna, cocain, jaborandi, but, ultimately, of the type or class to which it belongs, as when the virulent principle is exclusively confined to the seed, as in croton-oil. What could be more astonishing than the opium in a poppy-capsule? How has the plant come to tolerate, not to say to store up, and in the most concentrated form, so potent a principle—a principle which affects in the same soporific manner the entire animal and vegetable kingdoms, with the single exception of the poppy itself? Was the opium always thus tolerated? Was it never injurious to the plant? Was it always concentrated to the ovary? Is it un-reasonable to infer that strictly physiological in its end though the product may now be, and indispensable to the effective distribution of the plant, nevertheless, it may have been once upon a time, and for many ages, positively injurious and strictly morbific. It probably had, for a very considerable period, much the same effect upon the poppy as upon other living organisms, and was in reality, not a physiological, but a pathological agent, and constantly eliminated from the organism through the leaves or fading sepals or other deciduous structures. The highly concentrated form of such toxic principles, when exclusively confined to the seed or ovary, would in itself indicate alike a very gradual process of this concentration, and an equally gradual process of differentiation, which would be simul-taneous, on the part of the special structures involved in the capacity of storing it. In the seeds of the croton-oil plant or of the nux vomica, there is probably no larger quantity of the active principle than when, once, it was disseminated only through the leaves or bark, or through both structures. But in how concentrated and deadly a form does it now present itself! Any toxic principle, which is now exclusively deposited in the bark or leaf, serving at best but tempo-rarily to protect the individual from browsing cattle, may one day be still more concentrated and still further tolerated, and be found exclusively stored in the ovary or seed, and thus, ultimately, serving

to transmit and enlarge the species or class. The plant, which eliminates its toxic principle to the more transient deciduous structures,
is, perhaps, midway in this process of evolution.

But, in the vegetable kingdom, the micro-organisms which occasion
such products are, as a rule, not absorbed, and, most certainly, not
conveyed to the specific structures which store the products. The
bacterial life is even more strictly peripheral in site and activity
than the micro-organisms of tetanus, diphtheria, or erysipelas. If
plants are habitually surrounded by micro-organisms, and their roots
in constant vital contact with them, why should some of these never
take up their habitat in some special structure of the plant, and,
combining therewith, give rise to the ever-renewable elimination
characteristic of genuine " secretion " ? Why should the existence of
such micro-organisms in special structures be so altogether phenomenal, when their bacterial products or results are so common ?
It is no accident. As already shown, the absorbent corpuscles
of the entire living kingdom, whether of plants or of animals, are
more persistently phagocytic or microbe-devouring the lower one
descends the scale of organisation. The vegetable cells and the
primordial cells of the lowest animal forms, such as the sponge, are
in constant contact with micro-organisms, and depend upon their
phagocytic function for their very existence. As already stated,
it is in reality from such microbe-devouring cells that the phagocytic
function has been derived all over the amœboid or corpuscular order
of organism, even in the highest orders of the animal kingdom.
Micro-organisms, therefore, either in the immediate neighbourhood
of the lowest animal forms, or at and in the root-tissue of plants,
are as closely retained in their peripheral site and prevented from
intrusion into the organism as is the pathogenic micro-organism
of the preventive germ-disease of exclusively peripheral cultivation
by the leucocytes of the highest animal organisation.

Nevertheless, in the vegetable kingdom occasionally the micro-
organisms, themselves, penetrate into the tissues. And, what is still
more important, it is undoubted that these micro-organisms permanently reside and continue their bacterial agency in the vegetable
tissues which so absorb them. It would be difficult to exaggerate the
significance of this fact. It is probably one of the greatest discoveries
of our times. In respect of the direct and constant influence of
microbic life on plant-life, and in the interior of vegetable tissue, and
of the modifying power of such micro-organisms on even the simplest

ultimate elements of nature, it has been conclusively demonstrated by the late Prof. Hellriegel, assisted by Dr Wilfarth, that the papilionaceous sub-order of plants is capable of taking up and fixing in their tissues "the free or uncombined nitrogen of the atmosphere," and solely "*through the agency of the micro-organisms of their root-nodules*[1]." Apart from the brilliant elimination of argon by Lord Rayleigh and Prof. Ramsay, it would appear, from such a fact as this, that "the uncombined nitrogen of the air" is not so simple or so uncombined as had been for so long asserted. And, fortunately, Hellriegel's discovery has been demonstrated, over and over again, by subsequent research both in America and Europe, and is now well recognised by agricultural authorities.

How or why lupins, peas, beans, &c., should accumulate nitrogen, or from what source, "to render the soil more fruitful for the crops that follow," was an inscrutable mystery for ages. From the researches of Boussingault, and, still more so, from the very careful, combined work of Lawes, Gilbert and Pugh, it was deemed proved that, however such plants acquired and stored this important element, they were, *per se*, incapable of assimilating "*the free nitrogen of the atmosphere.*" And, without the specific micro-organisms in their root-nodules, or, in other words, if the plant itself be rooted in a soil without any, no such result takes place. Given the Hellriegel micro-organisms, however, then, through their perpetual agency in the substance of the root-nodules in which they reside, the free nitrogen of the air is being ceaselessly simplified or modified into some of its "allotropic" conditions, certainly into a condition which, so far as the plant is concerned, renders it easily assimilable. But for such micro-organisms and their ceaseless bacterial activity in the substance of the plant or in its plant tissue, there would be probably no papilionaceous sub-order, and but poor wheat-crops to follow, if any at all. As revealing the very wide possibilities of bacterial agency in the molecular transformations, chemical and vital, constantly going on in plant-roots and possibly other plant-tissues, this, without question, is a most important function. After such a revelation the discovery of a specific micro-organism with its bacterial agency in the root-tissue of the nux vomica or its environment would not be surprising. Nor would it be wonderful, if it should ultimately be found that, partly through the agency of micro-organisms, catalysis itself was due; and that likewise, were brought about the varying

[1] *Nature*, Nov. 7, 1895.

forms or modifications of, structurally, the same chemical compounds, such as the tartrates; or of the same element, such as carbon. In the same way, and through the same bacterial agency, even silicon itself, at least of the sandiest shores, might be transmuted into some of the carbon of which plant-structure is in so large a measure composed; for carbon and silicon are very closely allied elements; possibly with microbic agency, but "allotropic" or mutually transmutable forms.

Again, how has the nettle a poison-sting? What is this sting? Where or how did it get this venom-secretion? Is it in no way connected with bacterial activity, and in the tissues of the leaf? Strictly characteristic of the animal kingdom as is a secreting organ, or a very genuine physiological secretion of unlimited supply, it is not altogether unknown in the vegetable kingdom. In addition to the nettle, take, for example, the remarkable insectivorous order of plants. The Butterwort order constantly exudes from its stem and leaves a glairy, slimy juice which curdles milk, as is its time-worn country reputation, and, still more important, it dissolves and digests the curd and also many insects. The same is true of the Pitcher-plant, the number and variety of insects which it thus captures and devours being enormous. It is not less the fact in respect of the *Drosera* or "sun-dew" of our own moors. In this tiny plant we have a vegetable organism which constantly exudes through its leaf a peptic fluid, which differs very little, if in any essential particular, from the gastric fluid of an animal's stomach, and is quite as capable of digesting albuminous, organised material. Solely through this organ the plant subsists almost exclusively on insects and animal substance. The glittering globules of peptic fluid on the leaf attract and fascinate to their death insects, near and far. Place one of these, or even some particles of raw beef, amidst the sundewy globules, and the leaf will shut up and curl upon them, precisely like a sea-anemone; and, like the sea-anemone, it will dissolve and digest the whole of the animal substance before expanding again, but with a fresh supply of the glittering peptic globules. On the other hand, scatter on this dew the ash of a cigarette and the leaf will again close on the substance. But it will very soon reopen and get rid of the innutritious material, precisely as a sea-anemone will very quickly get rid of, and in the same way, a piece of cinder dropped between its tentacles. Moreover, and most significant of all, the supply of the peptic fluid, as the supply of the secretion in

S.   13 an anemone, is unlimited and ever-renewable, not in a fixed quantity as in the case of the croton-oil, the strychnine, or the opium in the seed or ovary of their respective plants.   Wipe with a camel-hair brush the secretion off the sundew leaf and in a short time it will expand once more and be as full of fresh, glittering secretion as before.   And this will take place if the peptic fluid be over and over again removed.   How has so insignificant a denizen of the moors acquired this remarkable secreting organ, with its unlimited, ever-renewable peptic fluid, so marvellously like that of the highest animal forms?   Why is the elimination of this peptic juice so unlimited, and likewise so immediate after its removal?   From these facts there can be no question that, however phenomenal in the vegetable kingdom, the leaf constitutes a secreting organ with a genuine secretion.

How has this been accomplished?   The attainment of such an organ even in plant-life, where it is so rare, is not wholly inexplicable. This anomalous secretion, now so invaluable to the plant, may in the first instance, and for a long period thereafter, have been virtually injurious, to be eliminated from the organism in and through the leaf, and elaborated through bacterial agency amidst the root-tissues in the marshy and highly decayed soil in which the plant solely lives, and where, without doubt, micro-organisms ever teem. And a specific micro-organism in the soil, capable of inducing such results even in the remotest tissues, may have itself at last invaded, or been taken up by, the absorbent cells of the root, and transmitted from these by a specialised train of the Gardner radiating-cells to the tissues of the leaf.   Even yet, however, and for many generations, or until sufficient specialisation of the leaf-tissues for the complete settlement of the micro-organism has been accomplished, the secretion may have been more or less injurious.   A time will come, however, when it will not be injurious, nor the micro-organism pathogenic, but quite the reverse.   Micro-organisms or their spores, as so frequently in the animal kingdom, may occasionally, even in the vegetable kingdom itself, be absorbed, and deposited in specific centric tissues, to germinate as in the most favourable nidus.   Certain it is that the Hellriegel micro-organisms in the root-nodules of the Papilionaceae are thus absorbed and habitually live in the tissues as in the most favourable habitat, converting, with and for the latter, the nitrogen of the air into absorbable nitrogen ;   the whole function in its final development being distinctly physiological.   If this transfer of a specific soil-micro-organism to tissues specialised for its reception does occur in plants, it must be extremely rare. On the other hand, so is the existence in the vegetable kingdom of anything like a true secreting organ. Thus, it is not beyond the range of probability that the specific micro-organism which induced, at the roots, a pathogenic product that for many generations was, without the micro-organism, eliminated to the leaf-structures and thus got rid of, has, in the case of the *Drosera* and every secreting plant, at length taken up its habitat in the specialised cells of the leaf. It might be conveyed thither through the absorbent cells of the root-tissues, and at last itself become, so to speak, a physiological micro-organism, to permanently induce the physiological secretion. By its habitual existence and activity in the specialised tissues of the leaf it transforms the latter into a very highly complex specific structure, very different from what it originally was, converting it into a genuine secreting organ. The leaf, now, both stores *and elaborates* the virulent principle, which is no longer pathogenic to the plant, but wholly physiological. It may have required an incalculable amount of specialisation to have effected such changes. This, however, is no objection. Evolution works on the intrinsic variability of living forms slowly, progressively and effectively, but with as silent harmony and with as great a total effect as if an invisible company of artist-spirits were habitually superintending the process.

Extraordinary as such secretions seem in respect of the vegetable kingdom, they are by no means uncommon in the entire animal kingdom ; in the latter, there are secreting organs everywhere. In the insect world, which, particularly in its embryonic stages, is so dependent upon the vegetable kingdom, and, significantly enough, is so intimately connected with the soil and the bacterial action incessantly going on in the soil, the attainment of toxic secretions is even of common occurrence. How many insects there are which are venomous ! Where or how have the gaudiest of caterpillars and maggots received their sickly secretions, in consequence of which the hungriest of birds will turn from them with shuddering disgust and dread ?

But, much higher in the animal kingdom, take the serpent's venom. Here is an appallingly virulent product which in a few hours, and in precisely the same way, is capable of destroying every animal but a venomous snake. As with the poppy or the nux vomica, the most insignificant of vipers will carry with impunity, and absolute immunity, in its venom-sac as much virus as will kill the most powerful mammal. And in this case, likewise, as most certainly in the insect world, the serpent-virus, however or wherever in the animal elaborated, is by far the most important weapon of offence and of defence which it possesses, and which has had everything to do with its keeping a place in the animal kingdom. So much so that it is hardly too much to say that, deprived of this formidable acquisition, the venomous order of reptiles would become practically extinct in a few centuries. Without its venom it would be one of the most harmless, possibly one of the most timid, creatures on earth, hardly less so than the "wild" rabbit itself. But it is important to note that it is only the most insignificant which are at all venomous, the giant-serpents and constrictors, such as the boa or the python, being stingless, and, in respect of their prey, as stealthy and butcher-like as the tiger itself. How did only the feeblest of serpents, and in proportion to its weakness, ever obtain so potent a virus, which has metamorphosed its whole existence?

The entire order, great and small, must at one time have been without the venom-secretion. Otherwise, there would be probably no member of the order which would not be venomous. Such a virus, therefore, must originally have pathologically affected the serpent as it pathologically affects every other animal to this day. How could so deadly a virus originate only in the feeblest of the race, except pathologically? And even to this day, how is it elaborated in such an animal, when it is no longer pathogenic, but genuinely physiological? Is it too hazardous to suggest that, as in the vegetable kingdom, and as probably in the insect-world, this virus likewise originated, pathologically, and to this day is elaborated, physiologically, solely through bacterial agency? If so, it was in the first instance a pathogenic product, and probably resulted from bacterial disease. The venom or virus was originated and specially elaborated in such an animal, and in the most hunted and weakest of the race, precisely because it was the weakest and most suffering of all animals; and because in this persecuted existence it was more and more driven to earth and to the richest haunts of pathogenic micro-organisms. For a very long period this most virulent product, however now elaborated, but in all probability still through bacterial agency, was, even for the serpent and preeminently, if not exclusively, for the weakest and the most hunted of the order, distinctly a pathogenic product. And it is only by a very prolonged process of specialisation of special tissues of the animal, with, possibly, a simultaneous process of differentiation of the pathogenic micro-organism itself to adapt it for living in the germinating tissues, and of subsequent concentration of its virus, that the venom has become capable of being tolerated by the animal and actually stored in a specific organ; and at last of being elaborated *in situ* by the specific micro-organism. In other words, this specific micro-organism has ceased to be pathogenic, and has at last made its permanent abode in the specialised tissues, to elaborate the venom in a physio-logical process indispensable to the animal's welfare. The pathogenic micro-organism has become really physiological: and its elaboration of venom in the tissues in which it is permanently located—the tissues being probably some highly specialised connective-tissue—has likewise become distinctly a genuine secretion, the whole apparatus being a complex secreting organ. But with such a natural history at what a cost of mere individuals must this acquisition have been gained! Nevertheless, however vast the loss, and for however long ages, surely it was not in vain. For, ultimately, how vast has been the gain to the species or type! How great the gain of such a secreting organ, even with bacterial agency, the persistence of the animal to this day proves, the entire animal kingdom being its enemy! In the animal and vegetable, not less than in the spiritual world, it is literally the scientific fact that the living organism is perfected only through suffering.

But, however the venom was originally elaborated, there can be no question that to the serpent itself it is now an absolutely harmless and physiological product, and secreted by special tissues in a genuine physiological process. It is a true secretion, not less so than saliva, pepsin, and bile ; but, in all probability, it is not nearly so old as any of these, and not anything like so established in the animal kingdom.

Now in the case of a rabid animal we have a rabic venom which is a toxic product of unquestioned bacterial agency. Like the serpent-venom, this toxic product is, all over the animal kingdom, still most poisonous. Will its micro-organism, however, always remain pathogenic? Or is this but a stage in its natural history, and particularly in the race of animals, the rabbit, where, at present, it is the most intensely pathogenic known in the entire animal kingdom? It is of interest in this connection to note that the rabbit, the most intensifying of the rabies-germ of all intensifiers, bears the same relationship to the great herbivorous race,—this entire class, as we shall see subsequently, being more or less capable of intensifying rabies on transmission,—that the smallest, the most persecuted and hence eventually the most venomous of serpents bear to the giant pythons and constrictors. As it so happens, the rabies-germ has by this time been serially transmitted through many hundreds of rabbits in the Pasteur Institut. With the result, that it has progressively increased in activity and germinating power, that its virus has progressively intensified in virulence, and that the disease has as steadily shortened in incubation. And this progressive intensification on transmission, so far as the rabbit is concerned, far from being fortuitous, is, as shall be shown, determined by fixed laws. The normal incubation-period of ordinary rabbit-rabies is "ten days." But by the serial transmission of this rabies through the rabbit there has been progressively evolved a rabies of nine, eight, or seven days' incubation ; and from this latter a six days' and a five days' rabies. If, however, this five days' rabies be still further serially transmitted, there is no reason why, according to the laws of progressive intensification, a rabies of one day's or even of half a day's incubation should not eventually be evolved ; for it has been established beyond doubt that there is no limit to the process of intensification.

In other words, there is no reason why the rabies-micro-organism, with its enormously intensified virus, should not in the final forms of the disease for the animal prove as rapidly fatal to all other animals as the venom of the serpent. Is it possible that the virus should ever attain such intensification, or its micro-organism such complexity of structure without modification? What have we already seen in the case of the malarial fever of the inhabitants of the tropics ? The same series of phenomena might occur in respect of rabies ; for both are preventive germ-diseases. In the long run the virus of rabies with its progressive virulence might, in a transmission of the disease through thousands of generations, excite and ultimately completely establish the phagocytic function of the leucocytes of the animal. By the attainment of this power, on its increase the rabies-micro-organism would be as progressively deteriorated and its virus correspondingly weakened, and the disease attenuated. Ultimately, the phagocytic power fully acquired would invariably destroy the micro-organism on infection, and the disease would cease. This may be the end of the malarial fever of the negro. Will it be the end of rabbit-rabies ?

The rabbit is too much of an intensifier of rabies for such a development ; it has no phagocytic or attenuating power whatever. Such development can, possibly, occur only in an attenuator, and in respect of exclusively the preventive order of germ disease. Hence, in the rabbit, or in any animal where phagocytosis in respect of rabies can never be established, the virus of rabies would only increase for every transmission ; there may be no limit to its intensification, and in time it would, certainly, be as virulent to all animals as the venom of a viper.   But if this were the case the rabbit-class, it may be said, would become completely extinguished ; so deadly a bacterial product, with its progressive intensification of virulence, sooner or later, exterminating the animal.   An entire species, however, is not to be extinguished so summarily.

The virus of rabies may continue to intensify in virulence as the micro-organism continues to be transmitted through the race. But whilst it continues to be more virulent for all animals, and at last as virulent as the venom of the serpent, it may likewise at the same time become steadily less virulent for the rabbit itself.   A condition of the blood, or of the connective-tissue which germinates the micro-organism, will be ultimately induced by the virus which will protect all tissues from the toxic effects of the virus.   This condition of the blood or tissues will at first and for many transmissions through the animal be essentially pathological, and the serum or blood-stream be germicidal, as in the case of tetanus or diphtheria and other preventive germ-diseases.   The effect of the virus of rabbit-rabies on the tissues and blood-stream may at first and for long be pathological ; but will this always be the case ?   In the long run, this pathological condition may become really physiological, and the blood-stream in no way injurious to the micro-organism.   Do we not see this in the serpent?   Its own venom, which kills every animal, and even some plants, is harmless to the serpent itself.

Again, the phagocytic power of the leucocytes never having been aroused by the virus in such an animal as the rabbit, the germinating tissues, after much modification on their part, may in consequence be ultimately converted into the most fitting and an habitual nidus of germination for the micro-organism itself.   Then, possibly after considerable simultaneous specialisation on the part of the micro-organism for its new home, there will be in the end an organic incorporation of the two forms of life into one complex, compound life within the organism, which will at length become even a most beneficial acquisition, and strictly analogous to the serpent's venom-secreting structure. The rabies-micro-organism, now a permanent physiological micro-organism of specialised tissues, will still elaborate virus, which will become a secretion as indispensable to the animal as the venom of a viper. Hence, it would follow that the rabbit, the most timid and "nervous" of animals, would, in spite of its many ages of hunted persecution, nay, in consequence of its very weakness, ultimately become possessed of an organ of offence and of defence, which would render it hardly less formidable to all other animals, particularly the hunting animals, than the most venomous viper. Is such a transformation of germ-disease, from a pathological to a highly specific, permanently physiological process, impossible in the animal kingdom?

If the serpent-venom differs from the virus of rabies in being physiological and not pathological, it differs still more from the toxic principles of plant-life, physiological in their results as these may be. For the venom is not only tolerated and stored in special tissues or organs, as the strychnine in the nux vomica seed, but it is actually elaborated *in situ* in these tissues. It is not merely a product of bacterial agency of fixed quantum and quality, retained in the tissues for physiological ends, but an unlimited, ever-renewable, genuine physiological secretion; as much so as bile, saliva, peptic fluid, urine, etc., which are certainly much older than the venom-secretion, as old as animal life itself, and therefore so completely established and physiological.

What, then, is even bile, peptic fluid, thyroid extract, or any other elimination from a genuine secreting organ? How has such an organ originated in the animal economy? Why does a renal-cell never elaborate pepsin, or a peptic-cell urea, or a hepatic-cell thyroid extract, or a thyroid-cell all such secretions, since one and all derive their characteristic eliminated products out of one and the same bland, uniform fluid, the liquor sanguinis? However harmless, or even beneficial, the secretion to the animal which secretes it, has it always been so physiological? Is it possible that all the physiological products and processes in the animal organism, without one single exception, are likewise of essentially bacterial agency. One and all of the specific secretions are, even as physiological and absolutely indispensable products and processes, but as so many fermentations; as much so as if or when they were pathogenic and distinctly injurious to the animal economy. The secretions with their most complex secreting organs may, then, be regarded as so many specific fermentations and fermenting nuclei. Have they been modified and developed from morbific into healthy, from pathogenic into physiological processes and products? A definite micro-organism, which was at one stage of the development so persistently pathogenic, may be now located in or permanently inhabiting each secreting organ or its tissues, and, in vital combination with the latter, at the source of its characteristic, unlimited, ever-renewable secreting power.

But no micro-organism has been found in such a site ; even less than in the plant-tissues amidst the soil. Nevertheless the Hellriegel micro-organisms in root-nodules are certain and undisputed. But if they exist, with such enormous and far-ranging benefit to the organism, in the root-nodules of a bean, they may well exist in the specialised tissue of the leaf of a "sundew," to give rise to its secretion ; and if in this genuine secreting organ, in the venom-secreting organ of the viper, and in all the secreting organs of the animal kingdom. A definite micro-organism may well exist permanently in every kind of secreting organ, and as the fundamental factor of its secreting process, without the micro-organism itself ever being necessarily detected, much less isolated. There is no positive or ocular evidence of the existence of very many of even the pathogenic bacteria. Yet no one doubts their existence. Now, if there is likewise a specific micro-organism, residing habitually in every secreting organ, it must be of the minutest, infinitesimal form. Manifestly enough, even by the side of such a micro-organism as that of rabies or of scarlatina, the bacillus of anthrax, of diphtheria, or of tubercle, is simply of colossal proportions, or as a palm by a tiny moss or a blade of grass.

"We cannot look forward," says Lord Lister, "with anything like confidence to being able *ever to see* the materies morbi of every disease of this nature (germ-disease). One of the latest of such discoveries has been that of Pfeiffer of Berlin of the bacillus of influenza, perhaps the most minute of all micro-organisms ever yet detected. The bacillus of anthrax is a giant compared with this tiny being. And supposing the microbe of any infectious fever to be as much smaller than the influenza bacillus as this is less than that of anthrax, a by no means unlikely hypothesis, *it is probable that it would never be visible to man*[1]."

[1] Lord Lister's *Presidential Address at the Liverpool Meeting of the British Association*, Sept. 16, 1896. (Italics not Lord Lister's.)

Nevertheless, infinitesimally minute though it be,—much smaller, apparently, than Pfeiffer's bacillus of influenza,—even the rabies-microbe may be a gigantic organism by the side of the physiological micro-organisms here assumed to be permanently located only in living secreting organs, and to be at the source of their secreting power. That they have not been detected, or even suspected, is, therefore, no proof that they do not exist in such tissue, and constitute with the tissue a specific secreting organ.

There are, then, it would appear, what one may term physiological, not less than pathological or pathogenic, micro-organisms ; and the former may be in reality but a modified and highly developed form of the latter, and by its constant life and activity in the specialised glandular tissues of secreting organs the cause of every physiological secretion without exception. Consequently, the physiological micro-organisms must far exceed in number and variety the pathogenic, and be but an ulterior and established form of the latter. But the attainment of one such result, or of one secreting-organ, however long in being acquired, and at whatever loss of mere individuals, would ultimately be the greatest acquisition which the type or race of animal could gain ; for it would be the acquisition of an absolutely new organ and function, and of an altogether new power. Life would be immensely enlarged thereby, and still more enlarged for every such secreting organ evolved.

We have seen of what lasting importance has been the attainment of one secreting structure and secretion in the nettle, in the sundew, in insects, even in the serpent. It will not be of any less significance in the lowest vegetable or animal organism ; for it will constitute a factor of vital importance in the organism's struggle for existence. Much more important, it would constitute the initial factor of a practically unlimited process of specialisation and evolution. The pathogenic product of bacterial agency, which has ultimately gradually become a distinctly physiological product, and the pathogenic micro-organism which has, itself, taken up its permanent place and passes its life in specialised tissues of an animal or plant, and, in vital combination and co-operation therewith, become physiological, will sooner or later, if not simultaneously, initiate even a rudimentary nervous system itself. This phenomenon is to be seen in a faint, elementary form in respect of the *Drosera* or sundew, and has been incidentally pointed out by Darwin[1] and

---

[1] *Life and Correspondence of Charles Darwin*, Vol. III.

other investigators. In the history of an animal organism, or in the evolution of even the animal kingdom itself, this fact is of enormous influence and importance. If two such secreting structures were evolved in an extremely lowly organised animal, they would, in due time, as the result of their very existence, be linked to each other by a rudimentary sympathetic nervous system. It is significant that all the secreting organs of even the highest animals are still thus chained by electric links, the sympathetic system being in every form of animal *par excellence* the nervous system of the secreting system. The existence of only one secreting organ in the lowest form of animal life, nay, in a plant-organisation itself, such as the sundew, would concentrate the general sensibility and irritability of the organism to the immediate region of this secreting structure and its bacterial activity, and specialise its elements of sensibility and con-tractile motion into genuine nerve-structures. Without secreting organs there could probably be no specialisation of a nervous system, and no evolution further than a plant-evolution. The attainment of one secreting organ, at whatever sacrifice of individuals, would in reality be the first step in the evolution of even the lowest forms of life to higher forms. Without micro-organisms in living tissues and as an integral part and parcel of the latter in constant vital co-operation, without their habitual existence and activity in the specialised tissues in which they eventually live, there could be no genuine secreting organ or secretion, and no other organisation but that of the lowest and simplest.

Is this, then, the end of bacterial agency in the animal kingdom? It is a grand end, and more constructive than destructive.

From the dawn of life the constant contest between the bac-terial and the cellular or amœboid forms could only lead, either to the ultimate extinction of one or other form of this primitive life,—which may have sometimes occurred,—or, and much more frequently, to an harmonious specialisation on the part of both forms, and on behalf of each other, which would be practically endless. With the arrival of micro-organisms on our planet came the possibility, not merely of germ-disease and suffering, but, through the suffering, of all evolution to higher forms. In every organism and everywhere in the living kingdoms a progressive adaptation of the most primitive antagonistic forms of life, with a constantly widening correlation of function, has proved a not less subtle factor of variation and evolution than the bitterest struggle for existence, and has moulded and ruled the living world.

CHAPTER XIII.

IS CANINE-RABIES THE PRIMARY FORM OF THE DISEASE IN THE ANIMAL KINGDOM?

WHAT is the origin of rabies in the animal kingdom?

It has been taken for granted, from time immemorial, that rabies is essentially a canine malady, and that, wherever in the animal kingdom it presents itself, it is invariably of canine source. And it has been further maintained, likewise from remotest ages, that the origin of the disease, even in the dog itself, is always "spontaneous." Having once arisen *de novo* in the dog, and through a definite set of morbid states exclusively characteristic of this animal, and which may at anytime or anywhere arise, it has been viewed as spreading from thence to all other animals; the rabies of every other animal being in point of fact virtually a canine-rabies, and nothing else.

The absolutely "spontaneous" origin of the malady, or of any germ-disease, however isolated or sudden in its first appearance, has been completely disproved by M. Pasteur's brilliant research in respect of "fermentation." There is no evidence of any such origin, but of the reverse. Were there, however, overwhelming proof, the explanation would not be adequate; for, in its turn, it is much more difficult to account for than the rabies, the mysteriously sudden outbreak of which it so plausibly "explains." Such an argument, as M. Pasteur has justly pointed out, "does *not* solve the difficulty, and wantonly calls in question the as yet inscrutable problem of the origin of life[1]."

The origin of life, as it so happens, is more enshrouded in mystery than the origin of matter or of force itself. The origin of consciousness, or even its precise bearing to the most highly specialised of

[1] M. Pasteur's Address at the International Medical Congress at Copenhagen, Aug. 10, 1884.

protoplasmic matter, is, even yet, inscrutable; being much further removed from the scope of scientific investigation than the origin of the so-called "fixed" stars themselves. A bordering realm of mystery enshrouds these problems, through which the most far-reaching scientific gaze gazes in awe. As an explanation of any kind of origin, or even any kind of ending, but particularly in respect of morbid processes, "spontaneity" conceals, rather than reveals, the true cause of such processes, and is but a good example of what M. Comte so happily termed "the metaphysical" mode of explanation. Most certainly, so far as interpreting the origin and nature of such a disease as rabies is concerned, this explanation is less satisfactory or even scientific than the ancient, much abused "theological mode" of the Middle Ages, which frankly attributed the malady to the presence of "an evil and unclean spirit." This, at least, completely accounted for the terrific tempest of the disease, and even for its mysterious "spontaneity." Moreover, it was nearly right; for the living organism has never been more possessed of *an evil and unclean spirit* than in the case of this appalling disorder.

The micro-organism of rabies is never *spontaneously* generated, or elaborated by a spontaneous set of pathological conditions in the dog or in any other animal. It is not a pathogenic micro-organism transmuted or "modified" from some other pathogenic micro-organism; much less from a physiological micro-organism, or from any normal animal tissue. Beyond question it is a specific existence, with a life-activity and a life-history of its own; and in its specific character it is introduced in infection into the system of every affected animal. If this microbe is so infinitesimally minute that its form and structure have not yet been microscopically determined[1], it is not of paramount importance. For its existence and even character, whatever its specific form, and as the *causa causans* of the entire malady, have been completely proved by M. Pasteur's crucial in-oculative methods of research, in spite of the fact that, as a micro-organism, it still remains nearly as invisible as when, long ago, it was deemed an evil and unclean spirit.

But although it has been absolutely disproved that the disease, or any germ-disease, has a *spontaneous* origin, nevertheless, wherever or however it presents itself, that it is fundamentally, and always primarily, a canine malady, has been by no means discarded.

---

[1] Since the above was written it has been identified by Prof. Sormani of Pavia.

On the contrary, this doctrine has been insisted upon by many authorities, and preeminently by M. Pasteur himself, as even a fundamental axiom in the interpretation of the malady.

" Dog-rabies, the *ordinary* rabies," *i.e.* the "furious," not the "dumb" or paralytic rabies, "is," says M. Pasteur, "*the only rabies.*" In other words, the rabies of all other animals are but varieties and modifications of this primary form. Again, "whether in dog, man, ape, horse, ox, deer, sheep, cat, rabbit, etc., rabies *comes from the bite of a mad dog*[1]."

In like manner, and with still more emphasis, Prof. Fleming states, "that if the canine species were *completely* freed from rabies, the disease would be *no longer known*[2]."

From such statements, therefore, it would appear that canine-rabies is the initial form of all others; and that, moreover, a rabies of the ordinary "furious," not of the extremely rare "dumb" or paralytic, character is the originating form, not merely in the dog, but, through the dog, in all animals. As opposed to what M. Pasteur has so justly described as the altogether exceptional form—the "dumb" or "mortal," or completely paralytic canine-rabies of 12 or 11 days' incubation in the rabbit—the ordinary "furious" or convulsive-rabies of the streets of 15 or 16 days' (rabbit) incubation is so characteristic of the dog in the most extensive outbreak, and, over any other "variety," so prevalent through the animal kingdom, that he has not scrupled to infer that this particular form of the disease is the initial, originating form of all others.

This (15 days') furious or convulsive-rabies is, it would appear, much the most prevalent form in the entire animal kingdom, because, as M. Pasteur has frequently explained, it is in reality "the most fixed" in type of any, and "the most stable"; "the fixed virulence of this ordinary canine-rabies having itself come to the present degree of *fixity*, after countless transfers by bites through past ages[3]."

The modifications of the canine disease, such as they are, would, accordingly, seem to be of the slightest and the most limited character.

" And the modifications, *which are very limited*, appear to depend solely on the varying aptitude for rabies of the different known races[1]."

---

[1] M. Pasteur's Copenhagen Address at the International Medical Congress, Aug. 10, 1884.

[2] Prof. Fleming's Address at the International Congress of Hygiene in London, Aug. 12, 1891.

[3] *Comptes Rendus*, Feb. 25, 1884.

If the ordinary rabies, so characteristic of the dog, has so slight and so limited a range of "modification"; if canine-rabies be so "sensibly one in its virulence" for every race of dog, and under every condition of infection; if it be as "stable" in form and enduring in type as would appear from such statements, there can be no question that the assumption of the clinical observers of the remotest antiquity was amply justified; that the disease is essentially a canine malady; and that it invariably takes its rise in the dog-race itself, being directly or indirectly derived from this animal, wherever else in the animal kingdom it should happen to make its appearance. Moreover, apparently, it takes its origin in the dog, not in the extremely rare and phenomenal "dumb" paralytic rabies of 12 or 11 days' (rabbit) incubation, but in the ordinary furious form, so prevalent in and so characteristic of that animal.

It is true that in every outbreak, however extensive, a convulsive-rabies of 15 to 18 days' incubation is the most common. But significant though this fact be, it by no means follows that this canine-rabies is therefore "one in *its* virulence," or "stable" in the form and structure of its special micro-organism, much less that it is the primary, originating rabies of all modifications of the disease in all other animals. Mere prevalence of any given form over another in any race of animal, much more in the dog, which, as it happens, is one of the most powerful attenuators of the disease in the animal kingdom, does not necessarily make that form a persistently stable and originating type even for the dog-race itself, or the special race of animal in which it happens to prevail.

By what standard, then, if not by its prevalence, shall the stability and the fixed form of the disease be measured? Take the signs and symptoms as a test. So far as these active, visible phenomena are concerned, it is notorious that there is no rabies, not even hydro-phobia (which, however, is confessedly but canine-rabies in man), which is more varying and variable; every other case, as M. Pasteur has shown, "presenting its own set of symptoms," and, it may be added, even its own sequence of these symptoms. There is well-nigh every modification of rabies to be met with in the dog, as in every animal equally capable of attenuating the disease on transmission. Viewed from the symptomatic aspect the canine disease presents itself by no means exclusively in the two unvarying types—the so-called "furious" and the so-called "dumb" or paralytic rabies— which have so long been solely delineated by the strictly clinical investigation, but in form after form, graduating and coalescing from the severest to the simplest. Thus, every "variety" of canine-rabies, may be allocated to at least one or other of the following groups.

Firstly, the disease may be paralytic in character from its outset to death, *completely paralytic*, or never varying in this character. This group is certainly the smallest of all, being, as M. Pasteur has so frequently stated, "rare in the extreme, and altogether exceptional." The more canine-rabies has a paralytic element, with its implication of the secreting organs, the rarer it becomes. So rare is it that probably in the most extensive outbreak of canine madness it does not occur in more than 4 or 5 per cent.

Secondly, the disease may be convulsive at the outset, but paralytic at the end, *i.e. partly convulsive and partly paralytic*, the former element intensifying into the latter. This important division in reality comprises by far the greater bulk of the infective forms of the canine malady; but, as it rises in the paralytic element and, consequently, in its infective rate, it becomes the rarer. Of this division,

A. The *paralytic* element may be much *the more prevalent*, the convulsive character occurring only in the preliminary stages. As the convulsive character prevails for some time the furious or aggressive tendency will present itself; and this form of the malady will, consequently, be commoner than the first; it occurs in probably at least 10 per cent.

B. The convulsive and the paralytic elements may be *tolerably equal features*, the former always first in point of time, and the latter never relapsing into the convulsive character. This group is yet wider in range. The infective rate will still be very high, because the paralytic element is pronounced through a considerable part of the disease; and as the malady is, for a considerable time, of a furious character this will materially add to the danger of infection. This group will consequently be distinctly larger than the last, and occur in probably 20 per cent.

C. The *convulsive* element may be much *the more prevalent*, only being transformed into a paralytic character at the later stages of the disease. As, however, the convulsive character is so pronounced for so long a time, and as there is the paralytic element with its infective rate, this group is the largest in range of any of this division, and probably occurs in at least 30 per cent.

Thirdly. The disease in the dog may be *convulsive* in character *from first to last,* from its onset to death; *completely convulsive,* and never varying in this character, the animal dying "furiously mad." Under this head comes a very large number of cases in an outbreak; but, as they are virtually without a paralytic element, they are the least infective of all, a maximum of the convulsive element, as we have seen, corresponding to a minimum infective rate. This division is the most common of all, and probably occurs in at least 35 per cent.

Here, then, we have not less than five different modifications of the canine disease, coalescing from their extreme forms into one another. Accordingly, there is nothing stable or fixed about the visible symptoms and signs of even dog-rabies itself, prevalent though it be. There is nothing more characteristic of the malady, whether it be viewed in its incubation or its symptoms, than its lack of character or uniformity, and nothing more invariable than its constant variability. "Every case shows, so to speak, its own set of symptoms."

But the same variability is not less obvious in respect of the characteristic lesions of the disease, every case presenting its own train of lesions. A completely convulsive-rabies may have no other visible lesion than the slightest "congestion" of the bulbar substance. A convulso-paralytic rabies will have this, and more or less disorganisation of the nervous axis. A completely paralytic rabies will have complete disorganisation of tracts of nerve-fibre, and degeneration of the intrinsic specialised tissue of every important secreting organ, from the salivary gland to the kidneys. The ante-mortem and the post-mortem phenomena of dog-rabies, far from being uniform or constant, above those of any rabies of any intensifier, are variable in the extreme. As an illustration take the foreign material found at times so copiously in the stomach at an autopsy. The greater the percentage of cases in any epidemic, where the merely furious symptoms prevail, the more will this extraneous material be found in the stomach, and in a quantity proportioned to the predominance of the convulsive elements (particularly pharyngeal) in the case. But in a dumb or profoundly paralytic rabies, these convulsive characteristics are reduced to a minimum, and, often enough, are wholly wanting. The more completely paralytic the disease the more passive the lesions, and, therefore, the less is foreign material to be seen in the stomach. How can an animal, which is so collapsed with paralytic rabies that it can barely swallow its own copiously-dripping saliva, and in which all aggressiveness or fury is well-nigh extinguished, tear and "bolt" "straw, hair, carpet, earth," even "pieces of zinc," as a very young dog suffering from "furious mad-ness" has been said to do[1]? The higher the percentage, therefore, where, after death, this extraneous material is found wanting, the more will it consist of the essentially paralytic as opposed to the completely convulsive form of rabies, the absence of such material being a very fair measure of the paralytic element in the case. Con-sequently, its absence is much more significant than its presence even in the largest quantities. Far from being an invariable phenomenon, or even peculiarly characteristic of canine-rabies, it is at best but an indication of merely the more or less convulsive or furious forms of the malady, and of nothing else.

Or, again, and as a still more crucial test of the "fixed" uniformity of the canine disease, take its infective rate. Is this any more constant than the symptoms and the lesions? The infective rate, as we have seen, is wholly due to the amount of paralysis in the rabies. If the disease is without paralysis, or altogether convulsive, the secreting system, but, above all, the salivary secretion, will be unaffected; the rabic condition of the saliva being a profound indication of paralysis, and particularly of the sympathetic nervous system. But the more paralytic the rarer it becomes, the com-pletely paralytic group of dog-rabies being altogether exceptional. Nevertheless, the salivary secretion of this group must be constantly rabic, and its infective rate, consequently, ranging from 90 to 100 per cent. The convulso-paralytic rabies, although still very high, must be much lower in its infective rate; where the paralysis is pre-dominant, ranging from 60 to 90 per cent.; where the paralytic and convulsive elements are equal, ranging from 25 to 50 or 60 per cent.; where the convulsive element is predominant, from 5 to 25 per cent. Lastly, the almost completely convulsive-rabies will range from *nil* to 5 per cent., the paralytic element, with its infective rate, being reduced to a minimum. It is the fact, and of common occurrence, that a dog may have rabies and, as we have seen, die of the disease "furiously mad," whose bite or bites, even when effective for infection, are not by any means invariably, or necessarily at all, followed by rabies or hydrophobia, the salivary secretion of such a case being from first to last devoid of infective material.

Nevertheless, it is unquestionable that there are cases of canine-rabies, in which the salivary secretion is always saturated with "virus"

[1] See Report to the Local Government Board concerning M. Pasteur's treatment against Hydrophobia.

and invariably rabic.   But it is admitted by every authority that such cases are rare in the extreme and quite phenomenal, being confined exclusively to the most profoundly paralytic or so-called "dumb" or "mortal" forms to be met with.   It would thus appear that the infective rate ranges from absolute *nil* up to 100 per cent.; the disease rising in infective rate with every rise of the paralytic element, this paralytic and transmissible form becoming rarer as a canine-rabies the more pronounced the paralysis and the higher its infective rate.   Conversely, the rabies, however profoundly paralytic to begin with, as it is transmitted through such an animal as the dog, progressively falls in infective rate with every decrease in the paralytic element, and as the disease more and more approaches a wholly convulsive character.   Far, therefore, from the infective rate being "fixed," constant and unvarying, it is not less variable than the symptoms and lesions, and for the same reason.   It is wholly determined by the amount of paralysis in the case; which, however, as the disease spreads through an attenuator is an ever-decreasing and varying amount.   How, then, in the face of such facts, can it be maintained that the canine-disease is at all "stable" or "fixed" in type; much less that it is so above that of all other animals?

Or, again, and even still more crucial, take the incubation-period as the test.   For it is a law, to which there is not one single exception, that the form or potency of any given rabies, canine or otherwise, is inversely as its incubation, the maximum of virulent intensity corresponding to a minimum incubation-period; or, conversely, that a maximum incubation-period corresponds to a minimum rabies, or a rabies of minimum intensity of virulence.   Now, if the ordinary (15 days') canine-rabies of furious character, as opposed to the altogether exceptional paralytic or "dumb" form, be as persistent in type as has been maintained, then, in accordance with this law, the incubation-period will most certainly be equally constant.   Is this, however, the fact?   Take hydrophobia, for example.   The extreme variability of its incubation-period has been notorious from time immemorial, ranging, as it does, from a few weeks to twelve or even fourteen months and more.   Surgeon-Major P. F. Frazer has narrated a case, of the authenticity of which there can be no question, where the incubation-period was "not less than 18 months[1]."   And there is one other remarkable case recorded (which is probably not altogether unique), of a boy in Bradford, in whom the disease did not supervene

---

[1] *Indian Medical Gazette,* June 1887.

until actually "*five years* after M. Pasteur's preventive treatment[1]," and had this been more severe and thorough it would probably not have occurred at all.   But this variability, so characteristic of man, is not less marked in the dog, the incubation-period of canine-rabies ranging from a few days to many weeks or even months.   It may be said that the subcutaneous infections inducing canine-rabies—and in Nature, it must be remembered, there are no other—cannot but result in ever-varying incubation-periods; for, as we have seen, even with the same virus-germ from the same rabid animal, the incubation-period varies in every case, according to the amount and according to the site of infection.   Such period, therefore, it may be reasoned, can be no adequate test of the real stability of the rabies induced. This is true; because the period taken up by the conveyance of the micro-organism from the site of infection to the cerebro-spinal substance, which is its sole seat of cultivation in the animal economy, is not, strictly speaking, the incubation-period proper of the disease, but what above has been termed a *pre-incubation period*.   Incubation proper does not begin until the micro-organism has been actually sown in the cerebro-spinal substance.   It follows, that in every case of rabies to be tested, it is of prime importance to reduce this pre-incubation period to a minimum.   And this M. Pasteur has most effectually accomplished by his "subdural" or *intracranial inoculation*; the rabies-microbe, by this means, being directly introduced into its specific centre of cultivation in the cerebro-spinal substance, incubation thereafter ensues more quickly and regularly than by any other incubation or infection.   How far, then, does this most infallible test demonstrate the stability and typical conformity of the ordinary (15 days') canine-rabies?

Take, in this connection, the experiments performed by Sir Victor Horsley for the Committee of Experts, appointed by the English Government to inquire into M. Pasteur's treatment.

"In the case of rabbits," says Sir Victor Horsley, "inoculated, by trephining, with the virus from dogs dying of rabies of the streets, *the incubation was from* 14 *to* 21 *days*.   In all these cases, the symptoms were similar to those produced by M. Pasteur's 'virus' (of the ordinary furious canine madness), and those of rabbits bitten by rabid dogs from the streets[2]."

[1] See *Lancet*, and *British Med. Journ.* for July 1887.

[2] Report to the Local Government Board respecting M. Pasteur's treatment of Hydrophobia.

But a series of "viruses" of even dog-rabies of the streets—which, in spite of an intracranial inoculation, ranges from 14 to 21 days' (rabbit) incubation—is surely, after all, not quite so "sensibly one in their virulence" as would at the first glance appear. A virus-germ which will rabidise a rabbit only after three weeks is a very different virus-germ in point of virulence and capacity of transmission from that which under precisely the same conditions of infection will rabidise the same order of animal in two weeks. Where, in such experiments, is there any evidence of persistency of form or unyielding uniformity of type? It may be objected that these experiments, significant though they be, were on too small a scale to be absolutely conclusive. But the limited range of the experimentation only proves the more conclusively the extreme variability of even the ordinary canine-rabies of the streets. For if a score of experiments with ordinary dog-"virus" will yield such diverse forms of the disease, even with the intracranial inoculation itself, this diversity will not be lessened, but quite the reverse, with many such experiments. And this, indeed, is precisely what one finds on turning to M. Pasteur's own most extensive range of experimentation.

"With the object of knowing," says M. Pasteur, "whether dog-madness *was always one and the same,* with perhaps the slight variations which might be due to the difference of race in diverse dogs, we got hold of a number of dogs, affected with ordinary street rabies, at all times of the year, at all seasons of the same year, and of different years, and belonging to the most dissimilar canine races." In each case, the canine-"virus" was intracranially inoculated into rabbits under precisely the same conditions of infection, and with the object of *proving,* rather than of revealing—for it was a fore-gone conclusion—the stability of the disease.

"The results were as follows : All the rabbits, from whatever sort of dog inoculated, showed a period of incubation which ranged between 12 and 15 days. Never did they show an incubation of 11, 10, 9, or 8 days; never an incubation of several weeks or of several months[1]."

Nevertheless, a canine-rabies of even 11 days is not unknown, and has been more than once noted by M. Pasteur in the course of his investigations; although, it is worthy of note and not without significance, that a canine-rabies of less incubation than this, or of 10 days, *i.e.* equivalent to that of the *normal rabbit-rabies,* much less of 9 or 8 days, is altogether unknown. On the other hand, a canine-rabies

[1] M. Pasteur's Address to the International Medical Congress at Copenhagen.

of 21 or 25 to 30, or even 40 days' incubation in the rabbit, if not of several months' duration, has likewise frequently enough been noted. The incubation-period would, therefore, appear to range from 11 and 12 up to 25 and 30 days; the most prevalent form being midway between these extremes, or, a rabies of 15 to 18 days' incubation. Where, however, is there any evidence in such facts of stability in form or persistency of type in respect of the ordinary canine-rabies over that of any other form of the disease?

Clearly enough, the modifications of dog-rabies, far from being "insignificant," are considerable. But even if they were as "limited" as assumed, it does not follow that "these slight variations may be deemed due to differences of race in the diverse dogs." There is no evidence of any "varying aptitude" in different dogs, but quite the reverse, the entire canine race being, above most animals, uniformly refractory to rabies. This fact was absolutely established by the investigations of Mr Dowdeswell, which have been already alluded to[1]. It is true that some breeds are more frequently affected with the disease than others, whilst some, again, there is reason to believe, practically never contract the malady. But, as will be seen presently, the breeds which are most frequently affected are so irrespective of race or of any special and intrinsic aptitude; most certainly, not because they constitute, *per se*, a fitter medium for the cultivation of the rabies germ—if anything, the reverse of this is likewise the fact—nor even because they happen to be dogs at all. If similarly exposed to the same risk, all the breeds of dog, probably all animals, would be quite as liable to incur rabies; and it is certain that whole classes of the animal kingdom—the entire division capable of *intensifying* rabies on its transmission—would be much more liable. Assuming, however, that there is a "varying aptitude," and that this is as solely due to a difference of race and breed as has been asserted, it is an aptitude absolutely contradistinct from that characteristic of such an animal as the rabbit. If such a liability exists in the dog, it exists in a form and a direction diametrically opposed to that characteristic of the vast *intensifying* division of the animal kingdom. In such an animal as the rabbit "the aptitude for the disease" is determined by the comparative and even superlative fitness of the animal as a medium for the cultivation of the rabies-germ. In the dog, on the contrary, such liability would appear to be characteristic

[1] "Investigations of Canine Madness," by G. R. Dowdeswell, F.R.S. *Trans. of Roy. Soc.* 1887.

of, if not induced by, its very refractoriness. Paradoxical as the statement would seem, the less liable the dog, as a race or breed, to, *per se*, initiate or elaborate the malady, or the more refractory the animal in itself to the rabies-germ, the more frequently it is found, as compared with all other breeds of the dog, to be affected with rabies. In other words, this "special aptitude" is characteristic only of those breeds or races which are the most pronounced *attenuators* of rabies in the dog-race itself. Why the dog-race, in spite of its extremely high *attenuating* power, as compared with other animals, or, still more remarkable, why the most refractory of dogs should, nevertheless, be the most liable, even of dogs, to contract the malady is, surely, not without significance in respect of the origin of the disease, and has as yet by no means received the attention which it deserves. Be this as it may, it can be unhesitatingly asserted that the varieties or modifications of dog-rabies, far from being strictly limited, are considerable, and that they depend, not upon any intrinsic or special liability to the disease of any given breed over another, there being an unvarying lack of any such liability all over the races, but wholly upon the amount of infection; which, however, varies, not merely for every race, but well-nigh for every case of the same breed. The most refractory variety or, in other words, the most potent attenuators of the dog-race, may in point of fact invariably receive the most frequent and, moreover, the most potent and massive infection. And this, as shall be attempted to be shown, there is good ground to believe is exactly what occurs in Nature.

The ordinary furious dog-rabies of, approximately, 15 days' (rabbit) incubation, in spite of its extreme prevalence, as a rabies, and of being so "diagnostic" of the canine race itself, cannot, therefore, be looked upon as a fixed entity or specific form, constituting it the originating rabies of all other forms of the disease. On the contrary, it would appear to be one of the least stable modifications of even dog-rabies. Probably from the very fact that it is but an intermediate or fading, if not one of the *final* forms of canine-rabies itself, it is so prevalent in and so characteristic of the dog-race as the most pronounced of attenuators.

Prevalent as this particular form is over the animal kingdom, it, nevertheless, cannot be the originating rabies, not merely in the animal kingdom, but even in the dog-race. For if this were so, it would be invariably attenuated out of existence with a very few transmissions through a pack of such animals. If a rabies of, relatively, so feeble a character were the originating form, and if the dog itself were the invariable starting-point of this initial rabies, then it would without question be constantly extinguished by the time that the mere fringe of a pack of wolves or dogs became affected. In such a case the disease would never really become epidemical. For if there be one fact which has been more conclusively demonstrated than another, it is the exceptionally high attenuating power of the entire dog-race.   There is no rabies, however potent or of however short an incubation, which on a serial transmission this animal will not *progressively* attenuate to zero or *nil*.   And a rabies of merely the furious or convulsive form, or of 15 days' (rabbit) incubation, it will thus attenuate in a very few transmissions.

This was very clearly shown by Magendie's experiments already referred to.   The initial dog-rabies in this case was not at all feeble, but highly infective; for no less than four dogs serially, or one after the other, were rabidised by means of it.   But, although all these animals were rabidised, the (initial) rabies became *progressively attenuated*, the incubation-period becoming for every transmission of longer and longer duration; so much so that even in four transmissions the original, highly infective rabies was attenuated beyond the possibility of imparting infection, at least through the medium of the salivary secretion.   From such evidence, then, if there were no other, it is certain that the rabies, which is transmitted through a series of dogs, however potent and transmissible and profoundly paralytic to begin with, is not only *progressively* enfeebled by such passages—and in strict proportion to these passages—but that, as a rabies, it is likewise thereby 'disintegrated ' in form, becoming an altogether lower and feebler "variety" of the disease. And the virus-germ of this degraded and disintegrated form, however apparently "fixed" or specific the disease from which it was derived, is not a mere *fractional virus* of the initial rabies.   After the disintegration of the initial rabies has been effected by its transmission through the dog, this attenuated rabies is incapable even in the most intensifying orders of the fraction's immediate restoration to the original.   Henceforth, the process of intensification must begin in the latter order of animal, but only in the latter, *de novo*, and as with a completed and perfect "variety" of the disease.   If this be true in respect of the most potent dog-rabies to be met with —of 12 or even of 11 days' (rabbit) incubation—how much more so of the "ordinary" dog-rabies of from 15 to 18 days!

But this *attenuating* process has been most exhaustively demonstrated in respect of the monkey tribe, and by no investigator in so masterly a manner as by M. Pasteur. It was, so to speak, only by accident that it was at length discovered by him that the monkey was an *attenuator* of the disease; and that there was, therefore, an *attenuating*, not less than an *intensifying*, division of the animal kingdom: the latter division, for reasons which we shall see presently, being very much vaster than the former; and the ape being, like the dog, but a very typical example of an attenuator. After M. Pasteur's absolutely conclusive demonstration of the fact, it is unquestionable that a virus-germ of even the most profoundly paralytic rabbit-rabies to be met with, or of only 6 or 7 days' incubation, when transmitted serially through a relatively very small number of monkeys, is thereby so progressively reduced in potency that it is at length transformed into a rabies of distinctly less virulence than that of the most ordinary dog-rabies of the streets, and with a (rabbit) incubation of considerably longer duration than 15 days. By the simple process of transmission through such an attenuator, it would appear that the most pronounced paralytic rabbit-rabies known is rapidly degraded or simplified into the feeblest convulsive dog-madness known. Nay, further, in an amazingly few passages—five or six—it is transformed into a rabies of so slight a form and of so feeble a potency that its "virus," even with the intracranial inoculation, is incapable of rabidising a dog itself.

"A very small number of passages from monkey to monkey," says M. Pasteur, "suffices to bring down the attenuation to a point at which the virus, injected hypodermically into dogs, never gives rise to rabies in them. *Intracranial inoculation, itself,* may now remain without effect[1]."

The rabies-virus, thus diminished in amount and simplified in structure, remains so for every animal in the animal kingdom—for intensifier and attenuator alike—and for every condition of infection. It is no mere *fractional virus* of the initial rabies, which may be restored to its original form on even a second passage through the rabbit. The initial rabies, in consequence of its transmission through such an animal has really become attenuated into an altogether new and inferior rabies; the virus-germ unit of which, although enormously reduced in potency and simplified in structure, is, nevertheless, so far as it goes, still structurally complete and whole. In this

---

[1] *Comptes Rendus*, May 19, 1884.

animal it is obvious from such experiments that there is no absolutely or even relatively "fixed" degree of potency for any rabies, *i.e.* persistent and identically the same for only a few transmissions; and that the ordinary furious 15 days' canine-rabies of the streets would be attenuated beyond the possibility of imparting infection through the salivary secretion in an incredibly small number of passages.

But, as already shown, it is certain that the same law which determines the attenuation of rabies in respect of the monkey also holds good in respect of the entire canine-species. It is, however, even still too often taken for granted that the bearing of the dog-race with respect to the rabies-microbe is similar to that of the rabbit, the guinea-pig and the very large class of animals which intensify rabies on transmission. After Magendie's experiments, which are not less conclusive in respect of the dog than M. Pasteur's in respect of the monkey, it is certain that successive passages through dogs will progressively diminish the virulence of every form of rabies without exception, not merely for dogs themselves, but also for monkeys and all animals, even for the rabbit or the most pronounced of intensifiers. Since this is the case, is it too much to assume that the ordinary dog-rabies of the streets of 15 days' (rabbit) incubation, when passed serially through only four or five dogs, will have become thereby *attenuated* into a rabies of 25 to 30 days' incubation; if in so effectual a transmission through such an attenuator it will not have become wholly non-infective and, thus, as an epidemical disease, practically obliterated? If such be the fact, this ordinary dog-rabies of 15 days' incubation, however characteristic it may be of the dog-race, or however prevalent over the animal kingdom, cannot be so specific a form of the disease as has been assumed; not anything like the most stable and transmissible form of canine-rabies itself. It is only an intermediate, or merely inferior and transient form in the process of attenuation and extinction. Still more important, it therefore cannot be the primary and originating form of the disease, not merely in the animal kingdom, but even in the dog-race. It follows that every outbreak of dog-madness, however extensive, and even in proportion to its extent, originates, not in a rabies of the ordinary furious form and of, approximately, 15 to 18 days' incubation in the rabbit, prevalent at last though this particular form may be in the outbreak, but invariably in a rabies of more or less pronounced paralytic character, and of not more than 12 or 11 days' (rabbit) incubation, however rare and altogether exceptional this form of the disease in the dog. This would be a rabies of the highest infective rate and of the largest possibility of transmission through the race, or through any such attenuator.

Thus, it comes to pass that even in dog-rabies itself, the more or less paralytic or "dumb" forms of shortest incubation, not the ordinary furious or convulsive forms, extremely rare and even phenomenal though the former be as compared with the latter, are the most important in every outbreak, for they cover and include every lower form; they are much the most persistent and "stable," and by far the most capable of transmitting the disease through the race. The very infectiveness of the salivary secretion in the "dumb" or paralytic canine madness would alone bear out this view; for, as already stated, the salivary secretion of a completely paralytic case is probably saturated with infective-material, never failing to rabidise. In the ordinary furious forms, on the contrary, the salivary secretion is often enough, as we have seen, wholly devoid of the virus-germ; in a considerable percentage of cases, as so clearly demonstrated by Dowdeswell, absolutely failing to rabidise even with the most crucial methods of inoculation.

But although in every outbreak the initial canine form is thus in every probability of a more or less paralytic, not convulsive type, a rabies of 12 and even 11 days' incubation rather than that of 15 to 18 days, and, therefore, capable of the longest transmission and the widest diffusion of any form of canine-rabies, there is no reason to suppose that rabies of the dog is, in itself, essentially a paralytic, any more than it is essentially a convulsive-rabies. In spite of the extreme prevalence of the disease in the dog above all animals—but it is not more prevalent in or characteristic of this animal than tetanus is prevalent in the horse, above all animals—there is no reason to believe that, whether in its convulsive or paralytic form, it is essentially a canine malady at all ; any more than it is a malady of the monkey or man or any other attenuator, or any more than tetanus is fundamentally a disease of the horse. Most certainly, as already stated, rabies does not take its rise in the dog or in any other animal spontaneously, or through any set of morbid conditions peculiar to the canine race, and which may at any time and under any set of circumstances occur. If rabies be fundamentally a canine malady, wherever in the animal kingdom it presents itself, and for this reason invariably taking its rise *in the dog,* and only this animal of all animals, how comes it to pass that the systematic use of a dog-muzzle practically abolishes the disease? Why should this procedure abolish it? Of the fact itself, however, there can be no question. The statistics on this head, as we shall see, are overwhelming and absolutely conclusive. After the very remarkable results obtained by the use of the dog-muzzle, and in this country mainly by the statesmanlike stability and scientific insight of Mr Long, there can be no doubt that, if as rigorously enforced over Europe as it has been all over Sweden and Germany, rabies would seldom if ever be met with. But what is to be inferred from this significant fact? If rabies, in whatever order of animal it should make its appearance, be *par excellence* a canine disease; if, consequently, the dog be invariably the *fons et origo mali* in the animal kingdom, and in every case without exception its primary source, why should the mere use of a muzzle, however thorough, not merely suppress the disease, but absolutely prevent the possibility of its arising in the dog? Were the malady a specific canine disease, depending exclusively on this animal for its origin and existence, and wholly on morbid or pathological conditions peculiar to the dog, then, as a matter of constant occurrence, the disease would crop up in this animal, in spite of the most rigorous enforcement of the muzzle or of any other form or amount of quarantine. This, however, is not the case. From this circumstance alone it follows that rabies is not essentially a canine malady, any more than it is a malady of the monkey or man; and that it does not necessarily take its rise, primarily, in this animal, in whatever other animal it should happen to originate. Clearly enough, so far as the dog-race is concerned, the disease, as in the case of the monkey, and in probably every attenuator, is extrinsic or acquired, not primary or dog-engendered; the *causa causans* of the malady, even the malady itself, being something altogether *ab extra* to the animal. As proved so conclusively by the use of the muzzle, if the animal were kept permanently freed from this assumed external source of rabies, rabies in itself would never develop intrinsically in the dog. It has never done so where a condition of isolation or protection has been maintained.

But it may be asked, Why, then, should the dog, one of the most potent attenuators of the disease in the animal kingdom, incur the malady so frequently as compared with all other animals? Why does it contract rabies, and, to begin with, invariably in so potent and so infective a paralytic form? Otherwise, it would never spread through such an animal. Where does this primary infective and pre-eminently transmissible form come from, if not from the dog? From the foregoing considerations, is it too much to assume that it is not really a disease of any attenuator, and does not take its rise in the attenuating division of the animal kingdom? Is it, then, essentially a disease of intensifiers, and does it invariably originate in the intensifying division of the animal kingdom? There is not a little evidence to establish such a view.

CHAPTER XIV.

RABIES, A GERM-DISEASE OF INTENSIFIERS.

In the monkey, the dog, and probably man, and in the entire attenuating division of the animal kingdom, every form of rabies on transmission becomes less transmissible and progressively attenuated to extinction. But when one turns to the intensifying division of the animal kingdom a very different spectacle presents itself. Here, the simplest and feeblest form, the virus-germ of which is incapable of rabidising the dog or probably any attenuator is, on transmission, progressively intensified; the animal's nervous substance, for reasons which will appear presently, affording one of the most favourable soils in the entire animal kingdom for the cultivation of the rabies-micro-organism. In this all-important property, the one class of animal would appear to be a complete contrast to the other. And if the dog may be taken as a type of an attenuator, the rabbit most certainly may be taken as the most perfect type of an intensifier. There is probably no animal, even amongst intensifiers, which is more delicately sensitive than the rabbit to the virus-germ of rabies. A virus-germ which will altogether fail to rabidise the dog, or probably any attenuator, with the intracranial inoculation itself, will never fail to rabidise the rabbit, even with the subcutaneous inoculation; and this most feeble rabies will be, sooner or later, transmuted on transmission into the most appallingly potent form of the disease to be met with.

Rabies, then, is to be viewed from two totally different aspects, according to the division of the animal kingdom, whether the attenuating or the intensifying, through which it spreads. The dispersal of the disease through the canine-race or any of the attenuating division may be likened to the flow of molten lava from an active volcano.

The further the lava spreads from its source, the thinner and the less active it becomes; till, speedily, it loses all activity whatever; the point of origin, from first to last, being the most potent centre of the entire flow. This primary, glowing centre may be compared with the highly transmissible more or less paralytic form of rabies which, as an infective nucleus, invariably initiates an outbreak of dog-madness, but which, sooner or later, on transmission as invariably dwindles into the widely-spread "furious" or convulsive forms, so characteristic of the dog. These latter at last become so reduced in potency that they are incapable of imparting infection, the salivary secretion not being charged with "virus." The dispersal of rabies through the intensifying division of the animal kingdom may, on the contrary, be likened to the spread of a fire through a forest or great city. However trivial in origin, the further it spreads the more massive and the more potent for destruction will the conflagration become, its potency increasing progressively with the spreading flames and for every transmission to a fresh centre. And this, again, is but to be compared with the more and more pronounced paralytic, infective forms which are invariably evolved, and progressively so, on a continued transmission of rabies through intensifiers. Any rabies of the slightest form will, in such an animal, in only a relatively few passages, become a rabies of more or less pronounced paralytic form, and of but 10 days' incubation—the normal rabies of the rabbit. In point of fact, in an intensifying race a slight rabies is, as an initial form, far more dangerous to the race than the most potent paralytic-rabies to be met with, because it is much more certain to be intensified and transmitted. A very profound paralytic-rabies, from the outset of the disease, all but extinguishes aggressiveness or "fury" in the victim; and this is the fact in respect of even the dog-race itself.

There is thus, it would appear, this remarkable difference between attenuators and intensifiers; the more purely convulsive a rabies to begin with in the former, the more certain is it to be rapidly extinguished on transmission; whilst the more feeble the rabies to begin with, the more certain will it spread through the latter and intensify in the transmission. Conversely, the more potent the rabies to begin with in such an animal as the dog or monkey, the more certain the possibility of infection, and the further will the disease be transmitted and spread; whilst, on the contrary, the more profoundly paralytic the initial rabies in such an intensifier as the rabbit or guinea-pig, the more certain is it to prostrate the animal beyond the possibility of aggressiveness; the disease, consequently, dying out with the death of the animal itself. The animal is as promptly but as thoroughly extinguished with its rabies, as is a house blown up by dynamite in the heart of a densely built city, without the neighbouring houses necessarily taking fire.

These facts are well seen in the entire herbivorous order, which, there is reason to believe, in reality wholly constitutes the *intensifying division* of the animal kingdom; and this is why, as a matter of fact, the intensifying division, as compared with the attenuating, is so very vast. The horse, the cow, the sheep, the deer, etc., when attacked by rabies of at all a potent and paralytic form, straightway retire to the obscurest solitude, and die prostrate without "fury" or aggressiveness. "Generally," says Prof. Brown, of the Government Agricultural Department, "*among herbivora*, cattle and sheep, etc., which are most often the subjects of rabies, the disease ceases with the death of the animals which were bitten[1]." And in the same report Mr Cope is careful to emphasise the same important fact. Thus, in referring to the phenomenon of rabies being transmitted from deer to deer, he characterises it as "a circumstance which is *extremely unusual in the herbivora*; the rule being *that only those animals of a herd which have been first bitten fall victims to the disease.*" This rule, however, holds good only in respect of the most potent and prostrating paralytic forms of rabies. With the feebler and the more purely convulsive forms the reverse of this is the law. A feeble rabies in this class of animal is hardly to be extinguished until a herd has been practically decimated, or until the initial feeble rabies has been intensified by its transmission through the herd into the most pronounced paralytic form, capable of killing outright the victim.

This is well illustrated in the outbreaks of rabies which occasionally take place in deer; but it is not less characteristic of all the herbivora, both great and small; and in no such outbreak has it been more marked and more scientifically recorded than in respect of the Richmond Park epidemic just referred to. The initial rabies in this case was unquestionably an ordinary canine-rabies, originated by the bite of some stray mad dog which had got access to the herd, as was conclusively proved by Sir Victor Horsley by means of an

[1] "Report respecting the Richmond Park epidemic of Deer-rabies, during the years 1886—7, for both Houses of Parliament," by Mr Cope and Prof. Horsley.

intracranial inoculation of the "virus" into rabbits. But this most ordinary rabies, as it spread through the herd, by no means maintained its primary canine or convulsive character. Most certainly it was not attenuated by the process. Mr Cope's delineation of the malady, as it presented itself in the Park and in a state of nature, is all the more valuable that it is a picture of the rabies at the outset of the outbreak; in this forming a striking companion-picture to Sir Victor Horsley's, which is a not less graphic clinical representation of the malady at the later and the latest stages of the outbreak, and as it presented itself in the laboratory. The contrast well indicates the difference which has taken place in the form and character of the initial rabies by its transmission through the herd, and proves beyond doubt that the deer are genuine intensifiers. At the outset of the epidemic there is no indication of pronounced paralysis or paresis with collapse. It is merely a convulsive or "furious" rabies, closely resembling that of the dog, even to the sticks and hair and other extraneous material found in the stomach at an autopsy. It is noteworthy, not only that the convulsive feature is the most conspicuous from the first, but that it is also the most pronounced till death; and that, in spite of their fury, "the animals keep their legs and graze and drink to the last." After a transmission of the disease through the herd of seven months, this is the form of rabies which presents itself to Sir Victor Horsley at the Brown Institute.

"When removed from the box in which it was brought the animal was very excited, but evidently very ill. Ap. 19, 9.30 a.m. When seen this morning, *it had not fed since admission*, and was lying on the ground, *apparently but semi-conscious*. When touched, it staggered to its feet, *markedly paretic in its hind-limbs*. It was, nevertheless, still very excitable ; for it flew at the stick, with which I touched it, with much fury. In doing so, however, *it fell down*, owing of course to the commencing paralysis. Ap. 20. Animal weaker, and still aggressive. *The hind-limbs were now obviously paralysed.* Ap. 21. The animal was now almost *completely comatose*; it lay on the left side with marked opisthotonic contraction of the muscles of the back. The least touch caused tetanoid spasm of the limbs on extension. *It, however, had not eaten anything since admission.* At 11 a.m. the animal suddenly died (cardiac failure, probably)[1]."

[1] Report, for both Houses of Parliament, of Richmond Park outbreak of deer-rabies. Italics not Sir Victor Horsley's.

Six or seven weeks subsequently, the rabies having been still transmitted through the herd, the paretic and paralytic features are more pronounced, and the disease even still more rapid in its course. From the outset of the malady, "the hind-limbs" are now "very much paralysed," and the general collapse extreme. Here, then, is clear evidence of the fact that the rabies, which has been at last evolved in the course of transmission, is a very different disease in point of virulence from that which initiated the epidemic. If wholly convulsive in character at the beginning, it has gradually become by transmission essentially paralytic. As the epidemic advances, the disease acquires a progressive increase of paralysis and paresis; and in many of its more pronounced features it recalls M. Galtier's classical delineation of rabbit-rabies even to "the constant, rhythmical chewing movement of the jaws." If, at the very end of the epidemic, the paralysis is not of so pronounced a character as in rabbit-rabies, it is progressively approaching it. There can, therefore, be little doubt that the deer-family—and if this, for the same reason every other of the greater herbivora—belong to the intensifying order of the animal kingdom. In spite of the most stringent precautions it was found all but impossible to stamp out the Richmond Park outbreak ; and but for the stern measures which were ultimately adopted—shooting the affected animals without an hour's delay—the malady would at length have completely stamped out the herd. And this catastrophe, before the systematic use of the dog-muzzle was thought of, there is reason to believe has occurred in some of the recorded outbreaks amongst preserved herds both in Germany and in England, and, possibly, is not a unique occurrence in nature. Had the disease in the Richmond Park outbreak intensified much further, or into the completely paralytic stage, characteristic of normal rabbit-rabies—as most certainly would have occurred had the transmission continued, and this, likewise, in all probability is no unfrequent occurrence in nature—the aggressiveness of the first cases would have been lost in sheer paralysis; and in this way, and by this most effectual method, the epidemic would have come to an end. Even the dog itself, when suffering from the most "dumb" or "mortal" madness of which the animal is capable, in consequence of the profound prostration and paralysis thereby involved, loses its "fury" and aggressiveness.

It would appear, then, that the paralytic rabies which is at last evolved by transmission through an intensifier actually defends from the disease the intensifying herd or class in which it occurs, at last stamping out the malady in so effectually stamping out the affected individuals. If this be so, clearly enough, in the most prolonged and extensive outbreaks, the disease, even in the most intensifying orders, has at last, likewise, a sudden ending; as summary as in the dog-race itself. Fortunately, therefore, in both intensifiers and attenuators, an outbreak comes at last to an abrupt finish, but in each case for diametrically opposite reasons. In intensifiers, such as the deer, it is due to the very intensification of the rabies involved in the process of transmission. This is even on the assumption that rabies in the herbivora *always* begins in the simplest convulsive (canine) form, as in the Richmond Park epidemic. But there is ground to show that this is not invariably the initial rabies. The disease may at once crop up in such an animal in a profoundly paralytic form, and, in consequence, the outbreak be extinguished immediately; as completely so, as in the case of an oak in a forest which is instantly blighted by a lightning-shaft, without the forest or even any other tree or shrub of the forest being necessarily involved in the destruc- tion. This may occur very rarely in the dog-race itself, the extreme severity of the malady in such a case, with a complete absence of " fury," preventing its dispersal, and even masking it as a " rabies."

But although the horse, the goat, the sheep, the cow, the deer are all more or less capable of intensifying rabies on transmission, these larger herbivora by no means constitute the most potent or the most noteworthy intensifiers. On the contrary, the smaller and even the smallest of this order are by far the most potent; the intensifying property of such animals being strictly proportioned to, and deter- mined by, their smallness and feebleness in the herbivorous class. Although the sheep, cow, horse, deer, etc., all in the long run thus intensify even the simplest convulsive-rabies to paralytic forms, this intensifying process is more rapid and effective, and much more methodically progressive, in such animals as the hare, the guinea- pig and the rabbit. But, again, of even these smaller herbivorous animals, there is good reason to believe that the rabbit is the most potent intensifier. In the entire animal kingdom there is no fitter medium for the germination of the rabific microbe; the intensifying property of this animal being, apparently, as endless as it is pro- gressive. In this respect, it is important to note that the dog (where the disease is, nevertheless, supposed so invariably to take its origin in the animal kingdom), or any other attenuator, or the deer, or probably any other intensifier, will not compare with the rabbit, not merely for testing purposes, but for yielding the preventive inoculation. The laboratory "vaccinal" material—and there is none other to be compared with this for unfailing efficacy—is to be obtained, not from the dog, but from the rabbit. A rabies-virus, from that of the lowest to that of the highest potency known, is only to be obtained, significantly enough, from the spinal marrow of the rabidised rabbit.

Consequently, M. Pasteur's group of "drying" marrows, with their progressively increasing virulence from that of zero up to that of the highest infective-rate known, may be viewed as a very microcosm of the disease as it exists in nature. In such a group—but only in this over any other in the animal kingdom—there is a representation of every known "variety," "type" or "modification" of rabies to be met with in nature. Every "virus" or rabies without exception, even the lowest and simplest, incapable of rabidising the dog or other attenuator, is intensified without limit in the rabbit. So much so that with only half a score of passages through such animals a rabies of so overwhelming a potency is produced that it will rabidise the very dog, which in the first instance it altogether failed to do, with the most paralytic form of the disease of which the animal is capable. If transmitted through a sufficient series of rabbits, the rabies will not only progressively increase in virulence, but its virus-germ will become more and more massive, stable and complex in form, ultimately far ahead of that of the disease from which it has been derived. However slight and insignificant may have been the original rabies-virus, in virtue of its transmission through such animals it will have become so magnified, so intensified in activity, so transformed and organised that, if once more retransferred to the dog race, from which it was derived,

"There is now produced," says M. Pasteur, "a dog-virus which, in point of virulence, goes far beyond that of ordinary canine madness." "So great is the acquired virulence," adds M. Pasteur, "that the new 'virus,' obtained from this dog, when injected into the blood-system of a fresh dog, *unfailingly gives rise to mortal madness*[1]."

Here, surely, is a very remarkable transformation, and as signifi-cant as it is remarkable. For this reason, just as the dog amongst attenuators is probably one of the best for studying the process of

---

[1] *Comptes Rendus*, Dec. 11, 1882.

attenuation, the rabbit, amongst intensifiers, affords by far the best ground for studying the process of intensification.

Innumerable experiments on this animal, bearing on the subject, have now been performed; the ordinary canine-virus of 15 to 18 days' incubation having been transmitted, serially, through hundreds of rabbits. The famous Melun series of M. Pasteur may be taken as much the most conclusive of any such experiments, being the most prolonged and gigantic transmission-test ever performed by a scientific investigator. Although begun with an ordinary canine-virus so far back as November 1882, the transmission is still being carried on in rabbit after rabbit in the Pasteur Institute in one continuous and unbroken succession. And, so far as intensification of the initial canine-rabies is concerned, with what results?

"Two rabbits were trephined and inoculated with the same dog-virus (obtained from the brain of a cow which had died of canine-rabies at Melun), and they showed the first symptoms on the 17th and on the 18th days, respectively, after inoculation. With the bulb of one of these"—presumably with that of the shorter incubation—"two more rabbits were inoculated, of which one took rabies on the 15th, the other on the 23rd day. The bulb-emulsion of the first of these two was injected into two more rabbits, still after trephining. One of these took rabies on the 10th, and the other on the 14th day. The bulb of the first one of these that died"—still that of the shorter incubation—"was again injected into a couple of new rabbits, which developed the disease in 10 or in 12 days, respectively. A fifth time two new rabbits were inoculated from the first one that died; and they both took the disease on the 11th day. Similarly, a sixth passage was made, and gave an incubation of 11 days. 12 days for the seventh passage, 10 and 11 days for the eighth, 10 days for the ninth and tenth passages, 9 days for the eleventh, 8 and 9 days, respectively, for the twelfth. And so on, with differences of twenty-four hours at the most, until we got to the twenty-first passage, when rabies developed itself in 8 days. And, subsequently to that, always in 8 days up to the fiftieth passage, which was only affected a few days ago[1]."

More than a year afterwards, which, of course, carries the process of intensification still further, we have another authoritative statement by M. Pasteur to the French Academy.

[1] M. Pasteur's Address at the International Medical Congress at Copenhagen, Aug. 11, 1884.

"After a number of passages (of the ordinary 15 days' dog-rabies) through rabbits varying from the twentieth to the twenty-fifth, the incubation falls down to 8 days, which remains the normal incubation-time"—*i.e.* for such a rabies—"*for the next twenty or twenty-five passages.* Then it reaches an incubation of 7 days, and recurring with striking regularity up to at least the ninetieth passage, which is the point we have reached at present[1]."

Or, again, at a still later date, take this general but very important statement.

"After a number of such passages have been made from rabbit to rabbit, the incubation goes down to 11 days; then to 10, 9 and 8 days in succession, remaining long enough at the last period. Long before reaching the eightieth or the hundredth passage, the incubation has already lowered to 7 days, without ever, even as an exception, going back to 8 days. It remains a long time at 7 days, only going down occasionally to 6 days. It is still 7 days at the present time, after the hundred and thirty-third passage. Can we, then, conclude that, in this direction at any rate, the 'virus' of rabies has come to a fixed period? Or will the duration of incubation go down *permanently* to 6 days, when the succeeding passages have reached far enough in our races of rabbits? Experience, alone, can decide the question[2]."

Experience *has*, even already, decided that there is no such "fixed" limit. A rabies of not merely 6 but 5 days has been actually attained; and there is no reason why, according to the systematic rate of intensification in the rabbit, a rabies of considerably less than half of this incubation, or of treble or quadruple this appalling potency, may not be one day reached and maintained on further transmission, to evolve a still more potent form of the disease.

There is, then, it would appear, no absolute limit to the intensification of the disease by the rabbit. Moreover, in this animal the process of intensification is not merely much more rapid but much more methodical than in the deer or any of the larger herbivora, if not possibly than in any other intensifier whatever. This process is by no means a haphazard one. On the contrary, it is regular and systematic in the extreme, and determined by fairly fixed laws; the fall in the length of the incubation, like the fall of the mercury in a barometer, being always in an inverse ratio to the intensity of the

---

[1] *Comptes Rendus*, Oct. 26, 1885. Italics not M. Pasteur's.

[2] *Annales de l'Institut Pasteur*, Letter from M. Pasteur to Prof. Duclaux, Dec. 27, 1886.

tempest which it so infallibly and so precisely foretells.   Thus, as we have just seen, in not more than half-a-dozen passages a canine-rabies of the ordinary "furious" form of 15 days' incubation, already makes for the very rare "dumb" or "mortal" canine-madness of pronounced paralytic form and of but 12 or 11 days' incubation.   And from this, again, the disease progressively intensifies to the completely paralytic form of 10 days, which is to be found as a *normal* rabies, significantly enough, only in the rabbit.

But, although this process of intensification proceeds without ceasing, from the feeblest and most insignificant form of the disease up to a 5 or probably a 3 days' rabies, if not possibly still higher, this progress, far from being irregular or in mere "leaps and bounds," is, after the primary normal 10 days' rabies has been attained, in a graduated ratio which may be absolutely relied on.   All through the process thereafter, up to the evolution of a 5 days' rabies, and in every probability, as time will show, very much higher, there are at stated intervals relatively settled stages.   Each of these represents a distinct, completed form of rabies with an incubation-period lasting for a definite number of passages, strictly characteristic of the stage, and determined by the number of transmissions which have been necessary to evolve it as a distinct form.   Thus, a virus-germ *unit*, if one may so term it, of, say, an hypothetical 5 microbe-form and force, capable of inducing a 15 days' canine-rabies, rapidly becomes on transmission a virus-germ unit of 10 microbe-form and force, capable of inducing the normal 10 days' rabbit-rabies; and this, again, but now most systematically and regularly, one of 20 microbe-form and force, capable of inducing a rabies of 5 days' incubation; and so on, until we reach a virus-germ unit of, it may be, 100 or possibly even 200 microbe-form and force, capable of inducing a rabies of but 1 or even half a day's incubation.   Moreover, it is to be noted, the higher the rabies thus evolved, or the longer the series of transmissions which this intensification has required, the longer will the rabies, as a distinct, uniform, completed form, be maintained on further transmission; the number of passages in which it will be thus more or less maintained depending upon the number of passages which it has taken to evolve it.   At the end of definite sets of transmissions there are, in spite of continued serial transmissions, stages of apparent changelessness in the induced rabies—but it is only apparent—this completed and relatively *fixed* form of the disease, with its temporary changelessness, lasting the longer the higher or more potent the form.

The whole process of intensification, therefore, from first to last, with the forms of the disease ever increasing in stability, potency and complexity of structure, is not merely an unending one, but is determined and graduated by sufficiently fixed rules. These may, perhaps, be broadly summarised as follows:—Firstly, there are periodically evolved definite and completed forms of rabies, from high to higher, the microbe-unit of which is the more organised, specialised and complex in structure, the more potent in virulent activity, the shorter in incubation, and the longer maintained, as such, the further the rabies is transmitted. Secondly, a rabies of any given form, up to the most complex, the most stable, and of the shortest incubation yet discovered, or probably yet to be evolved, is determined by, and, for its evolution, as a special rabies, solely dependent upon, the number of its transmissions through the rabbit. Thirdly, any given form of rabies, even the most potent and complex, which has been at last evolved by transmission, or yet to be evolved, will be maintained as such rabies, and at this stage, for a further number of transmissions more or less tantamount to the number of passages which it has taken to evolve it as this particular form.

These facts are well illustrated by M. Pasteur's investigation. Thus, even from the experiments narrated above, it is to be seen that, "after twenty to twenty-five passages through rabbits," the incubation falls down to 8 days. This is, however, it is worthy of note, "the normal incubation-time" for such rabies for exactly another "twenty to twenty-five passages," when a 7 days' rabies is occasionally evolved, and begins to be established. On the other hand, this 7 days' rabies maintains its 7 days' incubation for a still longer period, not indefinitely, however, but for a period commensurate with the increased potency of the rabies, and with the number of passages which have been necessary to induce it. And a 6 days' rabies does not begin to be rounded off or completely established until the 90th to the 100th passage, or, again, in a further number of transmissions which were in the first instance necessary to completely evolve the 7 days' rabies. According to this rate, a 5 days' rabies will not be fairly evolved and completed in form before at least the 180th to the 200th passage, or, again, in double the number of transmissions. And this is precisely what one finds to be the fact. The same may be formulated of even the possible forms of rabies which may yet be evolved: a 4 days' rabies not being fairly elaborated until from the 400th to the 600th transmission. The rate of progressive intensification would appear to be so, methodic that any given form or any given stage may be predicated with a certain assurance.

In accordance with such rules the intensification of rabies in rabbits, or in the most potent of even all intensifiers, and to the most virulent and the most complex possible forms, may perhaps be theoretically tabulated as follows:

INTENSIFICATION OF RABIES IN RABBITS.

Incubation-time					Number of transmissions					
A 10 days' rabies, beginning on					6th perfects on		10th and lasts to			12th
,,	9	,,	,,	,,	,,	12th	,,	,,	20th ,, ,, ,,	25th
,,	8	,,	,,	,,	,,	25th	,,	.,	40th ,, ,, ,,	50th
,,	7	,,	,,	,,	,,	50th	,,	,,	80th ,, ,, ,,	100th
,,	6	,,	,.	,,	,,	100th	,,	.,	160th ,, ,, ,,	200th
,,	5	,,	,,	,,	,,	200th	,,	,.	320th ,, ,, ,,	400th
,,	4	,,	,,	,, .	,,	400th	,,	,,	640th ,, ,, ,,	800th
,,	3	,,	,,	,,	.,	800th	,,	,,	1,280th ,, ,, ,,	1,600th
,,	2	,,	,,	.,	,,	1,600th	,,	,,	2,560th ,, ,, ,,	3,200th
,,	1	,,	,,	,,	,,	3,200th	,,	,,	5,120th ,, ,, ,,	6,400th
,,	$\frac{1}{2}$ (or 12 hours)		,,		,,	6,400th	,,	,,	10,240th ,, ,, ,,	12.800th
,,	$\frac{1}{4}$ (or 6 hours)		,,		,,	12,800th	,,	,,	20,480th ,, ,, ,,	25,600th

From experimental results, then, it is unquestionable that the rabies peculiar to the great intensifying order, which comprises by far the larger part of the mammalia, and particularly to the smallest and the feeblest of the herbivora, such as the rabbit, is a very different rabies in point of incubation, potency and transmissibility from that which is characteristic of the entire attenuating order, but, more particularly, of the dog-race. In the rabbit, the primary or normal rabies, *i.e.* the first relatively "fixed" form in the unending process of intensification which takes place in this animal, is, it is significant, a paralytic rabies of 10 or 11 days' incubation, not a convulsive or "furious" rabies of 15 to 20 days' incubation; which latter, however, as we have so repeatedly seen, is the characteristic rabies of the dog. A 15 days' rabies in the rabbit is still more phenomenal than a paralytic 11 or 12 days' rabies in the dog; and, unlike the deer or larger herbivora, such convulsive rabbit-rabies has never been met with in nature. Did it exist in nature, rapidly spreading epidemics of the disease through the rabbit would be of constant occurrence and still more obvious than in the case of the deer. This, however, does not apply to the paralytic 10 days' rabies, so characteristic of the animal, which, as we shall see presently, might well exist in nature, and not necessarily spread through the rabbit-race at all.

On the other hand, highly characteristic as a 15 days' rabies is of the entire canine race, it is not a "fixed" rabies in this animal;

no form of rabies is, not the most potent and paralytic. Prevalent, therefore, though it be in the race, this 15 days' rabies cannot be the originating form of the malady even in the dog. Only a potent, paralytic rabies of 11 or 12 days' incubation, rare though it really be in the animal, could spread serially through such attenuators for, relatively, a small number of transmissions. Hence, the originating form in the dog, which gives rise to anything like an extensive outbreak of the disease, must, as already shown, be of a more or less pronounced "dumb" or paralytic character, and of at least 11 or 12, not of 15 to 18 days' incubation, however rare the former, and however prevalent, ultimately, the latter.

It is owned that, normally, rabies is much more pronounced in the rabbit than in the dog, and in intensifiers than in attenuators. In the same way, it may be said, the germ-diseases of civilized life are found to be more disastrous amongst savages than amongst Europeans. But this is not the fact of all the germ-diseases of civilized life; only of the prophylactic germ-diseases. Smallpox or scarlatina, measles or whooping-cough decimates savage races. Because they are invariably so much more intense, are, then, these germ-diseases supposed to have arisen in the savage races? The reverse is the fact. These very diseases are now, comparatively, so mild and weak in Europe and America, because they have had their origin in, and have been so long transmitted through, the civilized races. Does not the same principle hold good of the convulsive-rabies of the dog as contrasted with the paralytic-rabies of the rabbit? The comparative mildness of the canine disease may really indicate a very prolonged process of modification through transmission of the pathogenic microbe. In the same way, the comparative feebleness of some of the germ-diseases of civilized life indicates their vast antiquity; whilst their intense severity in savage life indicates the absolute novelty of the diseases in such races.

But the mildest European germ-diseases which prove so disastrous to savages are, it is important to note, exclusively prophylactic, and have been passed from generation to generation for ages in Europe. Rabies, however, is not a prophylactic, but, as we have seen, in all probability a recurrent, preventive germ-disease; and preventive germ-diseases are as severe in civilised as in savage life, and as common in the latter as in the former. True, the ague of tropical races is distinctly feebler than the ague of European races in the tropics; and this is pre-eminently a recurrent germ-disease. But it is much more recurrent and much more prevalent than canine-rabies. Canine-rabies is, after all, a comparatively rare disease. The virus of ague, for so many generations incessantly affecting the negro-races, may have excited and, ultimately, established a phagocytic power with regard to the "paludal" pathogenic micro-organism. Only because the disease is so persistently recurrent, and has been so incessantly transmitted through the negro-races for ages, could its virus have, ultimately, induced a phagocytic protection. But the virus of canine-rabies has acted in no such continuous way on the dog-race, and for centuries upon centuries, without ceasing. The refractory or attenuating power of the dog may be, and probably is, due to its very high phagocytic power. But this phagocytic function is, clearly enough, not due to the rabies-microbe having been transmitted through the race for countless generations. There are other reasons for the stubborn refractoriness of the entire attenuating division of the animal kingdom. Thus, if canine-rabies, in point of virulence and intensity, is distinctly inferior to rabbit-rabies, and wholly because the disease has been transmitted through the race for so many ages, as it so happens, it is equally inferior or feeble in monkeys where it has not been at all transmitted. An ape from Africa will attenuate the disease, even the most profoundly paralytic-rabies, as powerfully and as rapidly as the dog. Yet, as a matter of fact, rabies does not exist, and has never existed, in Central Africa; and why this is the case shall be shown presently. Rabies is as new to the ape as measles or scarlatina is to the savage, or tropical malarial-fever to the European or American. Nevertheless, in the monkey, rabies is as slight and inferior as, normally, it is in the dog; and both animals so powerfully attenuate the disease for probably the same reason.

As, however, in either form, convulsive or paralytic, the disease is not essentially a canine malady, any more than it is a monkey germ-disease or that of any other animal equally capable of attenuating it on transmission; otherwise it would never be practically abolished by the mere use of a muzzle; and as it begins in this animal, however mysterious and sudden the origin, in the profounder, more paralytic and more transmissible canine varieties, where, one again asks, does the dog derive these primary, most potent and originating forms? Such a rabies is the rabies of the intensifying, not of the attenuating division of the animal kingdom. Does the canine disease in the first instance invariably come from the rabbit, or other such intensifier? Is there anything inherently improbable in such a view?

CHAPTER XV.

WHY RABIES PREVAILS IN THE DOG.

EVERY extensive or prolonged outbreak of canine madness must be originated, for the reasons alleged, by a more or less pronounced paralytic rabies of not more than 12 or 11 days' (rabbit) incubation, however exceptional this form of the malady in an epidemic. Without such an originating, highly transmissible form of the disease there could be no extensive outbreak in the dog. But, as just shown, this paralytic form is a rabies of intensifiers, not of attenuators, and, above all intensifiers of the feeblest and the most insignificant of the vast herbivorous order; and, again, even of this latter, normally that of the rabbit. Where, then, *except from some such intensifying animal as the rabbit*, does the dog-race so constantly incur in the first instance, if also so mysteriously, this profoundly paralytic and pre-eminently transmissible form? If this be the fact, it becomes at once comprehensible why the dog should be so frequently affected with the malady above all attenuators, in spite of the fact that it is, strangely enough, likewise above most animals, the most refractory to the disease. It follows that in every outbreak of canine-rabies the dog has, at first hand, received the disease directly from the rabbit, and from a 10 days' rabbit-rabies, or from some other of the most pronounced intensifiers. In other words according to this view, rabies is, primarily, a germ-disease of intensifiers, not of attenuators; in the latter it is always secondary and derived. And it so frequently occurs in some of the attenuating division, such as the dog, because it is so essentially a malady of *hunted* rather than of *hunting animals*: it is so prevalent in the latter, because it is in reality so peculiarly a disease of the former. Why, otherwise, on any other assumption, should rabies take its origin in the animal kingdom through the very animal which, of most animals, is alike the most stubbornly refractory to, and the most potent attenuator of, the disease?

Rabies, then, it may be inferred, takes its origin—in whatever way this may be occasioned—in the *hunted* rather than in the *hunting* division of the animal kingdom. And the realm of hunted animals comprises, as it so happens, the entire class of herbivora, from the greatest to the smallest; this vast class likewise constituting the entire intensifying division of the animal kingdom. Every species of hunted animal, even the highest and most powerful, such as the stag, the ram, the bull, is capable of intensifying rabies on trans-mission; but the more persecuted the animal, or the lower it is placed in the scale of the herbivora and, therefore, the more hunted even to earth and under the earth where pathogenic micro-organisms dwell, the more pronounced, significantly enough, is its intensifying property. On the other hand, the entire class of *hunting* animals is included in the attenuating division of the animal kingdom. Every order of hunting animal is capable of attenuating rabies on trans-mission. Nay, further, the more exclusively the animal relies upon hunting for its existence, the more pronounced will be found its attenuating and its refractory power. Consequently, if the disease crops up anywhere, however mysteriously, in the hunted division of the animal kingdom, much more, if it invariably originates for every outbreak of canine-madness in such intensifiers, then, the hunting division, and, above all such, the dog-race, cannot fail to acquire it, in spite of any amount of inherent preventive or refractory power.

But rabies is not confined to the exclusively hunting and the exclusively hunted classes; there is probably no animal which is not capable of being rabidised. Like erysipelas, diphtheria, tetanus, etc., and the large but exclusively *preventive* order of germ-disease to which it belongs, as opposed to the purely *prophylactic* germ-diseases, like smallpox, scarlatina, syphilis, anthrax, etc., rabies is capable of being imparted to probably every warm-blooded animal. Neverthe-less, it is manifest that, notwithstanding this very wide range of attack over the animal kingdom, so different from the prophylactic germ-diseases which are limited in the extreme, the disease is pre-eminently characteristic of, and, apparently, the most prevalent in, the canine-race, in whatever other class of animal it may make its appearance. It is dogs, wolves, foxes, not guinea-pigs, rabbits, deer, sheep, cows, or any of the herbivora, whether large or small, which are ever the conspicuous victims of the malady. But it by no means follows that the canine-race is inherently more liable to the disease than the herbivora. Without revealing any conspicuous outbreaks of rabies, the hunted animal may, nevertheless, be much more subject to the malady than the hunting, and, moreover, to its profoundest paralytic forms. That there are few or, often enough, no conspicuous outbreaks in the hunted class, and particularly in the feeblest and the most persecuted of them all, such as the rabbit, is no proof that the latter is not still more liable to the malady than the larger herbivora, where outbreaks (but of canine source) occasionally occur, and much more liable than the hunting class where epidemics are so frequent. For in this connection we have the one all-important habit, formed from untold ages, which is common to the wide diversity of the canine-race, from the wolf to the terrier, that they not merely live by hunting, but habitually prey on the most persecuted and hunted, and, therefore, the most potent of intensifiers. If rabies then be, fundamentally, a disease of the latter, ever cropping up in the animal kingdom from this source, however rarely, and however weirdly and mysteriously—all the more subtly and effectually if invariably in the "dumb" form—it would quite account for a prevalence of rabies in the canine-race; and, providing the originating rabies in the latter were of the "dumb" paralytic form characteristic of the former, it would also account for the disease in the dog, on its first appearance in an outbreak, being always of so high an infective-rate, and, consequently, so frequently epidemical in character.

But the dog is not the only hunting animal. How, then, stand the facts in relation to such animals? There is at least one familiar and well-known case, the cat. This animal is particularly prone to contract the malady; hardly less so than the dog itself, and, moreover, with a somewhat more potent rabies. But the cat is the only member of the great feline order which may be said to at all hunt, and, still more important, the very weakest and feeblest of the hunted classes. The tiger, the lion, the leopard, etc., do not hunt; but, by surprise, kill outright, and are admirably adapted for this purpose with almost an invisible form. All these, unseen, or in the darkness of night, approach in velvet-footed stealth, and spring on their victims like fiends. It is quite otherwise with the genuine hunting animal, which pursues its prey in the open glare of day with indomitable steadfastness; and its prey, as just stated, is the feeblest of the hunted classes, or, in other words, by far the most potent intensifiers in the animal kingdom.

Why, then, it may be asked, should the hunting animal itself be so refractory to rabies, and so necessarily attenuate the disease on transmission, whilst the hunted animal is so very much the reverse? Why should a rabbit's spinal marrow, for example, prove so fit a soil for the cultivation of the rabies-germ, whilst that of a monkey or a dog should prove quite the contrary? There is at least one striking and very fundamental characteristic to account for the difference which is common to every genuine hunting animal, and to every attenuator whether hunter or not, viz. extreme boldness and daring. But, as it happens, there is no surer or better indication of the strength and stability of the nervous system which are so essential to inherent refractoriness and to attenuating rabies. If indomitable courage or dogged tenacity of "pluck" be an indication of a strong, steady nerve, and if this, again, be taken as the *sine qua non* of the refractory or attenuating power, there is no intensifier, even the most powerful, such as the bull or stag, which will compare in this respect with any attenuator or hunting animal, even the most insignificant, such as a terrier. A terrier, in charge of its master's property, will boldly face the most brutal burglar, or even gang of burglars. A bull-dog will unhesitatingly make for and grip the most ferocious of bulls by the lip, and, although crippled and mangled, will maintain its grip with invincible tenacity. The paltriest pack of curs, nay, even one or two lean, starving wolves, will chase for miles and for hours the vastest herd of sheep, deer or cattle. And every order of animal, comprised in the attenuating division of the animal kingdom, whether a hunter or not, will be found on examination to be likewise characterised by the same unyielding daring, or, in other words, to be possessed of a nervous system characterised by the strength, stability and integrity so essential to the attenuation and the prevention of rabies. The monkey race may be taken as a good example. Clearly enough, the attenuating power of this animal, as of the dog, is due to no prolonged transmission of rabies through the race. It is due, in both cases, to the boldness and courage of the animals, which mean the most powerful of nervous systems. In the monkey they are hardly less pronounced than in the case of man himself. From the numerous observations on record in respect of this fact, there can be no question as to the exceptional strength and stability of this animal's nervous organization[1]. All these animals have more than the boldness of the lion or the tiger; for this daring is a growth of daylight, not of night or of darkness.

[1] See Darwin's *Descent of Man.*

If the vigour and stability of the nervous system, as a whole, and of the nervous substance in particular, are to be measured by such dogged daring, then, there is little wonder that such a class of animal should prove persistently refractory to rabies, or attenuate on transmission every form of disease. There is no class of animal whose nervous system or nervous tissue is less likely to yield a favourable "nidus" for the rabies-germ. A similar phenomenon is to be noted in respect of hydrophobia itself. The hydrophobia of a resolute, strong-nerved man is a very different disease from that of the timorous, irritable, broken-down "neurotic"; for the entire nervous system of the former is a very different structure with respect to the rabies-germ from that of the latter. Boldness and resolute endurance may, therefore, safely be taken as a reliable indication, not merely of the exceptional strength, but of the exceptional integrity of the nervous system and of the central nervous substance. But this central nervous substance, particularly the bulbar substance of the cord, is, it is certain, of all sites in the animal economy, the specific seat of germination of the rabies-germ. If this be enfeebled or in any way impaired, germination will in consequence be enormously aided and increased, like harrowed soil for the reception of the seed. If, on the contrary, it be exceptionally strong and sound, germination will be correspondingly hindered. In the latter case, if it be a feeble rabies-virus to begin with, or an insignificant infection, the rabies may be even altogether prevented by the refractory vitality of the animal. There is little wonder, therefore, in the fact that the attenuating division of the animal kingdom should comprise at least the entire order of *hunting* animal, whatever other order of animal it may happen to include.

Turning, now, to the *hunted* animal kingdom, a very different set of conditions presents itself. Why should the nervous organization of such an animal prove so favourable a soil for the rabies-germ? How comes the rabbit to be so fitted for germinating the rabies-microbe, and, above all even hunted animals, to be so sensitive to that of the feeblest rabies? If the property of *attenuation* be taken as a conclusive proof of the intrinsic soundness and strength of the central nervous system, the property of *intensification* may be viewed as an equally infallible indication of an intrinsic nerve-weakness and nerve-instability. According to the view here proposed, the rabbit is so sensitive to, and so profound an intensifier of, the disease because it is, and has been for so many ages, a pre-eminently *hunted* creature, perhaps without exception the most persistently persecuted of the entire hunted class; and because, in consequence, its nervous organisation has been rendered, even at its healthiest, permanently enfeebled and unstable. Consequently, the resisting power in respect of the rabies-germ is reduced to a minimum, and the incurring and the possibility of intensifying such a disease as rabies raised to a maximum.

In the "wild" state, it is hardly too much to say that the rabbit, as the most persistently hunted of animals, lives every hour in terror of its life. It is true that a hunted creature is blessed with a short memory; otherwise, brief as is its life, it would probably collapse sooner than it does. The memory of the acutest pains and agonies is, fortunately, very soon forgotten, even by the highest animals, including mankind; as, for example, in the case of toothache, neuralgia, renal colic, or even of parturition itself. It is the memory of pleasures and delights which lingers so long, and which expands and idealises, as it lingers, like a sunset glow. But, short as is the memory of the hunted animal with respect to past danger, it is ever forcibly reminded of the peril of forgetfulness. A deer, a sheep, a hare or a rabbit is constantly on the alert for the approach of a hunter, and admirably provided by Nature and organic experience for detecting its lifelong enemy. Suspicious, timid, "nervous" in the extreme, and constantly exposed to the possibility of prostrating nervous shock, a "wild" rabbit, or any other equally hunted creature, lives a large part of its life in avoiding or evading this shock. Day after day this dread persists, and in some measure even when the animal is in repose. But what strain to the nervous system is involved in this lifelong dread! Above all, what acute tension must ensue in the actual moment of pursuit! and in the life of such an animal such alternate tension and shock are of frequent occurrence. Under such strain it is little wonder that the life of the entire herbivora or hunted class is relatively so short, and that the brevity is even in proportion to the extent of this constant stress on the nervous system. In like manner, but from a totally opposite cause, the intense excitement of hunting must also tend to shorten the life of the hunting class. For, as a matter of fact, the more specially hunting and the more specially hunted class of animals are by far the shortest-lived of all vertebrated animals, even when they live their "allotted span." Compare, *e.g.*, the life of a rabbit and that of a pike in a pond, or the life of a dog with that of a parrot. It would probably be impossible to exaggerate the prostrating terror which takes place in the actual moment of the pursuit of a hunted creature, even when it makes its escape; but especially when there is no escape and no capacity of "standing at bay," as is the case with the smallest herbivora. The prolonged torture of a semi-comatose mouse on the part of a cat is a spectacle fit only for the darkest depths of Inferno. The anguish of a rabbit which is ferreted from hole to hole, or imprisoned in a hiding-place by a relentless terrier, can never possibly become stale. The long-pursued hare, which, at last, unable to escape, giving up its run for life, crouches down with quivering ears drawn back to eye the panting greyhound immediately behind in its murderous leap, is a picture which, once seen, for blended pathos and savagery haunts one for life.

The horror which a hunted animal has for a hunting is constant and unalterable, and begins with its very birth; it is a congenital dread. As indicating this deeply-rooted terror take the case of a flock of sheep in a park madly massing together from every quarter at the sudden sight in their midst of a Skye-terrier! Absurd, even ludicrous as the spectacle looks, it is not unique in the animal king-dom, nor even inexplicable. It is in point of fact strictly analogous to the dread which the human race feels with respect to the serpent. Suddenly place the tiniest of snakes, even if it be a harmless one, on the carpet of a drawing-room, where there is a party of ladies and gentlemen, and the scene of the sheep, scampering from the puniest of dogs, is exactly repeated! The sheep, with probably every other hunted creature, has likewise the same horror in respect of the serpent. And even in the gambols of the lamb, with the curling fling of its hind legs as it bounds in the sunshine, there is evidence of a very ancient and most profound provision against the insidious bite of both the dog and the serpent.

The same thing is seen in sheep following a bell-wether, one after another to hundreds, over an extended crook, and keeping up the vault long after the stick has been withdrawn. This singular habit has been noted and moralised over, from time immemorial, by moralists of every grade of wisdom and genius. But grotesque as it seems, its *raison d'être* is most certainly not merely to afford the moralist with an apt illustration. Whatever it may be on the part of man, it by no means follows that, mechanical and thoughtless as it would seem, it is so very absurd on the part of sheep. Any habit which has become ingrained through so many millions of generations, in spite of constant human protection, is for the lasting benefit of the animal. Let a bell-wether or any other single sheep, whether bell-wether or not, of a flying flock, at whatever rate the latter is driving before a few dogs or wolves like a fleecy cloud before a gale, suddenly leap into the air, at the same time swiftly flinging its hind feet in the curl characteristic even of the lamb, what is there surprising, much less absurd, in the fact that every approaching sheep which has seen this sudden bound should likewise spasmodically vault into the air exactly at the same point and in the same fashion, if, as it should so happen, there has been coiled at this very spot *a snake*, ready to dart at the sheep, or which in point of fact may have actually darted at the first passing animal? To the whole coming flock in its headlong flight there could be no more effective signal as to what danger is at hand, and precisely where the danger lies. If this be so, the habit is not without use in the welfare of the race.

Probably the "shying" tendency of the excitable young horse has arisen in the same way. And it is not merely over an outstretched stick that the sheep's impetuous vault is to be seen. Anything which remotely suggests the likeness or presence of a serpent will produce the same effect. Even an outstretched stick may do so; and, for this purpose, the more crooked the stick the better. But a bit of coiled rope lying in the way of a driving herd will give rise to the same apparently senseless leap. And in this connection it is not without practical interest to note that, when a small flock of sheep is embarking on a steamboat in the lochs, it is no uncommon occurrence for one suddenly to leap overboard, clearing the gunwales at a bound, to be instantly followed by every one of the flock. Is it possible that here, too, a coiled rope is the cause of the frantic leap, being mistaken, in the excited state of the animal, for the sudden glimpse of a coiled adder at close quarters? If this be so, would it not be advisable on such occasions to conceal all such ropes with tarpaulin? Nor is a spiral fling of the hind limbs peculiar to sheep, which is so admirably adapted for eluding the sudden bite of either serpent or dog; and for this sudden snap the mouths of a hound and a serpent are marvellously alike. It is characteristic of the entire hunted class, both great and small, but particularly the latter or the most persistently hunted of any. And, as indicating its vast antiquity as a habit, it is, as already stated, specially notable in the young in their gambols. But of no hunted creature is it more characteristic than the rabbit.

16—2

The mere sight or even suggestion of a dog or serpent agitates the sheep, the hare, the rabbit, and every excessively hunted creature as no other spectacle on earth does. In the "wild" state, not one of these ever gets accustomed, much less callous, to the sight of the hunting. But this perpetual dread must ever act as a strain on the nervous organisation of the animal, to unsettle and deteriorate it in proportion. The influence of this unceasing tension on the nervous system must be debilitating in the extreme, and constantly undermining its resisting power with respect to such a germ-disease as rabies. How, under such circumstances, could the central nervous substance of a hunted animal fail to prove, and in proportion to its persecution for untold ages, by far the most favourable soil in the entire animal kingdom for the germination of the rabies-microbe, more especially since it is the fact that the rabies-germ is a micro-organism of nervous substance, *and of no other tissue*, pre-eminently of *enfeebled* nervous substance?

And if one turns to even the *hunting* class, itself, there is evidence of the same law at work. In proportion as the nervous system of such animals is deteriorated and enfeebled the rabies is pronounced and severe, and far more often paralytic than convulsive in character. As we have already seen, this is obvious even in the case of hydro-phobia. It is the haggard, careworn being, with the scared, *hunted* look of insomnia and increasing dread, who, alone, develops paralytic hydrophobia. And this is not less true of the exclusively hunting animal. As it so happens, there are at least two important members of this class, the fox and the cat, which are also hunted animals. The fox's life is hardly more tolerable than the hare's or rabbit's; and to make it at all successful in its struggle for existence the animal needs all his subtle cunning and intelligence. But, out of doors, the cat is not much freer from persecution, as is evidenced by its peculiarly slinking, sneaking gait. Beyond its own immediate home there is no more suspicious, "nervous" creature. It trusts few strangers, and no dog, and looks for (and receives) persecution every-where. Hunters although both these animals are, so far as rabies is concerned what is the result of this persistent persecution? What form of rabies do they habitually present? As compared with that of the dog or even the wolf, the normal rabies of the fox is notoriously more dangerous and distinctly more potent; the bite of the rabid fox, attenuator as it is, requiring the promptest and severest pre-ventive treatment, and often, in spite of this, ending in paralytic hydrophobia. The normal rabies of the cat, which is also an attenuator, is even still more potent, the incubation-period, if not so short as that characteristic of the rabbit, being invariably somewhat shorter than that characteristic of the dog. This was very ably and conclusively demonstrated by Sir Victor Horsley for the British Commission appointed to examine M. Pasteur's preventive treatment, in respect of the attendant, Goffi, from the Brown Institute, who was bitten by a rabid cat. In spite of the inoculative treatment at the Pasteur Institute this unfortunate man died of " paralytic " hydrophobia. But, by the incubation-test in rabbits, the disease was proved to be, not M. Pasteur's *rabbit-rabies*, incurred at his laboratory through the treatment, as had been so dogmatically and so malignantly asserted, but *cat-rabies*, incurred at the Brown Institute; the incubation-period being longer than that of rabbit-rabies, but distinctly shorter than that of ordinary dog-rabies[1]. The bite of a rabid cat, therefore, not less than that of the rabid fox, and both more than that of a rabid dog, requires the promptest and the strongest inoculative treatment.

After such facts, does it not follow that the persecuted, *hunted* existence peculiarly determines a capacity for developing or intensifying or even initiating rabies? Given the rabies-germ in the central nervous substance of such an animal, the micro-organism could not fail to germinate, and in the most persecuted and hunted of such animals to germinate to its utmost capacity. Does this never occur in nature? Finding not merely the readiest but the fittest of all organised soils in the deteriorated nervous substance of a hunted animal,—and the more intrinsically enfeebled and unbalanced its nervous system, the better the soil,—is it too much to suggest that it is pre-eminently in such an animal in the entire animal kingdom that rabies takes its rise? If this be so, the disease is most certainly initiated in intensifiers, not in attenuators; it takes its origin in hunted, not in hunting animals, and, again, of all hunted animals, in all probability chiefly the rabbit, as the most persistently persecuted of any. Consequently, the animal has become probably the most potent intensifier of the disease in the animal kingdom.

Now, it is again necessary to emphasize, as it is hardly possible to exaggerate, the importance of the relationship which hunted animals, as a whole, but, above all, rabbits, as the most persistently hunted, bear to dogs, wolves, foxes, etc. and to the entire attenuating class of

[1] See Report to the Local Government Board, respecting M. Pasteur's treatment of hydrophobia.

animals which live by hunting. Could any relationship be more direct
or more constant and close? But if rabies be primarily a disease of
the hunted order of animal, it follows, as already shewn, that the
dog, as a hunter, is ever exposed to the risk of incurring the malady;
and more so than any other attenuator which is not a hunting animal.
Consequently, even although itself most refractory to rabies, it will
be the most frequently attacked by rabies of all attenuators.

On the assumption that the rabbit, as the most persistently persecuted of the intensifying order and, consequently, the most potent
of intensifiers, occasionally incurs the disease in nature altogether
irrespective of the dog-race, what would be the result were a hunting
dog to come suddenly across such a rabbit, that is to say, one which
at the moment of the onslaught was actually suffering from the
disease? Could the dog, in at least a certain, possibly phenomenally
small, percentage of cases, fail to incur the malady? And as connected with this possibility it is not without significance, and has an
important bearing on the transfer of the disease to the dog or other
hunting animal, that all such animals, at the final fatal leap, unerr-
ingly seize the rabbit or the smallest of the herbivora, not by the
body or at haphazard, nor by the leg or hamstrings, as in the case of
the horse, cattle, sheep, or deer, or the larger herbivora, *but invariably
by the nape of the neck.* Terriers clutch rats by the neck, and instantly shake them to death ; often in so doing, and therefore causing
instant death, crushing the cervical vertebræ into splinters. In like
manner, the cat at once springs at the cervical site of a guinea-pig,
and also often enough splinters the vertebræ into fragments. A
case of this kind, one of my son's pets, once came under my notice;
the smash of the nape of the neck on the part of the cat was so
considerable that, when the poor guinea-pig was released, which was
almost immediately, it was found to be paralysed ; and some of the
splinters of the vertebræ that protruded were extremely sharp.
Again, it is notorious that wolves, foxes and dogs, on the hunt for
themselves, will at once proceed to devour their captured prey ; and,
in the case of the smaller herbivora, the first point on which they
seize is likewise, invariably, *the nape of the neck.* Here, too, and
even still more frequently, the cervical vertebræ, with its enclosed
spinal substance, is mangled into pulp. But, above all other hunted
animals, this holds good in respect of a hare's or a rabbit's neck ;
it is invariably thus more or less torn and crushed, the vertebræ
and its spinal substance being often comminuted into a splintered
mass.

This cervical site, however, it is important to note, is not merely the most vulnerable point, so far as the rabbit or hunted animal is concerned,—which is fortunate for the unfortunate creature,—but in a case of rabies, or of the captured animal actually at the time suffering from the disease, it would likewise prove the most dangerous and infective site, so far as the dog or hunting animal itself is also concerned. In the violent *crunch* of the cervical vertebræ and its enclosed spinal substance, the highly vascular gums of the hunting animal, whether dog or cat, must occasionally be at least slightly punctured by some of the splinters. It is surprising how frequently this trivial accident occurs with dogs, even in ordinary domestic life, when munching the bones of a fowl or a rabbit; the very smallness and slenderness of the bones apparently conducing to such splintering and puncturing. Occasionally, a splinter will stick tenaciously between the teeth until forcibly dislodged by the animal itself, and some considerable time after the accident has occurred. This is particularly noticeable in the cat, but it is by no means rare in the dog also. Thus, on one occasion, I removed from the upper jaw of a friend's terrier a sharp fragment of bone, a piece of a rabbit's vertebra, which was tenaciously impacted between the teeth, *and had been so for three days*, with considerable abrasion of the gums, in spite of the animal's violent and most persistent efforts to dislodge it. And in both animals such an accident must be still more frequent, if not comparatively common, in the "wild" state, where there is far more savage and violent hunger to induce it.

Now, on the certainty that puncturing of the gums takes place in this manner, however rarely, infection on the part of the hunting animal could hardly fail to take place, providing the hunted animal, whose cervical vertebræ have been thus so effectually splintered and comminuted, has been suffering at the time from rabies. For, as we have repeatedly seen, the spinal cord, and above all sections of the entire cerebro-spinal substance, the *bulbar* and spinal substance enclosed within the cervical vertebræ, or, in other words, in the immediately subjacent region of *the nape of the neck*, constitutes the specific seat of germination of the rabies-microbe. Nay, further, it is certain from M. Pasteur's experiments that the "rabies-virus" from fresh rabbit-cords, *i.e.* immediately after death, is, of any stage after the death of the animal, at its strongest and most intense virulence; for, in even a day or two's exposure of the cord, the virulence is very materially diminished, the rabic condition progressively diminishing every hour. But this rabies-virus in the bulbar or spinal substance will not be less virulent, but, on the contrary, possibly very much more so, and, consequently, still more infective, whilst the animal is still alive and labouring under the disease. Probably only at this stage is the "rabies-virus" invariably at its maximum of virulence and infectiveness for the case, and in no region of the entire cerebro-spinal system will this maximum be more centred than in the bulbar or spinal substance within the cervical vertebræ. It is precisely at the moment and at the stage of the disease when the spinal substance is in its most rabic condition that it is so torn and mangled by the hunting animal, and at a point of the spinal substance itself which is the most rabic of the cord.

On the certainty that the bulbar or spinal substance within the cervical vertebræ is the specific seat of incubation of the rabies-germ in the animal economy, and, further, that the hunting dog in its ferocious onslaught of the rabbit as of all the other inferior hunted animals, and, particularly, of the nape of the neck of such animals, is occasionally punctured in the tissues of the gums by the splintered fragments of vertebræ, and on the assumption that rabies is essentially a disease of the rabbit and takes its rise in this animal, it follows that the dog could not possibly escape, at least occasionally, direct infection. The infection, moreover, is in a site of the dog hardly less fatal or less certain to impart the disease than the intracranial inoculation itself; and, with a rabies-virus of the most potent paralysing form, at the maximum intensity point of infectiveness. Would it be surprising under such circumstances if the attacking dog or hunting animal should be occasionally infected; and, when so, invariably with the worst, the most transmissible, the most pronounced "dumb" canine-madness to be met with,—a form of the canine disease of 12 or even 11 days' (rabbit) incubation, not that of 15 to 20 days? One or two such cases cropping up "sporadically" and simultaneously in a district would be quite sufficient to initiate a widespread epidemic of canine-rabies.

By a puncture, scratch or abrasion of the gums in the manner here suggested, however slight the wound and however rare, a direct inoculation of virus-germ into the hunting animal would take place. For by such a mode of infection the rabies-germ would be immediately introduced into the lymphatic system of the mouth and palate, by which however it would be directly conveyed to the higher tracts of the cerebro-spinal and sympathetic nervous tissue, and, above all, to the bulbar substance; nearly as directly so as by M. Pasteur's subdural inoculation itself. However apparently slight, there could therefore be no infection or no site of infection more fatal. What, at times, could be more apparently trivial than the scratch or puncture which gives rise to tetanus-infection? It is true that a puncture of the gums at all noticeable does not always take place in such cases; otherwise, canine-rabies would probably be a more prevalent disease than it is. But in a thousand cases of such puncture, possibly one inoculation of the gum, with effective infection, might be quite sufficient to account for the prevalence of the disease as it actually exists. The dumb or profoundly paralytic cases of dog-madness, which initiate an outbreak, would alone represent such cases; and these are "altogether exceptional," there being, it would seem, probably not more than 4 or 5 per cent. in the most extensive epidemic. Unfortunately, the possibility of such infection on the part of dogs, either whilst a rabbit is still suffering from rabies, or even when the animal has just died from the disease, has, so far as one can gather, not been experimentally tested. This has to be regretted, for the results elicited, whether negative or positive, would be not merely of theoretic but of great practical value.

Nor is this all. So far it has been assumed that the hunted animal, whilst attacked, has been actually labouring under the disease, and that, therefore, the rabies micro-organism in the spinal substance of the seized animal has germinated to its full capacity. But, as we have also seen, for a very definite period prior to the outburst of the morbid phenomena, the rabies-germ has already settled and copiously germinated in the spinal substance. It is unquestionably the fact that the rabies-germ, received in infection, has not reached the cerebro-spinal substance through the entire *pre-incubation period, i.e.* the period of conveyance of the micro-organism. It is certain, too, that through this whole stage it has undergone no incubation or germination whatever, but rather the reverse. Hence, it is only during this *pre-incubation period* that the inoculative preventive treatment is of any avail. Until the rabies-microbe has reached and settled in the spinal substance incubation proper does not really begin. But having been once conveyed to this structure, it immediately sets in, and lasts till the full germination of the micro-organism has been accomplished, or till the advent of the disease. No stronger proof of the existence of the rabies-germ in the spinal substance and of its active and progressive germination in this structure for a definite time prior to its culmination in the disease could be afforded than by the fact that in hydrophobia the inoculative treatment is found to be of little or no avail *twelve* or even *fourteen days* before the disease declares itself. The same will hold good of the rabbit or hunted animal, but for a still shorter pre-incubation-period. The cerebro-spinal substance of such an animal, as compared with that of man or the dog or of any attenuator, is, as we have already seen, so favourable a soil for the settlement and the cultivation of the rabies-germ that the latter will germinate in this structure most copiously at the earliest possible moment, the entire pre-incubation-period being reduced to a minimum.

Hence, for possibly five or six days before rabies declares itself even in such an intensifier, the cerebro-spinal substance must already be disseminated with the rabies-germ in actively-incubating centres, and yet the animal be apparently in its normal health ; for, as yet, no virus has been eliminated in the case. Now, suppose a rabbit to be captured by a hunting animal, when the rabies-germ has extensively germinated in the spinal substance, and without as yet having elaborated its virus, it is conceivable that a ravenous dog may be occasionally infected, by the method already described, even at this stage, or a few days before the disease has actually declared itself; the rabies-microbe in the cerebro-spinal substance is on the point of rabidising the rabbit itself. How long before the disease fairly sets in this may occur, or even if at all, it is impossible at present to definitely say, for hitherto it has not been tested. But the *normal* rabies of the rabbit is, as we have seen, a 10 days' rabies. If, therefore, we assume that the genuine incubation-period of such a rabies, as opposed to the mere pre-occupation-period, is at least five days, if not longer, here, even before the advent of the disease, is an appreciable interval for the possibility of infection on the part of the dog or hunting animal. At all events, so far as the infected rabbit is concerned, it is certain that the rabies-germ is disseminated and probably copiously germinating in every direction in the spinal substance, but particularly in the bulb and the cervical sections of the cord, sooner than in any other infected animal, and at least for a space of some days before the disease actually declares itself, the pre-incubation-period in such an animal being reduced to a minimum. It is perhaps safe, therefore, to assume that if such a rabbit be seized by a hunting dog, and with the ferocity characteristic of the hunting animal, the possibility of infection, even at this stage when the rabies-microbe in the spinal substance of the hunted animal is in its most active, germinating condition, is by no means merely problematic.

CHAPTER XVI.

HOW RABIES ARISES IN INTENSIFIERS.

How does the statistical investigation bear out the theory before us? The conclusion from a statistical survey of the disease, which hitherto has been universally arrived at, is that rabies is essentially canine in character, and also invariably canine in origin.

"The dog," says Professor Fleming, "is certainly the animal which is by far the most frequently attacked of all animals." So prevalent is the disease in this animal over all others, that Professor Fleming has not hesitated to further infer that "it is, therefore, exceedingly probable, nay certain, that if the canine species were completely freed from rabies, *the disease could be no longer known*[1]."

It is beyond doubt that the dog is the animal which is the most frequently attacked with "*furious*" rabies. But that, above all animals, it is the most frequently attacked with rabies itself, particularly with "*dumb*" or paralytic rabies, and the most transmissible of any even in the dog, is a very different statement, and open to question. Nevertheless, viewing the hunting animal in the light of the theory suggested above, the statistics which Professor Fleming has amassed are very important and of deep significance. Thus, it is certain that, prevalent and difficult to stamp out though it be, rabies can be, and has been over and over again, completely checked and suppressed by an adequate protection or isolation of the dog-race.

"That the disease can be limited, or altogether suppressed, by the enforcement of proper measures (such as the use of the dog-muzzle) there is an abundance of evidence to prove. Sweden, Norway, Switzerland, Baden, Prussia, Bavaria, Wurtemburg, and other countries

---

[1] "The Propagation and Prevention of Rabies," by Geo. Fleming, C.B. and F.R.C.V.S. Paper read at the International Congress of Hygiene in London, Aug. 12, 1891.

have been freed from it by such measures. In Vienna, we are informed that rabies was entirely suppressed by eighteen months of stringent muzzling; but in the summer of 1886 the muzzling order was rescinded. In the following year rabies became epizootic, and the muzzle had again to be worn; with the result that the malady soon subsided and disappeared....In Sweden rabies was at one time a somewhat common disease. But on muzzling being enforced, and the importation of dogs prevented, *rabies has been unknown for many years; and no deaths from hydrophobia have occurred since* 1870[1]."

These are great protective results to be obtained by so simple a means as a muzzle, which, in itself, is by no means so irritating or "cruel" as the habitual use of an iron bit and a bridle. But what do they imply? Not, certainly, that the disease is primarily and wholly a canine malady, or invariably of canine source, wherever it appears. Apart from their practical value, which has been so universally demonstrated, it is obvious from such evidence that rabies is not peculiarly a canine disease, and that therefore it does not necessarily take its rise in the animal kingdom through the dog. Were this the fact, the mere use of a muzzle, or any form of quarantine, however "stringent" or prolonged, would neither wholly abolish the disease when it was rife, nor, when it did not exist, prevent its sudden and irregular rise in the animal in country after country. It unquestionably does so. It is therefore clear from such evidence that the liability of the dog to incur the malady is extrinsic, not intrinsic, being solely determined by the animal's exposure to infection; or that the rabies to which it is exposed, and which it incurs, is at least primarily a disease altogether *ab extra* to the dog-race. This is strikingly demonstrated in the case of Holland, as contrasted with the neighbouring state of Belgium, where the muzzling order has not been in force.

"In Holland, before 1875," says Professor Fleming, "rabies was prevalent to a very serious extent. But in June of that year the use of the muzzle was ordered; with the result that in the autumn the number of cases fell to 41. In the next whole year they were 55. In 1877 they were 14. In 1878 they were 4. And in 1879 they were 3. These (latter), and the cases which have since been reported, *only occurred in or near the frontier of Belgium*, in which country the

---

[1] Prof. Fleming's Paper read at the London International Congress of Hygiene.

muzzle is not in use, though rabies is always prevalent. To such a degree, indeed, does the disease exist in Belgium, that in 1889 there were brought to the Veterinary School at Brussels no fewer than 94 rabid dogs[1]."

It will not be denied that, after the muzzling order was enforced in Holland, the dogs of that country were not, *per se*, just as liable as before the order was enforced to develop the disease, and just as inherently subject to rabies as the dogs of Belgium which were not muzzled, and where in consequence the animals were being "continuously contaminated all over the country by the scourge." Even the one or two cases which kept cropping up, but only on the borders of Holland, in spite of the most stringent muzzling, were certainly contaminated from the same (Belgium) scourge. If there were no other evidence than this, then, it is clear that rabies is not intrinsically a canine malady, but that the dog derives the disease, even primarily, from an external source, the initial and primary forms of the malady in an epidemic being peculiar to, and taking its rise in, an altogether different order of animal.

But again, even in countries such as Belgium where there is no muzzling order, or such as England, where the order (except Mr Long's) has been but irregular and transient, it is found that all breeds of dogs, although inherently equally capable of incurring rabies, do not as a matter of fact equally often contract it. This, again, there is good reason to show, is due to the circumstance that all breeds are not by any means equally exposed to the same risk of infection. What dogs, then, in particular, are found to be most affected? Unfortunately this point, likewise, has hitherto not been sufficiently, or even specially determined; what evidence there is is somewhat meagre. Thus, in the Report to the Local Government Board, whilst there is a sifting scrutiny of nearly 100 cases of hydrophobia, quoted verbatim from M. Pasteur's own journals, and of 150 other such cases, tabulated in an abridged form from the same source, with the exception of two or at most three cases,—all, singularly enough, "terriers,"—there is not a hint as to the particular breed of dog which imparted the disease[2]. The animal itself is simply dismissed with the remark that it belonged to the person bitten, that it was one of a gang, that it was young, or that it was "on

---

[1] Prof. Fleming's Paper read at the London International Congress of Hygiene.

[2] Report to the Local Government Board respecting M. Pasteur's treatment of hydrophobia.

the loose," etc. But that it was a spaniel, a poodle, a sheep-dog, a bull-dog, a Newfoundland, etc. is ignored. In M. Pasteur's own invaluable communications, too, unfortunately, the same omission is to be noted. It is sometimes merely casually mentioned that a "mountain-dog," or a "farm-dog," or a "wandering dog" was the factor of the hydrophobia to be cured. What information of any value does the phrase "wandering dog" convey? All rabid dogs, except those suffering from the most pronounced paralytic or "dumb" canine-madness, are wandering.

Fortunately, however, there is not wanting a certain amount of evidence bearing on the subject. In the Report to the House of Lords in respect of the surgical (local) treatment of rabic wounds, it is assumed that ill-fed, homeless mongrels are the main medium of the propagation of the disease, if not likewise its sole source in the dog-race[1]. But the transfer of the micro-organism or the capacity of infection is by no means confined to such animals. Most certainly the disease, however severe in these—and it will be severe in them for the same reason that it is severe in the fox and in the cat—does not originate in the foul-eating habits of such animals; it does not necessarily originate in this class of dog at all. The semi-putrid garbage on which the unowned mongrel subsists is not the habitat of the rabies-germ. On the contrary, after only a week's exposure the most rabic rabbit's cord, teeming from end to end with the micro-organism, has lost its virulence, and directly putre-faction sets in has entirely lost the rabies-germ; the latter having died, or begun to die, immediately on the death of its victim. In dead matter, however organised, or "fresh," and however nutritious, it has been found impossible to cultivate the micro-organism; putrid or decaying animal matter would probably instantly destroy it. Thus, there is no evidence that the dogs of the East, which nevertheless so wholly feed on garbage and decaying animal refuse that they con-stitute by far the most effective scavengers of the country, are particularly often affected with the disease. The reverse of this would appear to be the fact. The putrid filth on which they revel with such repulsive gusto, and which renders the Oriental dog every-where so odious (for this reason, no doubt, the dog is always referred to with such contempt in the Bible and the Koran, hardly less so

---

[1] Report to the House of Lords respecting the surgical treatment of rabidised wounds.

than in the case of swine), destroying the rabies-germ rather than proving a medium of its cultivation; and, therefore, if anything, protecting the animal from infection rather than inducing it. The rabies-micro-organism is pre-eminently a micro-organism of *living* if of enfeebled nerve-tissue, not of *dead*, much less of putrid or decaying matter. And the dog which presents the disease most frequently and in by far the severest forms, and consequently "propagates" it most effectually is, there is reason to show, of the purest breed, the cleanest habits, and of the strongest and healthiest organization. How or why should this be so? One would naturally expect the ill-fed, ill-treated mongrel, if rabies were essentially a canine malady, to be the primary source of the disease in at least the dog-race itself.

It is true that all dogs are capable of taking and of imparting rabies; but it is also certain that all dogs are not equally often affected with the disease. This, as we have just seen, is sufficiently obvious from the use of the muzzle itself, which, in abolishing the exposure to infection, or reducing it to a minimum, practically abolishes the disease. But these facts are still more strikingly borne out by the statistics of the Battersea Dog's Home, and, on a still larger scale, of the London police authorities. In these records the animals, destroyed on account of rabies, have been, fortunately, fairly well tabulated according to breed or race. And from these lists the dogs which would appear to be most frequently affected comprise, significantly enough, such breeds as the following:—the terrier, the collie, the sheep-dog, the retriever, the spaniel, and the hound, in all their varieties and sub-varieties. These constitute much the greater percentage of the canine victims of rabies. On the other hand, the following breeds are more or less conspicuous for their absence, and some of them entirely so:—the Newfoundland, the mastiff, the bloodhound, the staghound, the St Bernard, the poodle, the bull-dog, the pug-dog, etc. But why should the former class of dogs, as contrasted with the latter, so frequently incur the disease? It is not because they are intrinsically more liable to the malady, but, much more probable, because, as it so happens, they are the only genuine *hunting* dogs. Still more important, of all dogs, they are, significantly enough, the only hunters of the rabbit and of the smallest and feeblest of the herbivora, or what one may perhaps term *minor* hunters. Even sheep-dogs and collies and "farm-dogs" are inveterate hunters of the rabbit and hare. An intelligent shepherd of long experience once assured me in the Argyllshire Highlands, that, all through the winter and the earlier months of spring, sheep-dogs of neighbouring farms occasionally evince a strong tendency to gather together and to hunt in small packs. When they return they are usually shot, not merely for fear they should attack sheep at the lambing-time,—a very reasonable fear,—but because this very habit proves them to be erratic and wholly unreliable; and frequently, if not shot, they become mad.

Thus, then, assuming the disease to take its rise in the rabbit, such hunting breeds, above all dogs, cannot fail to incur it most frequently; and the healthier, the more vigorous and the purer the breed, and the more exclusively it is a minor hunter, the more certain will it be exposed to the risk of infection. Moreover, in spite of the animal's exceptional refractoriness, the more profound and paralytic will be the rabies thus at first hand incurred, or the more will it approach in form that characteristic of the rabbit. On the other hand, such breeds as the Newfoundland, the St Bernard, the mastiff, the staghound, the bull-dog, the poodle, the pug-dog, etc. are so freed of rabies, because, strictly speaking, they are not hunting dogs, at least of the smallest of the herbivora; most certainly they do not hunt the rabbit. In like manner, dogs living habitually on board ship, or in a kennel as watch-dogs, whether or not they belong to the hunting class, there is good reason to believe, never incur the disease. And the same holds good of even the wild dog, the fox, the wolf, and the wild cat when they are confined in a menagerie or a zoological garden; no case of rabies has ever been recorded in such confinement. But, according to the theory before us, this is necessarily so ; because such breeds, or these particular animals, are never really exposed to infection. Hence it would appear that the less exposed the dog-race to the possibility of such infection, whether from habits or mode of life, not less than from the use of a muzzle or from any other form of quarantine, the more certain will be the absence of rabies.

It may be objected that the special hunting dogs, here referred to, are more frequently attacked with rabies than either the non-hunting or the major-hunting breeds, not so much because they so habitually attack the rabbit and the smallest herbivora, which is undeniable, as because they are in reality the most numerous. Is this so? The same line of argument has been applied in the hypothesis that rabies originates in the animal kingdom, and even in the dog-race itself, exclusively through the *male* dog, and, mainly, from *sexual* restrictions ! But the male dogs are attacked in the greatest numbers because they are more numerous than the female;—at least this is certainly the case in respect of the domestic dog. There is, however, no inherent reason why the female dog should be, *per se*, less liable to rabies than the male, but rather the reverse. Does the same line of argument apply to the hunting as opposed to the non-hunting dogs? Are there, for example, more greyhounds than bull-dogs or pug-dogs? Are there more terriers or collies than poodles, Newfoundlands or mastiffs? Are, then, Newfoundlands, St Bernards, poodles, bull-dogs, pug-dogs so very rare? Even if these breeds, as compared with the genuine hunting-dog, were as rare as assumed, which, however, is very far from the fact, why should rabies be so extremely uncommon, and the mortality from the disease of so low and insignificant a percentage, in the former as compared with the latter? There is no such discrepancy between female and male dogs. There is no such diversity in respect of the rabbit-race, or any class of animal capable of intensifying the disease. If it be the fact, as has been so often unhesitatingly asserted, that rabies is *par excellence* a canine disease, and invariably takes its origin in the dog itself, why should not the disease be as common, or the mortality as high, in one breed as in another when both are equally numerous? The one order of dog is as capable of being rabidised, or of taking rabies, as the other. There must, then, be some very special and constant reason why rabies is so prevalent in the hunting as compared with the non-hunting dog.

From this circumstance, therefore, apart from the evidence furnished by the use of the muzzle, it is also clear that rabies, even canine-rabies itself, is not essentially a canine malady, but that it is derived by the dog from a source in the animal kingdom which is altogether *ab extra* to the dog-race. Hence, the disease, first incurred in an extensive outbreak, is always so unlike "the ordinary" dog-rabies of the streets. It is profoundly paralytic and capable of a prolonged transmission even through the dog; for it is in reality the rabies of a *hunted*, rather than of a *hunting* animal; of an intensifier, not of an attenuator; of the rabbit, not of the dog.

But if rabies takes its origin in the rabbit, or other equally *hunted* animal, how comes it to pass, when the disease crops up in this animal, however "sporadically" or mysteriously, that it never spreads? One never hears of an outbreak of rabies in the rabbit. Until comparatively a few years ago, when M. Galtier first demonstrated its existence, it was unknown, even unsuspected, that the rabbit was affected with rabies at all. But, according to the theory before us, rabbit-rabies must be of at least occasional occurrence in nature; not less uncommon than the profoundest "dumb" or paralytic dog-rabies, seeing that every extensive outbreak of dog-madness takes its rise in this form and from this very source. It must be of even somewhat more frequent occurrence; for not every case of rabbit-rabies occurring in nature would necessarily give rise to dog-rabies.

There would be great force in this objection, if rabbit-rabies were, to begin with, invariably of a *furious* and aggressive character. But, unless directly derived from a canine-rabies, it is never really so. The furious rabies thus induced is in no way to be distinguished from, and has all the characteristics of, the ordinary furious rabies of the dog, including even the aggressiveness, and the foreign material found in the stomach at an autopsy, just as is likewise the fact in respect of the deer and the larger herbivora. In each of these cases, the furious rabies is the canine disease, or but a 15 days' rabies, and nothing else. And, as we have seen, it will take at least ten transmissions through the rabbit of this convulsive canine-"virus" before the rabies normal to the rabbit, *i.e.* a 10 days' paralytic rabies, is fully established. A furious or convulsive rabies, then, so far as the rabbit is concerned, is an altogether abnormal rabies, solely derived from a canine source; and for this reason this form of the disease in the rabbit is so phenomenal even in the laboratory, and so absolutely unknown in a state of nature.

If, assuming the disease to exist in nature, rabbit-rabies were, to begin with, always of this furious character, and the animal invariably as aggressive as the mad dog, there can be no doubt that the disease would spread through rabbits with every outbreak, and far more seriously, for a very much longer time, and in a very much wider range than in the case of the dog or any such attenuator; just as a rabies of this character and origin spread with such unceasing and increasing potency through the Richmond Park deer in the epidemic of 1886-7. In every case of the malady, however feeble and obscure to begin with—and the more feeble the initial rabies in the rabbit the more certainly would it spread—there would always be a very obvious and an extensive outbreak of rabbit-rabies in the district. But this, as just stated, is far from being the fact. No such outbreak has ever been known. Consequently, if the rabbit incurs rabies for itself and through its own conditions of existence, and apart altogether from the dog or any other animal, the originating form of this disease cannot be the furious or aggressive rabies of 15 days' incubation. If rabies takes its origin in this animal, it must, on the contrary, do so as a paralytic *rabbit-rabies* of 10 days' incubation, not as a canine-rabies; a paralytic, not a convulsive, rabies being the normal form of the disease in the rabbit. But a profound paralytic rabies, whether in this or in any other animal, is devoid of aggressiveness or "fury." If the dog, suffering from the furious rabies which is so character-istic of the animal, may be said to be *mad drunk* with the "virus," the rabbit, suffering from the profound paralytic rabies which is so peculiar to it, may, still more strictly, be said to be literally *dead drunk*. The animal is much too seriously prostrated by the disease to be capable of attacking any other animal, and is but able to stagger or drag itself to the nearest hiding-place to lie down and die. This is obvious even in the dog itself, when the animal is suffering from the most pronounced "dumb" paralytic madness of which it is capable. A dog, under the influence of this rare form of canine-rabies, will shun all other dogs or all other living creatures, and, dazed and bewildered, will stagger to the nearest solitude, con-scious only of approaching death, being, likewise, *dead drunk* from the appalling virus. But if this be true of a hunting animal, and of the most potent of attenuators, how much more true of a hunted! If this be the case in respect of the dog, how much more so in respect of such an animal as the rabbit!

As we have already seen, the rule in the entire herbivora is, "that only those animals of a herd which are first bitten fall victims to the disease[1]." They die without fury, almost without notice. An aggres-sive element in the rabies normal to the entire intensifying division of the animal kingdom is conspicuous for its absence; and, in con-sequence, an epidemical outbreak, even in the larger herbivora, is rare in the extreme. This, however, is more especially the case in respect of the feeblest and the smallest of the herbivora. It is questionable if an epidemical outbreak ever occurs in such animals; and not without reason. The more persistently persecuted and hunted the animal the more potent is it as an intensifier, and the more profoundly paralytic will be the rabies which is normal to it; consequently, the more devoid will be such rabies of any aggressive element whatever. The rabbit, suffering from its own specific rabies, is in no sense "furious"; but, as M. Galtier from the first

[1] See Report to the Local Government Board on outbreak of rabies in the Richmond Park herd of deer.

clearly pointed out, it is all through the disease "*extremely* quiet and low-spirited; and, as a rule, *it does not even try to bite*," being totally unable to so. Now on the assumption that rabies takes its rise in the rabbit in the paralytic form which is normal to it, it is not surprising that, under such circumstances, the disease does *not* spread through the nearest colony of rabbits, and does not constantly, or in point of fact *ever*, assume an epidemical character. From the beginning of the disease till death the animal will be so stricken down by the malady, so collapsed with the paralysing virulence of the rabies, that, even were it so disposed, it would be incapable of attack. So complete is the collapse, that it is doubtful if the animal could impart infection even amidst the most swarming colony. Hence, the proposal to exterminate the rabbit of Australia with rabbit-virus, much more with canine-virus, is untenable ; for, directly the profoundly paralytic rabies characteristic of the animal was established by transmission, the disease would summarily die out with the prostrated and utterly paralysed individuals. A rabbit affected with such a rabies would be, even in a crowded colony, as suddenly and as singly and completely struck down as a pine-tree in a forest by a lightning-shaft. And the very gravity of the malady, in thus so effectually destroying the individual, would protect the entire colony with which it lives, and prevent any outbreak whatever.

It is this very severity of the disease with the complete collapse and speedy death attending it, which has in all probability hitherto *masked* it in the rabbit for so many centuries. Nor is this surprising. Precisely the same thing has occurred in respect of paralytic as opposed to the ordinary convulsive hydrophobia. Until M. Pasteur conclusively demonstrated the existence of this form of the malady, it was absolutely unknown for at least twenty centuries of the most penetrating clinical observation. And even in recent years it has been mistaken by experienced physicians for, and actually registered as, *Landry's Paralysis* or "the acute ascending paralysis[1]." If, however, this be true of hydrophobia, which has been under such close and constant scrutiny for many centuries, it surely may well be true of the profound paralytic rabies normal to rabbits. For as a matter of fact this is more blighting than the severest *paralytic hydrophobia* to be met with ; and, moreover, if it exists in nature,

[1] See Report on M. Pasteur's treatment to the Local Government Board, where a case of this kind is alluded to.

it has never been studied, never even been looked for. The intense severity of rabbit-rabies might, therefore, well mask it from the observation of the keenest investigation, and the profoundly paralytic form of the malady, with its corresponding collapse, might completely prevent it from spreading through other rabbits, all aggressiveness or possibility of attack being thereby wholly eliminated. If so, a rabbit thus affected might die in the most crowded colony of rabbits without necessarily imparting the disease. Certainly, it has nowhere been recorded that paralytic rabbit-rabies has been spread from rabbit to rabbit and by each other in the laboratory itself, even in a hutch of rabbits. But, unfortunately, this experiment, likewise, has not hitherto been specially tried. Surely, however, the point is a very practical one, if not for man's sake (who, apparently, is not worth considering) at least for the sake of the dogs and rabbits themselves.

Now, granting the possibility of at least the occasional occurrence of the disease in the rabbit in nature in its *normal* paralytic form, and derived from a source altogether irrespective of the dog-race, it is not surprising that the dog, above all animals, should be so frequently infected with rabies, from this very animal, and, *always primarily*, with the severe "mortal," highly transmissible canine-madness so closely resembling the normal rabbit-rabies, and which gives rise to every extensive outbreak of the canine disease. In this connection it is important to note that the "dumb" madness which initiates an outbreak of dog-rabies is always as mysteriously sudden in its appearance as it is rare in its occurrence. When, it may be for years, there has been no rabies whatever in a district, a dog all at once turns up with this particularly severe form of the malady; or, possibly, a few such dogs at different points of the district simultaneously turn up, each infecting, with an infective-rate of from 95 to 100 per cent., or well-nigh every living creature it meets and attacks, as in the terrible case at Deptford, referred to by the Committee appointed by the Local Government Board. Such an animal, or a small group of such cases scattered over a district, would constitute the glowing nucleus of an outbreak which would extend for miles over the country, and if unrestrained, as by the use of the muzzle, would last probably for years. But sudden as is the appearance of such a case, or even a small crop of such cases, it is not a spontaneous outbreak, due to any intrinsic morbid conditions ; for these dogs, far from being diseased, are quite the reverse.

Otherwise, the mere use of a muzzle could not prevent this any more than the ordinary "furious" madness from constantly occurring, but rather the contrary. It does, however, absolutely prevent it. And for this reason in such countries as Sweden and Germany, where the dog-muzzle has been so persistently enforced, the disease has been completely abolished. If this paralytic canine-madness of highest infective-rate, and which is the initiating rabies of every extensive epidemic, be rendered impossible, all other forms of canine-rabies are abolished; for this potent and most transmissible initial form, as already pointed out, covers and includes one and all.

Again, it is surely significant that canine-rabies is a disease *of the country* much more than *of the towns and cities*, if, indeed, it does not exclusively take its rise in the country. Statistics, such as those of the London Police journals (which through the kindness of Sir Charles Warren I was permitted to examine), would, alone, seem to indicate that an outbreak of canine-rabies invariably reaches the towns and cities through the suburbs and from the surrounding country districts, seldom or never the surrounding country districts from the cities.

But this is still more fully revealed in the case of Berlin. "In the city of Berlin special regulations are in force. In consequence of a severe outbreak in the year 1852, during which 107 dogs were destroyed as rabid, the Royal Police issued a decree to the effect, on July 2, 1853, that all dogs should be provided with a wire muzzle positively preventing the animal from biting; and to empower certain persons, appointed by the police for that purpose, to seize and destroy all dogs not so muzzled, and, when the owners could be found, imposing a fine of 10 thalers (£1. 10s.) or a term of imprisonment. In the year following this decree only one dog was killed as rabid, against 97 in the previous year[1]."

Although this universal muzzling of the city dogs, but most certainly not at all of the country or even suburban dogs, was immediately, it was by no means permanently effectual. Further police action had to be taken.

"The decree (of 1853) still remains in force, but does not seem to have been effectual in preventing the recurrence of epidemics of rabies; for the number of dogs killed as rabid, which up to 1863 had not exceeded in any year nine, rose progressively in the succeeding years, till in 1868 the number had reached sixty-six, declining

[1] Report of the Royal Commission on Rabies in Dogs, 1887.

again to seven in 1870, only to increase in 1872 to sixty-nine. In 1875, however, a law was passed, extending to the whole of Prussia, for the suppression and prevention of animal diseases; which provides that all dogs suspected of rabies shall be immediately killed, as also all animals which it is evident have been bitten by rabid animals; and, also, that all dogs in a district which has been infected by an outbreak of rabies shall be confined or, when abroad, both muzzled and led. The Technical Section of the Veterinary Board in Berlin are of opinion that the passing of this law, and not the existence of the muzzling-order in that city, is the cause of the extinction of rabies in Berlin. No case has occurred there since 1883[1]."

From such results it is clear that the German Government was amply justified in at last passing a measure, whereby *all the dogs of Prussia* should be muzzled; and that the muzzling of the animals in the suburbs and country districts not merely reduced the rabies in Berlin, but very soon abolished the disease from the city. The protection from the muzzling-order was in the first instance much too local and limited; nor did the disease arise in the city. Hence, if the country districts and outlying suburbs are sufficiently protected by the dog-muzzle there probably would be comparatively little fear of rabies cropping up in the cities proper. Under these circumstances it is surely of much more importance to enforce a muzzling-regulation for lonely *country districts* rather than for crowded towns. Unfortunately, from first to last, the rule has been quite in the opposite direction.

That the country districts are the primary starting-points of rabies is still further, if not conclusively, evidenced by the fact that such animals as the wolf and the fox are so frequently affected with the disease, of the entire dog-race perhaps the most frequently attacked. These animals do not frequent cities or towns; nor do they incur the disease of themselves in zoological gardens or in confinement. Why should this be the fact, if rabies is really a canine-disease, and especially a canine-disease of cities and towns? It is so, simply because, on the contrary, it is in the country, not in the towns, where dog-rabies is primarily contracted. And in such solitudes it is invariably in the first instance contracted in its severest and most infective forms, and entirely through the hunting pursuits of the dog-race. It is so essentially a disease of the country, because in

[1] Report of the Royal Commission on Rabies in Dogs, 1887.

all probability it is essentially a disease of *hunted* animals; and, of all such animals, pre-eminently the rabbit.

And there is not wanting a certain amount of collateral and corroborative evidence, which may be briefly indicated. Thus it would appear that the occurrence of dog-rabies is not altogether irrespective of season. It is most prevalent and most severe, not, as so usually supposed, in summer and early autumn, or the so-called dog-days, nor in the very depths of winter, but, curiously enough, *in the spring*. Unfortunately, however, this observation, likewise, has not been sufficiently extended. Nevertheless, what slight evidence there is, is not without value and extremely significant. The following Table, published by Dr Pasca, of Milan, may be taken as an indication of the general facts.

> In March, April, May, there were 35 cases of canine-rabies.
> In June, July, August, there were 14 cases of canine-rabies.
> In September, October, November, there were 25 cases of canine-rabies.
> In December, January, February, there were 14 cases of canine-rabies.

Why should dog-rabies be so prevalent in the spring as compared with any of the other seasons, actually 40 per cent. of the cases occurring at this time? What is to be inferred from so marked an occurrence? Assuming that in every outbreak the dog, in the first instance, directly received the disease from the rabbit, and in its severest, most transmissible form,—for here, unquestionably, the initial form must have been very infective,—there is nothing remarkable in the phenomenon. On the contrary, it is precisely what might have been looked for. The primal infection for the outbreak, with the occurrence of the pronounced paralytic or "dumb" canine-madness, would probably take place from about a month to six weeks before the disease actually broke out, even "sporadically," in the dog. That is to say, this originating infection would have occurred in the depth of the winter or, at latest, at the very end of this period, when, on the theory before us, the disease really broke out in the rabbit. If this be so, it is not, apparently, an accident that dog-madness is the most severe and infective, and the most prevalent in spring. The very severity of the initial forms of canine-rabies during this season, with their similarity to rabbit-rabies, is, therefore, significant in the extreme.

Again, it is, surely, not without significance that both hydrophobia and canine-rabies are unheard of in certain countries, where, nevertheless, the dog-race abounds, and has abounded for untold ages.

What countries or districts in particular? There is reason to show that they are the countries and islands *without rabbits*, yet where the dog-race is plentiful. This holds good of the Arctic Circle, of deserts, of large equatorial and southern territories, or where the rabbit, as it so happens, does not exist. "In the Azores, in Madeira, in St Helens, and in Sumatra, rabies is absolutely unknown[1]." In such places the rabbit is also quite unknown; but the dog-race abounds, and has abounded from time immemorial. In every country where the rabbit does not exist canine-rabies has been, and is, conspicuous for its absence; as much so as in the case of a wolf or a fox in a zoological garden, or of a dog on board-ship or when kept permanently chained to a kennel.

"Rabies," says Mr Kerslake, "has occurred frequently in Egypt and along the northern coast of Africa; but it has never crossed the deserts; and the other regions of this vast continent have hitherto enjoyed perfect immunity from this terrible scourge, although every village and settlement swarms with dogs. The immunity of Cape Colony has been so perfect as to give rise to the idea that some climatic influence operates there, and that a rabid dog has only to 'sniff the air' of the colony to be cured[1]."

Again, to take one vast and well-known example; canine-rabies has never been seen or known in Australia or New Zealand;— "rabies," says Mr Kerslake, "is absolutely unknown in Australia, New Zealand, and Tasmania"; and until recently in these territories the rabbit has, likewise, been unseen. Nevertheless, the dog-race has abounded in the land, and has been imported from Europe for generations.

But it may be said, and with justice, that in at least recent years the rabbit has made its appearance in the Australian world, and that rabies in any form, canine or rabbit, has not at all supervened. The rabbit has recently multiplied all over New Zealand and the Australian colonies as it has never multiplied, even in Europe; to such an extent, indeed, and with such rapidity and prolific vigour,—comparable to the thistle-seeds of the old country in Pampas,—that in a few years it has become a formidable pest. It has taken such possession of the new land that it has already been found impossible to exterminate it, or even to keep it in check. Every kind of

---

[1] *Hydrophobia, its Cause, and Prevention by Muzzling*, by Mr Kerslake, Hon. Sec. to the Society for the Prevention of Hydrophobia, 50, Leicester Square.

restrictive measure, with Government awards of high value for the best proposed measures, has been employed, but in vain, to exterminate the animal. In spite of this very massive invasion, however, no one has heard of canine-rabies, or yet met with one single case of hydrophobia. How in the face of these facts can it be suggested that the rabbit is probably the animal which originates the disease in the animal kingdom; and that from the rabbit the dog primarily and directly derives his "dog-rabies"? If this be true, why has canine-rabies not broken out in the Antipodes?

If the rabbit has not initiated rabies in Australia, it is most certain that neither has the dog; and the dog is no mere recent arrival in the colonies, not so recent as the rabbit. If the disease originates in the dog-race it would have cropped up long ago even in Australia. It would have done so, altogether irrespective of its swarming colonies of rabbits, and long before rabbits arrived in the land. But if, on the other hand, rabies is fundamentally a rabbit-disease, and invariably originates in this animal for every outbreak of canine-madness, why has canine-rabies or hydrophobia not, at least recently, made its appearance? Precisely because Australia is a new, fresh world; because New Zealand has suited the rabbit like a very paradise. The conditions of its existence are more favourable here than probably in any other part of the world. For this reason, the animal has so prodigiously multiplied and so firmly established itself in the land. To judge from the Government Reports, drawn up by special Commissions, if the rabbit in New Zealand suffers at all it is from plethora, not from starvation. Still more important, it enjoys comparative, if not constant, freedom from all persecution, and is not subjected to the incessant misery of a hunted existence. So much is this the fact that it does not even require to burrow under the soil, and live in, so to speak, a seething grave like its European ancestors. In such a land, and under such circumstances, its life is equable, singularly free from its worst and most harassing enemies, and, for a rabbit, possibly well-nigh perfect; its ailments, such as they are, arising, mainly, from gluttony and satiety. It is not presumed that in such an environment a rabbit would develop or initiate rabies anywhere, even in Europe. The rabbit which in a European country would originate rabies in the manner suggested by the present theory is a very different animal with respect to the rabies-micro-organism and to the incurring of the disease. Its conditions of existence, its vital power, and its nervous substance can only be adequately described as in every way a contrast. The morbid conditions necessary for the inception and settlement and the most favourable development of the rabies-germ in the cerebro-spinal substance of the rabbit as a persistently hunted creature, and which, as we have seen, are by no means phenomenal in Europe or other rabies-infected regions, are completely absent in the Australian colonies. Were these morbific conditions as wholly wanting in Europe as in New Zealand, rabies with hydrophobia would probably also never be seen. In spite, therefore, of its swarming shoals of rabbits which, within recent years, have so firmly established themselves as natives, it is not surprising that rabies has not yet presented itself. It would be quite an anomalous accident if it should appear; for the conditions necessary to the origination of the malady are, in such rabbits, altogether wanting. So long as these conditions do not exist in New Zealand there is little likelihood of rabies making its appearance in the country; even if the entire Australian continent should be at length overrun with the animal. The snakes and venomous vipers of the country may in such an event, and probably will, enormously increase in numbers, and possibly in size, but rabies will not necessarily arise. The very absence of rabies of any kind, canine or rabbit, in such favourable conditions for the life of the rabbit, is therefore an argument in favour of rather than against the theory here suggested.

Assuming rabies to be a rabbit germ-disease, much more than a canine-disease, does it, then, arise *spontaneously* in the rabbit? If by this be meant that the rabies-germ, with its 10 days' paralytic rabies so characteristic of this animal, is, so to say, the spontaneous product of a very definite set of morbid conditions which at any time may occur, there is no proof of any such origin. The disease originates spontaneously in no animal, whether attenuator or intensifier, in the dog or in the rabbit. In every animal the rabies-microbe, which is introduced in infection, is the *causa causans* of the disease. With this infection, if sufficiently large, rabies even in the monkey or dog, or the most potent of attenuators, is inevitable. Without this, not any amount of paralyzing shock, as from a disastrous accident, will produce canine-madness or hydrophobia, and no set of morbid conditions, involving the spinal substance, even in the rabbit, or the most pronounced of intensifiers will ever, *per se*, cause rabies. To test this possibility, experiments of a crucial character, in respect of the spinal substance of the dog, have been performed; but they have never produced anything like rabies. No railway shock or concussion, however disastrous to the cerebro-spinal substance, has ever once ended in hydrophobia. The condition of the nervous system, but especially of the nervous substance, determines, on infection, the character of the rabies induced; but it never causes or induces the disease. So much so that it may be said that, whilst rabies is in reality a germ-disease of nervous-substance, it is pre-eminently a germ-disease of enfeebled and deteriorated nervous-substance, or of the nervous system in a state of shock and collapse.

If not a spontaneous product from intrinsic morbid conditions, where and how does the rabbit receive the rabies-microbe? Under what set of conditions does this most deadly of all pathogenic micro-organisms find an entrance into the animal's system, and settle so speedily and effectually in its cerebro-spinal substance as in by far the most favourable germinating-ground in the entire animal kingdom? As we have repeatedly seen, the rabbit, even above all hunted animals, is capable of intensifying the rabies-germ on transmission. But it does not follow from this fact, significant though it be, that every rabbit will constitute an equally favourable ground for the germination of the micro-organism. Given the existence, in even large numbers, of the micro-organism with its spores in the immediate neighbourhood of the animals, it does not follow that it will necessarily find in one and all an equally ready entrance to the cerebro-spinal substance, in which tissue of the animal economy it is alone capable of germinating. Persistently hunted, and correspondingly deteriorated in its nervous system, though the rabbit be, there is probably not one in a thousand, possibly in many thousands, which will present all the conditions necessary for the origination of the malady. The rabbit in which the rabies-germ at all naturally finds entrance, and whose cerebro-spinal substance affords the most favourable germinating-ground, is in all probability, as compared with its normal vigorous state, or as compared with that of the bulk of its fellows, in a deplorable condition; it may be half-starved, possibly even maimed and enfeebled to the last degree. But these conditions must be extremely rare. The disease in the rabbit, consequently, must be far from common. Were it as rare, however, as the most pronounced paralytic-rabies of the canine-race, which is questionable, it would be sufficient to account for every extensive outbreak of dog-madness.

On turning to the closely allied malady, *tetanus*, one may see a set of conditions which in all probability determines the occurrence of rabies in the rabbit, altogether irrespective of its connection with the dog-race. Thus it is alleged by surgeons of the highest eminence that, like gun-shot wounds, *frost-bite* is, as we have seen, a very frequent initial factor in the production of tetanus, "one of the commonest of all." It is unquestionable that the tetanus-bacillus must be introduced directly through the skin, as in frost-bite, or the disease will never be incurred. But a mere abrasion or puncture is quite as effective for infection, and still more common. The same holds good in respect of rabies; a subcutaneous or submucous infection is the preliminary *sine qua non* of the malady in all animals, there being no such disease as "idiopathic hydrophobia," any more than idiopathic tetanus.

Again, if the introduction of the bacillus into the subcutaneous areolar or connective-tissue determines the occurrence of tetanus, in all probability the condition of the nervous system at the time of this infection, and all through the incubation-period of the disease, de-termines the *character* of the tetanus which is at last evolved, and even the length of the incubation. A state of nervous shock at such a stage is, there is very good reason to show, a most dangerous, if not hopeless complication ; and which, it is to be feared, is too much ignored in the preliminary investigation and treatment of an accident which is likely to end in this dreadful disorder. If at the time or in the course of the accident, however trivial, whereby he has been infected, the sufferer has undergone the most extreme dread or anguish, in itself involving complete nervous collapse, the shock, how-ever apparently brief, is a very profound and lasting factor in the development of the tetanus induced. Take, as an example, the case of a workman who has been caught by a belt of machinery and swung round the entire works with no other apparent injury than a crushed finger or thumb. What anguish must the man have suffered during this accident ! Again, it is notorious that, although both exist in precisely the same inclement conditions, the wounded of a de-moralised and routed army are more prone to tetanus than those of the conquering. But the same holds good, even still more emphati-cally, in respect of rabies, for it is still more a germ-disease of the nervous substance. A state of *nervous shock* at the moment of infection, and all through the pre-incubation and incubation periods of the disease, as in the case of the sleepless dread of the worn-out "neurotic," after being attacked by a mad dog, is a deplorable complication, against which even the most heroic inoculative treatment is probably of no avail.

But, to revert to the case of frost-bite as an effectual and very frequent occasion of tetanus, suppose that such an accident has occurred to a careworn woman, or a delicate girl, or, still worse, a child who at night has lost her way on a mountain-path in a blinding snow-storm. No solitude could be more bewildering and overpowering even to a strong man; the child being hunted to death, so to speak, by the primeval elements of chaos. Could any set of conditions be more likely, than this terror-stricken wandering, to produce collapse of the entire nervous system; a collapse, moreover, which would be by no means merely momentary? Suppose, further, that in this desolate, most prostrating wandering, *frost-bite* of the fingers or ear-tips should supervene, it is clear that no possible set of conditions could be more favourable to the inception and evolution of tetanus, assuming that the child has been at length rescued and carried home, providing that the tetanus-bacillus is not far from such a home, or even from the shepherd's warm enwrapping plaid. Will the tetanus-bacillus, or its spores, be far from such a household? Badly drained, ill-ventilated stables and huts, gardens and farmyards are, it is notorious, a very special haunt of the tetanus-bacillus; it is probably never absent from such sites. In this case, likewise, tetanus is pre-eminently a disease of *the country*, rather than of the city or town. Be this as it may, it is certain that of all subcutaneous wounds, frost-bite is one of the most effectual for the ingress of such a micro-organism; for by the wound the bacillus is directly introduced into the subcutaneous connective-tissue in which, as it so happens, it alone germinates. Under such circumstances, would it be surprising if, in due course, our frost-bitten child should incur tetanus, and with her nervous collapse speedily succumb to the severest form of the malady? Precisely the same series of phenomena is to be noted in respect of the tubercle-bacillus and the incurring of tuberculosis, as also of the diphtheria-bacillus and the incurring of diphtheria, and of many other such preventive germ-diseases. Two conditions would appear to be essential to contracting the malady; the presence of the specific micro-organism which, alone, induces the disease, and hardly less important, a definite set of morbid conditions on the part of the infected, constituting a harrowed soil for the seed, in consequence of which the full germination of the micro-organism, and the character of the disease, are mainly due. And in the case of tubercle and cancer as well as of tetanus and rabies and all preventive germ-diseases this harrowed soil is hereditary. From M. Pasteur's exhaustive research it is certain that these conditions hold good of rabies, not less than of tetanus, tuberculosis, diphtheria, erysipelas, and all the other strictly *preventive* germ-diseases to which rabies belongs.

Again, the tetanus-bacillus is not by any means the only pathogenic micro-organism which haunts, with its spores, badly drained soils and their ill-ventilated, badly lit surroundings. It has this feature in common with the entire group which induces preventive germ-diseases. Thus the specific micro-organism of erysipelas, of diphtheria, of tubercle, of pyæmia, of probably pneumonia, of possibly acute rheumatism, and of many others, have, in every likelihood, their primary habitat in badly drained soils; it may be a special kind of soil for each micro-organism. And it is further worthy of note that every one of these finds its special seat of cultivation in the living economy, not in the highly specialised leucocytes of the marrow of bones, of lymphatic glands, and of the spleen and circulation, as in the case of the genuinely prophylactic germ-diseases, not in any specialised secreting-cell, but in the connective-tissue, the most elementary and the least specialised in the entire economy. And here, again, as we have seen, the same holds good of rabies. It is perfectly possible, if not certain, that its micro-organism, like that of tetanus or that of any of the entire preventive order, has likewise its primal habitat in some specific badly drained soil. Supposing this to be the case, is it too hazardous to further suggest that, precisely as the tetanus-bacillus frequents, and is probably never absent from, badly drained stables, gardens and farmyards, or the haunts of the larger herbivora, so in like manner the rabies-microbe with its spores may probably never be altogether absent from the soil of a badly drained, ill-ventilated warren infested with rabbits, or from the haunts of the smallest herbivora? Here, it may be, is a medium, peculiarly fitted for the earth- or soil-life of the rabies-germ. If this be so, in what condition must a warren be, swarming with rabbits in the depth of winter?

It is true that, when it can get such, the rabbit selects a sandy soil in preference to any other, probably because it is easier to burrow, but possibly also because it is more porous and (unknown to the animal) proves better fitted for drainage. Whilst pathogenic liquids or products might unquestionably drain effectually through such a soil; on the other hand, it is not less true that micro-organisms or their spores might for this very reason be all the more copiously and tenaciously retained. If, therefore, the rabies-microbe, like the micro-organism of so many germ-diseases to which in every important feature rabies is so closely allied, has its primal habitat in the soil, it may well be that it is specially in that of a warren crowded with persistently hunted rabbits, or amongst the smallest and the very feeblest of the herbivora; and just as the tetanus-bacillus so specially frequents with its spores the immediate and habitual surroundings of the larger herbivora. On this assumption, the existence of the specific micro-organism itself in the immediate surroundings of the rabbit favourable for its reception would thus be assured.

But were the soil and air of their surroundings teeming with the micro-organism or its spores, providing the rabbits were sound and vigorous, rabies would not necessarily ensue, any more than tuberculosis is necessarily incurred by the attendants of a Consumptive Hospital, although the air of the wards or even of the pulmonary tubes of the attendants may be crowded with the bacillus of the disease; or any more than diphtheria is necessarily contracted by the children of the most crowded board school, although the air of the class-rooms may be more or less charged with the spores of the malady; or any more than tetanus is necessarily incurred by the horses of a stable, although the air may be constantly charged with the bacillus or its spores. In rabies, likewise, as in all preventive germ-diseases, before not merely the inception and the settlement, but the most favourable germination of the rabies-microbe can take place, there must be, to begin with, a definite set of morbid conditions on the part of the rabbit itself. Do such conditions, however, never actually and naturally arise in the rabbit in the course of its hunted life?

Suppose that in the depth of an exceptionally severe winter the struggle for existence in the case of the rabbit is extreme and, for even so persecuted a creature, altogether phenomenal; and that, in consequence, it is underfed and reduced to the extremity of misery for food, being, nevertheless, constantly subjected to the hunted persecution which is its fate. Even of a closely packed warren of such animals, however, all will not be equally weak and deteriorated, or equally prone to take rabies; and, providing there be no abrasion, puncture, or wound for the free admission of the rabies-germ or its spores, the feeblest will not necessarily take rabies. But let a solitary rabbit on the search for food be exposed to a winter-storm for hours with the thermometer below zero, the animal in its starved and weakened condition might well incur, in one of its unhappy expeditions, *frost-bite* in the tip of the ears, or in the foot or toes. On limping back, thus frost-bitten, into its hole, prostrated from cold, hunger and dread, would it be surprising, from what we know of tetanus and other preventive germ-diseases, if the rabbit incurred rabies? Again, one asks, could any set of conditions be more favourable to the inception, the settlement, and the most perfect incubation of the rabies-germ? Providing the rabies-microbe or its spores are in the warm, steaming soil around the rabbit, why should they not gain access into the tissues of this frost-bitten ear, just as the tetanus-bacillus gains access into the collar-abrasion of an over-worked, enfeebled horse, resting for a day or two in a badly drained, ill-ventilated stable? But the introduction of the rabies-germ through this site, or such direct infection of the ear-tissues, would be as unfailing in its results and as prompt and severe as M. Pasteur's intracranial inoculation itself. A paralytic rabies of certainly not more than 10 days' incubation,—in other words, the rabies *normal* to the animal,—would be the inevitable consequence. No more favourable site for infection exists over the entire peripheral area, internal or external, mucous or cutaneous; it is more favourable, because still nearer the bulbar substance, than the vascular tissues of the gums of the dog or cat. Is there anything inherently improbable in such an origin?

It is true, that an occurrence of the kind here assumed, even in the most hunted and prostrated rabbit, must be very rare. But, as already stated, it is probably not more phenomenal, possibly somewhat less so, than the occurrence of the most pronounced "dumb" paralytic madness in the dog. It may be that not more than one in a thousand of the most enfeebled rabbits would thus incur the disease; any more than one in a thousand of the children at a crowded board school would necessarily incur and initiate diphtheria from the spores of the bacillus floating through the air of the schoolrooms. But in respect of rabbits and rabbit-rabies, this proportion, small as it is, would be quite sufficient to account for the recorded prevalence of pronounced paralytic rabies in the dog, and therefore, for every very extensive outbreak of the malady which occurs in that animal.

From these and the foregoing considerations is one, then, not justified in inferring that rabies takes its origin in the animal kingdom,

s.

18

not in attenuators, but in intensifiers, not in the *hunting* but in the *hunted* order of animal, not in the dog, as for so long and even yet assumed, but pre-eminently in the rabbit? If this be the case, and as it is in full accordance with the experimental investigation of germ-disease, it becomes comprehensible why the systematic use of the dog-muzzle should reduce the occurrence of canine-rabies to a minimum, and even altogether suppress it with hydrophobia. But it follows that, to completely eradicate it, the dog-muzzle must be employed with unvarying thoroughness, and both universally and permanently. Without this, canine-rabies with mysterious sudden-ness must ever and anon recur, particularly, if not exclusively, in country districts.

INDEX

Absorbent corpuscles of circulation, 98, 119, 122, 125, 133, 134

Acute or wholly paralytic rabies, 51—53, 208

Aërophobia, 41

Afferent or sensory system of nerves, fundamental seat of disturbance in rabies, 36—45

Ague, 147—152; a recurrent, centric germ-disease, non-prophylactic, 148; morbific results of its virus, irrespective of fever, 116; significance of its characteristic periodicity, 149

Ague of negro, 176, 177; as a final form, 181, 234, 235

Alcohol, a typical virus, 106; morbific results of, when protecting from intoxication, 114, 116; graduated accumulation of, *sine quâ non* of alcoholic protection, 109, 110

Alcoholic immunity, amount of, test of drinking habit, 107; its simultaneous morbid effects, 116

Alcoholic protection, evanescence of, 111

Alcoholism, 106—110; its alliance to rabies, 107—109; acute form, important half of germ-disease, 106; chronic or long-standing, protecting from intoxication, 114

Amœboid cells, behaviour of, to toxic material, 163; vegetable, 162, 163

Amœboid order of cell, 158, 162, 163; of connective-tissue, absorbing the micro-organisms of centric preventive germ-disease, neither as phagocytes nor as germinators, 121; its relation to pathogenic microbes, of a threefold character, 134; its phagocytic function, 158, 162; as cause of the external or exclusively peripheral germ-disease, 90, 100; of the prophylaxis of the prophylactic order of germ-disease, 139, 157, 168; of the ultimate attenuation of the excessively recurrent preventive germ-disease, 180

Analgesia, with extreme prostration, fundamental feature of paralytic rabies, 36, 38, 39, 40, 41

Anfractuous circulation of invertebrate, retained in vertebrate, kingdom, 145

Annales de l'Institut Pasteur; Metschnikoff's theory of the vaccinal element, 169; Pasteur's, 170

Anthrax; Pasteur's research on, 101, 102; a germ-disease, prophylactic, 101, 139; its modified micro-organism, as eliminated from a gelatinous medium, 172; a triumph over the prophylactic order of germ-disease, 101; a vaccination, 101, 102, 172; in frog, cold-blooded and, artificially, warm-blooded, 134

Anti-toxin or serum treatment, 159; its value in preliminary and intermittent stages of germ-disease, 131, 159; its failure, when used late, 160, 168

Areolar spaces of lymphatic system, subcutaneous and subvenous, its limits, 145

Ascending neuritis, rabies as an, 92, 94

Ascending or intermittent paralytic rabies, 51

Attenuating power in rabbits, possible consequences of its absence, 199

Attenuating power of dog, 216, 218; of the monkey, 217; proof of intrinsic soundness and strength of central nervous substance, 240, 255

Attenuation of rabies, 4, 84—87, 215

Attenuators or attenuating division of

18—2

animal kingdom, 5, 204—221; characterised by exceptional strength and integrity
of nervous system, 239
Attenuators' rabies, convulsive and convulso-paralytic, 208, 209; secondary and
derived, rather than primary, 220, 235
Attraction of phagocytes or amœboid order
of cell, succeeding repulsion, vital and
permanent, 163, 164, 165

Bacillary products as the cause of germ-
disease, 106, 107
Bacillus anthracis, as a prophylactic micro-
organism, modifiable, 101, 102
Bacterial agency, in living tissues of plants,
191, 195; indispensable characteristic of
vegetable and animal kingdoms, 181;
in relation to allotropic forms and conditions, 185; to catalysis, 192; to the
mineral as well as the vegetable kingdom,
185; to the removal of dead animal and
vegetable matter in soil, 184
Bacterial life, cause, direct or indirect, of
the pre-digested pabulum of plants, and
of their toxic principles, 185; in relation
to the evolution of secreting organs,
179—203; more extrinsic or peripheral
in plants than in animals, 181—191
Bacterial zone of the soil, 186
Bactericidal qualities of the serum of a
protected animal, 159; may be occasioned
by infinitesimal quantum of bactericidal
material, 173; peculiar to the preventive
order of germ-disease, 159; cf. also
Germicidal
Bark of furiously mad dog, diagnostic, 39
Belladonna, 186
Bell-wether; his *raison d'être*, 242
Berlin muzzling of dogs, its results, 262, 263
Bert (Paul), on rabies-virus of salivary
gland, 7; of the bronchial mucus, 9
Bignami, on causation of ague, 148
Bite of rabid dog not necessarily rabic, 2,
3, 11, 209
Blood-stream and lymph-stream, the routes
of conveyance of the rabies-microbe, 96
Blood-stream of rabidised animal rarely
rabic, 96; only in respect of an intensi-
fier, 145
Blood-system, two currents, its liquor san-
guinis and its wandering amœboid cells,
96; corpuscular system of, germinating-
soil of prophylactic order of micro-

organism, 96; phagocytic in respect of
preventive order, 135, 162
Bouchard, on rabic condition of lymphatic
glands, 9; and lymphatic fluid, 145
Boussingault, on incapacity of Papilionaceous plants to assimilate free nitrogen
of air, 192
Bradford case of hydrophobia, its extremely
prolonged incubation period, 212
Brown, Prof., on cessation of rabies in
herbivora with death of victim, 224
Brown-Sequard on rabies as "an ascending
neuritis," 34, 45, 92
Bulbar nerves supplying glosso-pharyngeal
region, 45
Bulbar nerve-tissue, theoretic and practical
importance of, as a primary site, 28
Bulbar rabies, 28, 29
Bulbar substance, the most constantly implicated by rabies-microbe, at the end of
incubation, 27, during the disease, 25, in
death, 23, 24; containing the microbe in
every stage of growth to decay, 124
Bull-dog's tenacity of "pluck," 239
Burdoni-Uffreduzzi of Turin, on rabic condition of pancreatic gland, spleen, and
liver, 9
Butterwort order of plants, its peptic power,
193

Cancer, a peripheral and centric germ-
disease of a connective-tissue nidus, 144
Canine character and source of rabies, 204,
206
Canine-rabies, 24, 223; convulsive in
character and diagnostic of attenuators,
23, 24, 141, 142; extreme rarity of a
wholly paralytic element in, and in
that of attenuators, 2, 16, 18, 210, 211;
extrinsic in source rather than intrinsic,
220; fading, final form, 181, 234; initial,
originating form of rabies examined,
204—210; initial form of, of an outbreak paralytic and the most transmissible; why, 238; not necessarily canine,
221; of country districts rather than
of the towns, 262; canine or convulsive
rabies more dangerous to the intensifying division than profoundest paralytic
rabies, 223, 224; more phenomenal in
rabbit than the completely paralytic
rabies in dog, 233; aptitude for, contradistinct from that of rabbit or intensifiers,

214, 215 ; serial transmission of, through rabbits, 198 ; signs and symptoms of, however prevalent, no test of its typical stability, 207 ; statistics of infective, of Battersea Dogs' Home, and of the London police authorities, 255

Cat, the, as a hunter, 238

Centric germ-diseases, 137—141 ; preventive and prophylactic, 138, 139, 140; former, germinating exclusively in centric connective-tissue, 138, 141, 142 ; latter, exclusively in wandering, corpuscular system of circulation, 139, 140

Centric nervous substance, specific seat of germination of rabies-microbe, 240

Cerebro-spinal infection in completely convulsive, in convulso-paralytic, in completely paralytic rabies, 23, 25, 28, 53 ; cerebro-spinal system, as offshoot (differentiated) of sympathetic, 61

Cervical site, the, seized by the hunting class, the most infective, 247

Chemiotaxis, characteristic of amœboids of animal and vegetable kingdoms, 163

Circulation, anfractuous, of invertebrate, retained in vertebrate, kingdom, 145 ; cf. also Absorbent corpuscles, Blood-stream, Blood-system

Comité d'Hygiène, on variability of rabies-infection, 11, 33

Completely convulsive rabies, bulbar in site, 50, 128, 209; non-infective by salivary secretion, 53, 210 ; viewed with tetanus, the sensory lesions of former, the motor of latter, 37

Comte's metaphysical and theological modes of explanation, 205

Connective-corpuscles of peripheral connective-tissue, absorbents of preventive micro-organisms, 121, 141, 144; media of conveyance of rabies-microbe, 96, 98, 125 ; not of germination, 133, 135, 137; the more they abound, the more favourable the site for infection, 144, 145

Connective-tissue, the lower, or simpler in structure, the more favourable to the germination of the preventive order of micro-organisms, 153

Connective-tissue, peripheral and centric, seat of germination of the entire preventive and recurrent order of germ-disease, 136, 141, 146, 152, 153 ; gelatinous composition of, 154

Connective-tissue, composition of, of interstitial framework of centric organs, and of synovial membranes and sacs, 142

Connective-tissue of spleen, as site of germination of malarial fever, 151 ; of cerebro-spinal substance, as that of rabies-microbe, 154

Connective-tissue, the most lowly organised in animal frame, 153 ; the least injured by a virus, and the most fitting germinating soil, 153 ; the seat of germination of the preventive order of germ-disease, 137, 138, 144—147

Conveyance of preventive micro-organisms, mode of, favourable to their deposit in the connective-tissue of centric structures, 144

Conveyance of rabies-microbe, mode and route of, to cerebro-spinal substance from periphery, 90—98

Convulso-paralytic canine-rabies, 208; its infective rate, 210

Cope, on cessation of rabies amongst deer with the death of victim, 224 ; on deer-rabies at outset of Richmond Park epidemic, 225

Croton-oil, as a product of plant-life of bacterial agency, 189; primarily, as a pathological, ultimately, as a physiological product, 190

Darwin, on specialised sensitiveness of sundew, 202 ; on exceptional strength and stability of monkey's nervous organisation, 239

Dead micro-organisms, after a germ-disease, or after preventive inoculations, as "the vaccinal matter," 169

Dearth of germ-disease in animal kingdom, and of toxic principles in vegetable kingdom, where dearth of micro-organisms, 184

Death inevitable in even slightest convulsive rabies ; why, 23

Death, sudden, of reinoculated dogs, but not from rabies, 114, 115

Deer-rabies, 225, 226

Deptford case of convulso-paralytic canine-rabies, 17, 261

Descending neuritis, the character of rabies, 45, 94 ; its virus-germ being centrifugal, not centripetal, 94

Desiccation of rabic nerve-substance kills, progressively, its rabies-germ, 124, 170

Differentiation of specific plant-tissues for toxic principles with synchronous concentration of latter, 190

Diminution in amount and potency of rabies-microbe during pre-incubation period, 95, 123, 124

Diphtheria, a preventive germ-disease, 90, 91; of peripheral connective-tissue cultivation, 93, 135

Diphtheritic membrane, 136

Dispersal of rabies, its character, through canine-race, 222; through rabbit or intensifiers, 223

Dog, as an attenuator of rabies, 208—228; contracts rabies, irrespective of race or breed, and of any intrinsic aptitude for the disease, 214; liability of, to rabies diametrically opposite to that of intensifiers, 214; its significance on origin of rabies in the animal kingdom, 215

Dog, folly of summarily destroying a suspected, 2, 3, 4

Dog, the, of the East, 255

Dog-race, intrinsic liability to rabies of, examined, 215; cf. Mongrel-dogs

Dog-race, bearing of, to rabies-microbe, contrasted with that of rabbit, 216, 218, 239

Dowdeswell's investigation of canine-rabies, 16; on refractoriness of dog to rabies, 214, 219

Dread after dog-bite, predisposing cause of intensification of hydrophobia, 3—5; the persistent feature of hydrophobia, 44

Drosera, evolution of the secreting organ of, 193—195

Drunkenness, its "mad" and "dead" varieties, 107

Duboué, on rabies-virus in salivary glands, 7; on rabies as "an ascending neuritis," 92

Dumb or paralytic canine-rabies, 39, 107, 208

Duration of protection from rabies-virus, or from inoculative treatment, its character and mode of protection, 105, 111, 112

Efferent or motor nerves, at their roots in spinal substance, special seat of disturbance in tetanus and in strychnine-poisoning, 40

Elephantiasis and its connective-tissue element, 147

Elimination of the virus of a pathogenic micro-organism, an irregular process, but final, 128; more or less sudden and simultaneous, 131; occurring neither during pre-incubation nor incubation periods, 125, 126, 127

Elimination of bactericidal material in blood-stream, or establishment of a bactericidal condition of specific tissues, pathological, 174

Elimination, ever-renewable, special character of a secreting organ, 191

Environment, immediate, of plant-roots, natural habitat of micro-organisms, 183

Erichsen, on fear of swallowing in hydrophobia, 44

Erysipelas, a preventive germ-disease, 90, 93; recurrent, 117; of peripheral connective-tissue cultivation, 134, 135

Evolution, exclusively on intrinsic modifying variability of living tissues, 195; of a pathogenic to a physiological microorganism, that of rabies, 198, 200; to higher and complex organisation, from attainment of secreting organ, 202, 203

Extension or migration of rabies-microbe through nerves, 45, 92; when it occurs, 94

Face and neck, why exceptionally dangerous sites of rabies-infection, 34

Farm-yards, badly drained stables, gardens, natural "home" of tetanus-bacillus, 91

Fermentation, bacterial, 181

Fibrocytes or connective-corpuscles derived serially from vegetable cells, 158; less phagocytic with respect to preventive micro-organisms than leucocytes or lymphocytes, 136, 137, 144

"Fixed," so-called, character of ordinary canine-rabies, 215, 218, 233, 234

Fleming, Prof., on canine character and origin of rabies, 206; his statistical investigation of canine-rabies, 251, 252, 253

Flügge, on tetanus-infection, 91

Fol's discovery of the rabies-microbe, 86

Foreign material in stomach at autopsy, 209; its meaning, 210

Fox and the wolf frequently contract rabies, why, 263; and an "immune" animal resists the disease, 97, 157

Fractional virus-germ of rabies, 82, 83; restored to its completed virus-germ on a second transmission through an intensifier, 83

Frazer's, Surgeon-major, case of hydrophobia, prolonged incubation period, 211

French Commission on Pasteur's experiments before them; the positive and the negative results disclosed, 12, 13

Frost-bite, as a condition of tetanus, 90, 269, 270; as a possible condition of rabies, 272, 273

Furious, or wholly convulsive, canine-rabies, 38, 209; abnormal to rabbit, 258

Galtier, on rabies-virus in bucco-pharyngeal mucous membrane and in lingual glands, 9; in parotid and salivary glands, 7; on rabbit-rabies, 40; on its copious salivary secretion, 5, 41

Galton, Sir Douglas, on "light from the sky" as bactericidal, 183

Gamaleia, on rabies, as an ascending neuritis, 92

Gardner's connecting-cells of a plant, 182, 186; as a specialised train, for conveyance of nutritious material and of toxic products, 187; and, very rarely, even of special micro-organisms, 194

Gelatinous composition of connective-tissue, peripheral and centric; its significance in the germination of micro-organisms, 154

Gelatinous substance, film of, around connective-corpuscle, 144; possibly around red blood-corpuscle, 144; its significance in absorption of the preventive micro-organisms, 144

Germ-disease, of exclusively centric connective-tissue cultivation, alone possessing a pre-incubation period, 122; dearth of, in animal kingdom, 184

Germ-diseases, either preventive or prophylactic in type, 99—118; of the Middle Ages mainly prophylactic; and their attenuation on transmission, prophylactic, 103; order of, to which rabies belongs, 99—117

Germicidal principle in serum; as a product of the pathogenic micro-organism? 170, 171

Germicidal property of plasma sanguinis and of specific tissues, 159, 160, 172; unproduced in dead tissue; inference, 172, 173; why germicidal, 168, 169, 173; cf. also Bactericidal

Germinating-tissue of stubbornly recurrent preventive germ-disease, ultimately specialised into a nidus for the pathogenic micro-organism, 199, 200

Germination, exclusively in fixed connective-tissue, characteristic of the preventive order, peripheral and centric, 139; exclusively in interior of the wandering absorbent corpuscles, characteristic of the prophylactic order, 121, 122, 139, 140; of rabies-microbe, exclusively in nervous substance, 19—32, 127; in the connective-tissue of nervous substance, 154; only after pre-incubation period, 127

Gilbert, on incapacity of Papilionaceous plants to assimilate the free nitrogen of the air, 192

Glandular system rabidised from centric nerve-source, 19; after, not before, incubation, 93

Golgi, on the causation of malarial fever, 148

Goulstonian Lectures on "the chemical pathology of diphtheria," by Sidney Martin, 171

Hellriegel micro-organisms in root-nodules of Papilionaceous plants, 192; their influence and significance, 192, 194

Hemp, Indian, 182

Hens and birds, their characteristic rabies, 16; of lumbar site and of intermittent paralytic character, 26, 130

Herbivora, the intensifying division of the animal kingdom, 5, 198, 224, 226; their feebleness determining the intensifying property, 227, 228, 229, 230

"Histology of the cell-wall," Gardner's research, 186

Horsley's, Sir Victor, delineation of deer-rabies at end of epidemic, 225; his experiments with dog-virus on rabbits, 14; testing the incubation period of canine-rabies, 212; the special rabies of the Richmond Park deer outbreak, 223, 224; of the attendant Goffi who died of paralytic hydrophobia in spite of inoculative treatment, 245

Humoralists, on germ-disease, 160 f.

Hunted animal, why its nervous organisation so fitted for germinating the rabies-microbe, 240—245; and that of a hunting animal so ill fitted; yet rabies so prevails in the dog, 236—250; horror of, for the hunting, 242, 243, 244

Hunted class of animal, comprising the entire herbivora, 236, 237; relationship of, to the hunting class of animal, 245—250; liability of, to rabies, without conspicuous outbreaks of the disease, 238

Hunter, John, on refractoriness to rabies of dog, and of man, 10, 11; his estimate of the mortality of ·hydrophobia examined, 11, 12

Hunting class of animals, attenuators of rabies, 237

Hunting and non-hunting dog, 256, 257

Huxley, on red blood-corpuscle, 149

Hydrophobia, but a canine-rabies in man, 8, 207; a convulsive swallowing, 44; its fundamental lesion, a specific poisoning of the sensory side of the cerebro-spinal axis, 41, 42; of a strong-nerved man, a very different disease from the paralytic hydrophobia of a neurotic, 240; unamenable to inoculative treatment twelve days before the advent of the disease, 27, 250; dread after dog-bite, 3—5, 44; terror predominant feature of, 42; thirst in, 52; cf. also Canine-rabies

Hyperæsthesia with intense excitability the fundamental feature of convulsive rabies, 36—39, 41, 43

Hypertrophied connective-tissue of spleen in malarial fever, 151; of testicle in leprosy or tubercle, 147, 151, 153

Hypertrophy of connective-tissue, increasing its adaptability for germinating the preventive order of micro-organisms, 151

Identity, with specific character, of micro-organisms of the prophylactic and of the preventive order, 180

Idiopathic hydrophobia, 269; tetanus, 91, 269

Immune animal, or natural protection, 113

Immunity, general, of the preventive germ-disease, contrasted with prophylaxis, 129—169; how induced, 130, 134, 168—175; contrasted with specific prophylaxis, 157

Incubation of prophylactic and of peripheral preventive micro-organisms, immediate and regular, 121

Incubation period and symptoms of convulsive and paralytic rabies, fundamental difference between, 38—43, 223; between tetanus or strychnine-poisoning and rabies, 133

Incubation period of rabies, genuine, opposed to its pre-incubation period, 122; as normal and unvarying as that of tetanus, 122

Incubation period of rabies and of centric preventive micro-organisms delayed and irregular, 127—131; extremely prolonged, 212; latency of, 127, 128; of ordinary canine-rabies, 74, 206, 214, 233; its irregularity in canine-rabies, 97, 211, 212, 213; of ordinary rabbit-rabies, 74, 223, 233; of hydrophobia, 211; inversely as the potency of the disease, 95; a law of germ-disease, 211; the Pasteurian period of germ-disease, iii

Infection of cerebro-spinal axis during pre-incubation, and incubation periods, 20—35; of the bulb, or the superior or anterior tracts of cerebro-spinal axis, 23—28; of the lumbar swelling, or the inferior or posterior tracts, 26, 28, 32, 71; of the dog or the hunting animal in the later stages of incubation, 249, 250; risk of, from profoundest paralytic rabies, during latest stages of incubation, 28; sites of, 26, 34

Infective rates of completely convulsive, of convulso-paralytic, and of completely paralytic rabies, 208, 209, 210; determined by amount of paralysis in case, 19, 210, 211

Influenza maligna, as a recurrent germ-disease of the centric preventive order, 141

Infusorial monads of sponge, 162

Inoculation, intravenous, M. Pasteur's experiments, 96; in relation to the lumbar-swelling and to the development of intermittent paralytic rabies, 71; subdural, as test of incubation period, 212

Inoculations, intracranial and intravenous, 212; the former, feebler in its results than intravenous or subcutaneous, why, 69—72

Insectivorous plants, 193

Insects, their venomous secretions, why, 195—197

Instability of canine-rabies, 207—219

Intensification of rabies on transmission, 4, 84—87, 222—233; through rabbits, methodic, progressive, and endless, 228,

231, 232, 233; table of, by its transmission through the rabbit, 233; laws of, 232; illustrations from M. Pasteur's investigation, 232, 233

Intensifiers, the, or the intensifying division of the animal kingdom, 5, 222—235; their special rabies, paralytic, and of the cerebro-spinal and sympathetic systems, 28, 52, 53, 55

Intensifying property, an infallible indication of intrinsic nerve-weakness, 240

Intermittent character of rabies-saliva, 12, 14; of the rabies of hens and of birds, why, 26, 27, 51; similar to the intermittent character of ague, pyæmia and of many preventive germ-diseases, 26, 130

Intermittent rabies, an ascending paralytic rabies of lumbar-swelling infection, 72

Intoxication; cf. Drunkenness, Mad

Jenner's vaccine, 118; his vaccination the *beau-ideal* of prophylaxis, 104

Juniper " essence," 182

Kelvin, Lord, on origin of living forms on earth, 183

Kerslake, on the regions where rabies does not occur, 265

Klein, on the occasional phagocytic power of the tubercle-bacillus, respecting its absorbent corpuscle, 152

Koch, on causation of malarial fever, 148; on the spores of the paludal microorganism in the intimate tissue of the spleen, 150; Koch's tuberculin, or the virus-elimination of the *Bacillus tuberculosis*, 67, 91, 106, 131; his tuberculin-test, as one of the most infallible in research, 107, 132, 147, 173; in bloodstream, as a cause, even in infinitesimal amount, of the elimination of the virus of germinating *Bacilli tuberculosis*, 131, its significance, 173; as an analogue of what occurs in the final outburst of every germ-disease, 131; in very graduated course, likewise protecting against tubercle, 110

Kölliker, on the relation of the sensory or posterior nerves to the sympathetic ganglia, 61

Lankester, Prof. Ray, on modifying influence of vaccine on small-pox, 105

Latency of pre-incubation and incubation periods, why, 127, 128

Laveran, on causation of ague, 148

Lawes, on the incapacity of the Papilionaceous plant to assimilate free nitrogen of the air, 192

Leopard, lion, tiger, or the giant *Felidae*, not genuine hunters, 238

Leprosy, a germ-disease of a connective-tissue nidus, 847

Leucocytes and wandering corpuscular cells of the highest animals, peculiar to the lowest planes of animal organisation, 163, 167; lineal descendants of vegetable cells, 158; seat of germination of the prophylactic micro-organism, 139, 162; phagocytic, even in respect of the prophylactic order of micro-organisms, after germination in their interior, 162; normally so in respect of the micro-organisms, which germinate exclusively in connective-tissue, 135, 162

Leucocytic system, limitation of, as a cause of prophylaxis, 165, 166

Liability of dog to rabies diametrically opposite to that of intensifiers, 214; its significance on origin of rabies in the animal kingdom, 215; of the hunted classes to rabies, without conspicuous outbreaks of the disease, 238

Liability to a preventive germ disease increased after protection, 117

Life, organic incorporation of primitive forms of, into one complex compound life within an organism, 199

Ligament, tendon, bone, connective-tissue structures, 143

Limitation of leucocytic system as a cause of prophylaxis, 165, 166

Limited range of the prophylactic order of germ-disease over animal kingdom, its extreme significance, 103, 104; a clue to prophylactic investigation, 102, 119, 162

Liquor sanguinis, a uniformly-flowing stream, 97; its influence in conveying the virus and the rabies-microbe to the cerebro-spinal axis, 96, 97; its bactericidal condition, after protection, 168—175

Lister, Lord, on Gardner's researches in respect of " The histology of the cell-wall," 186; M. Pasteur's experimentation regarding the superabundance of micro-organisms in overcrowded life, vegetable and animal, 184; the invisible minuteness of many specific micro-organisms, 201; his antiseptic treatment, 118; in the suppression of pyæmia and germ-disease, particularly preventive, 146

Living, not dead, tissues, constituting a germicidal condition, and eliminating a germicidal principle into the blood-stream, 173

Local Government Board, report to, its definition of the protective and the preventive properties of the rabies-virus, 105; on the alleged averting of small-pox by vaccination, 106; on the prophylactic character of Pasteur's treatment, 104; on Pasteur's statistics of canine-rabies, 253

Long's, Mr, influence in suppressing the canine-rabies of England, 220, 253

Lords, report to House of, respecting the surgical treatment of rabic wounds, 254

Lower or posterior extremities, a less important site of infection than upper or anterior, 26

Lumbar-swelling, as a primary centre of the rabies-microbe, 24—28

Lupus, 131, 137

Lymphatic stream, an important relic in the vertebrates of the invertebrate circulation, 145; a medium of conveyance of rabies-microbe and of the preventive micro-organisms, 98; through its wandering connective-corpuscles, the most direct route of extended infection in preventive germ-disease, 137

Lymphatic system; its fluid, even of an attenuator, never failing to rabidise, 145; observations of Galtier and of Bouchard, 9; cf. also Areolar spaces

Mad drunkenness, 107

Madness, canine, "furious" and "dumb," 107

Magendie's transmission experiments of canine-rabies through dogs, 15, 216, 218

Malarial fever, as a germ-disease of the spleen, 150; of the negro or of tropical natives, as a fading, final form, 181, 198

Malarial micro-organism in blood-cells, Manson's chart, 148

Mannaberg, Manson, and Marchiafava, on the causation of malarial fever, 148

Manson, on the degenerating and degenerated forms of the paludal micro-organism in blood-cells, 149

Marrow of bones, lymphatic glands and spleen, as the sources of the phagocytic leucocytes, 140

Marrow of bones as osseous lymphatic glands, 166

Martin, Sidney, on the chemical products of pathogenic micro-organisms, 171

Measles, why prophylactic, 179

Medulla oblongata or "bulb," as the prime seat of germination, 24, 25

Melun series of rabies-transmissions through rabbits, 229, 230

Memory of pains soon forgotten, of pleasures lingers and expands, 241

Metschnikoff's observations on *Daphne*, 134

Microcosm of rabies as it exists in nature in the drying marrows of rabidised rabbits, 228

Micro-organism, of every preventive germ-disease, unmodifiable, 101—106; law of the virulent results of a pathogenic, proportioned to its incubation, 211; law of the protection afforded by a virus, 109

Micro-organisms; their agency in plants and animals, its enormous importance, 192, 203; in plants, extrinsic, 191; very rarely centric, or directly in plant-tissues, 191; pathogenic and physiological, 202; latter far more numerous than the former, 202; located in secreting organs, and at the source of their secretion, 201, 202, 203; associated with rabies-microbe in rabic saliva, 8; transmuting agency of, in mineral or inorganic as well as in organic substances, in gases and elements of the atmosphere, 184

Micro-organisms of rabies, centrifugal in growth rather than centripetal, 94; equal, as monads, in germinating capacity, 81, 86; individually, unmodifiable, 86, 88, 101—106; pathogenic, but in the most persistent intensifiers ultimately may become physiological, through specialisation of germinating tissues and of micro-organism, 199

Minuteness of the rabies-microbe, extreme, 87, 202

Modified form of a prophylactic micro-organism, 167, 168; retaining the prophylactic property of the virus-germ, of which it is a modification, 84, 156

Modifying character of the individual micro-organism, peculiar to that of the prophylactic order of germ-disease, 87, 88, 89

Mongrel-dogs, as the source of rabies in the dog-race, 254

Monkey of tropical Africa, a most potent attenuator of the rabies-microbe, 181, 217

Monkey-rabies, a convulsive rabies, and as a final form of the disease, 235

Morphia-solution, absorbed by root-tissues, conveyed to remotest structures, 183

Mortification or necrosis, as a predisposing cause of tetanus, 90

Mosquitoes, the mode of conveyance of the paludal micro-organism, or the means of infection of malarial fever, 148

Mumps, an exceptionally prophylactic germ-disease, 166; why, 179

Muzzle; in suppressing the canine disease; significance of the results, 220, in Sweden and in Germany, 262

Natural preventive conditions, extrinsic and intrinsic, 10

Nerve; fragments of, peripheral terminations, occasionally found rabic, 93; function of sensory, blended with that of sympathetic, 62

Nerve-instability of the hunted class, 241; essential to the intensification of rabies, 245

Nerves, cf. Afferent, Bulbar, Centric, Cervical site, Efferent, Peripheral, Pneumogastric, Sciatic, Spinal, Terminal

Nervous substance, in the motor, the sensory, and the sympathetic systems, not alike sensitive to the virus of rabies, 54, 55

Nervous system; its vital influence in specific centres on the leucocytic system of animals, 164; in the establishment of specific phagocytosis and in the production of prophylaxis, 164, 165, 167; condition of, determining the character of tetanus and rabies, 269, 270

Neuroglia, a most primitive connective-tissue structure, 142, 143, 144; as specific

site of germination of the rabies-microbe, 154

Nocard's dialysis of rabic salivary secretion, 7, 98

Normal, convulsive canine-rabies, 21, 214; as sensibly one in its virulence and germinating capacity, considered, 81, 82

Normal hydrophobia, the convulsive rabies of the dog, 41

Normal rabbit-rabies, 21, 40, 213, 231; the paralytic rabies of intensifiers, 27, 28, 40, 41, 233

Normal tracts of migration of the rabies-microbe after infection, and after incubation, 93—95, 119—135

Nux vomica, its strychnine, 187; of bacterial agency amidst root-tissues, 192

Onsets, sudden, of virus, a series of, necessary for the full induction of rabies, particularly in its intermittent forms, 128; likewise characteristic of many preventive germ-diseases, 131, 159, 160

Opium in the poppy as a product of bacterial agency, 190

Organ in plant or animal, storing a virulent principle, specialised for storing, not elaborating it, 188

Organism, plant or animal, perfected through suffering, 197

Origin of consciousness and life, increasing mystery of, 183, 205; of elementary nervous system from attainment of secreting system, 202; of rabies in intensifiers, 251—268; of secreting-organ in plant and animal, 200, 202; of serpent-venom, through bacterial disease, 196

Origin, spontaneous, of canine-rabies, considered, 204, 205

Outbreak, extensive, of canine madness originating from a paralytic, not a convulsive, rabies, 218, 219

Paludal micro-organisms in blood-cells, degenerated and degenerating, 149

Paralytic element, importance of, over the convulsive element, even in canine-rabies, 19, 219; in rabies, surety of a rabic salivary secretion, 56

Paralytic hydrophobia, 244

Paralytic rabies, involves the cerebro-spinal and the sympathetic nervous systems, 50, 51, 128, 208; extremely rare in the dog, 2; the most stable and the most capable of transmission through the dog of any form, 219; the initiating canine-rabies, 218, 219, 234, 237

Paralytic, convulso-, canine-rabies of high infective rate, at Deptford and Pantin, 14, 17, 208

Paralytic, profound, rabbit-rabies, 40; the most persistent and specific variety, 77, 230—233; its extreme severity masking it as a rabies, 260; its rarity in nature, 268, 273

Parotid glands,—rabic, 7, 93

Pasca's seasonal statistics of canine-rabies, 264

Pasteur, on canine character and source of rabies, 201, 206; cerebro-spinal infection of canine-rabies, 23; constantly rabic condition of the bulb as compared with the salivary secretion, 20—35; why selected for experimental purposes, 35; on dog-rabies, as "the only rabies," 206; desiccation of rabic marrows, 170; fermentation, and spontaneous generation of rabies, 202, 204; intensifying property of the rabbit, 229—232; intermittent rabies of the hen, 26; intracranial, intravenous and subcutaneous inoculations, their difference in imparting the disease, 70; lumbar-swelling, as a primary seat of the intermittent paralytic rabies, 71; massive infection in blood-stream, with occasional protection, 129; monkey, indicating the animal's superlative attenuating power, 217; peripheral sites of infection, as determining factors of the sites of cerebro-spinal infection, 29, 30, 31; quantitative character of protection from rabies-virus inoculations, 109, 111; quantitative character of the rabies-virus-germ, 68; of intravenous and subcutaneous inoculations, as compared with the intracranial, 72; rabic condition of the blood, 9; its extreme rarity as compared with that of nervous substance or of salivary secretion, 9; rabbit, indicating the animal's superlative intensifying property, 228, 229, 230; refractoriness of the dog and the possibility of escape from infection, 14, 15; subdural inoculation as testing the incubation period of ordinary canine-rabies of the streets, 213, 214; variations in the length of incubation from diminution in an initial virus-germ, 78; various forms of rabies, induced by various amounts and sites of infection at the periphery, 29—33; various sites of the cerebro-spinal substance as seats of germination, 22—29

Pasteur's discovery of the rabies-microbe, 87; his research, i—iv; initial experiments from salivary gland of a girl who died of paralytic hydrophobia, 7, 8; his treatment of anthrax that of a prophylactic germ-disease, 101; and of the entire realm of germ-disease that, either of a preventive or of a prophylactic order, 118; of rabies, as a germ-disease, of essentially prophylactic type, 101; being in reality that of a genuinely preventive germ-disease, 110, 118; his views of the germ-diseases "common to man and animals," 102; of the nature of the "vaccinal matter" in drying rabic marrows, 169

Perfume of flowers and leaves, 185

Peripheral infection, most regular, 30; nearness of, to cerebro-spinal axis the more effective the rabies induced, 69

Peripheral terminations of nerves, as the starting-points of propagation of the rabies-microbe, 93, 96

Persistency of recurrence, for many ages, of a preventive germ-disease, in the attainment of prophylaxis, 176, 180; or, failing prophylaxis, in the establishment of a secreting-organ, 199, 200, 201

Persistency of virulence, test of a typical rabies, 76

Pfeiffer's microbe of influenza, 87, 201

Phagocytes, lineal descendants of amœboid order of cell in plants and in lowest planes of animal organisation, 158; attraction of, succeeding repulsion, vital and permanent, 163, 164, 165

Phagocytic function common to the amœboid order of cell, 158, 162, 163; very special, 165—168; oldest function of animal organism, 158, 167; as a cause of prophylaxis, 166; of its persistent endurance, 166; of prevention itself, after prolonged recurrence of a preventive germ-disease, 175—177, 198—200

Phagocytic prophylaxis as a probable ending of the malarial fever of the negro, 147;

and a possible ending of rabbit-rabies, 198

Phagocytosis or microbe-devouring, 157—159, 165, 167; characteristic of prophylactic order of germ-disease, 167; physiological, not pathological, 165; vital and permanent, not mechanical nor chemical, 163, 165

Physiological accumulations of toxic products in a plant, fixed in amount and unaltering in character, 190

Physiological micro-organisms, as ultimate evolution of the pathogenic, 201, 202

Pitcher-plant, 193

Plants, active principles of, significance of their elimination to deciduous structures, 182; insectivorous, 193

Pneumogastric nerve, rabic, 93

Pneumonia, a pulmonary erysipelas, 135

Poppy, European and Indian, 186

Power, on wounds favourable to tetanus, 90

Predigestion by micro-organisms of animal and vegetable matter in soil, 184

Pre-incubation period, importance of, for inoculative treatment, 97; and for research, iii

Pre-incubation period of rabies, 119—127, 212; a process of conveyance by connective-corpuscles, 120; its varying duration, and why, 120—122; through the pre-incubation period no germination, 123, 124; no virus eliminated, 125; latency of, 127, 128

Preventive conditions, intrinsic, of the animal kingdom, 11, 34; extrinsic, 10, 34

Preventive germ-diseases, 99, 100; exclusively cultivated in fixed connective-tissue, 131—142; of external or peripheral connective-tissue cultivation, 134, 135, 136, 139; of universal (peripheral and centric) cultivation in connective-tissue, 137, 142, 162; of exclusively centric or internal connective-tissue cultivation, 141, 142; their primary habitat in badly-drained soils, 271; liability to, increased after protection, 117

Preventive inoculations as potent after as before incubation, 105; their protection quantitative, 105, 110, 156, 157; unenduring, and essentially pathological, 174, 175; the germ-disease recurrent, 175, 177

Preventive micro-organism, law regulating the germinating site of, and determining the special tissues which its virus deteriorates, 152

Preventive order of germ-disease of widest range over the animal kingdom, 183; recurrent, 176; cf. Onsets

Prophylactic order of germ-diseases, 100—116, 138; centric, never peripheral, 138, 139; limited range of, over animal kingdom, its extreme significance, 103, 104; a clue to prophylactic investigation, 102, 119, 162; deterioration of, through transmission for many ages, 179; of likewise the excessively recurrent preventive germ-disease, 180, 181; phagocytosis in both cases determining the attenuation, 181

Prophylactic, as compared with the preventive order of civilised life, exceptionally disastrous amongst savages, why, 234

Prophylactic property, a highly specialised function in leucocytes, 103, 163, 165, 167; permanent and vital, 165, 167

Prophylactic treatment, clue to possibility of a, 102, 103

Prophylactic virus-germ, simple, not quantitative, 88; individually, most modifiable, 89; may be modified into a vaccination, 89; the individual prophylactic micro-organism, compared with rabies-microbe, 88, and with micro-organisms of the preventive order, 102; prophylactic micro-organism, amount or site of, does not determine the character of the disease, 87, 112

Prophylaxis, how occasioned, 140, 159, 162, 163, 167; characteristic of prophylactic order of germ-disease, 167; may be also induced by the continuous, recurrent action of a preventive virus, 176

Protection from a prophylactic virus-germ, enduring character of, 112; the vital nature of its prophylaxis, 175

Protection from rabies-virus, its evanescence, 111

Protection of preventive class of germ-diseases, evanescence of, 111, 112

Pugh on incapacity of Papilionaceous plant to assimilate the free nitrogen of the air, 192

Pyæmia, a preventive germ-disease of universal connective-tissue cultivation, 137, 138, 146; site of infection in no way determines character of the disease, 137

Quain's Anatomy, on the bulbar nerves, and their origin in the bulb, 45; disparity of size between anterior and posterior roots of spinal cord, 48, 49; the motor roots and their freedom from ganglia, 59; the sensory roots and their incorporation with the ganglionic system, 59; the special connective-tissue structure of the interstitial framework of centric organs, of synovial membranes and sacs, and of valves, 60

Quantitative character of rabies-virus, in the production of the disease, and of prevention; Pasteur's experiments, 64—80, 109—111

Quantitative virus, not virus-germ, and of a preventive germ-disease, alone producing prevention, 156

Quantity of the rabies-microbes of which it is composed constituting a virus-germ unit, 88, 89; this, in specific types of the disease, specialised and organised to its full possibility, 82, 84, 89

Quantity of tetanus-bacillus in peripheral connective-tissue sufficient to tetanise, infinitesimal, 125; of rabies-microbe varying and various, 62, 64

Rabbit, the best ground for the study of intensification, 229; the most potent intensifier, 222, 227, 228; possible consequences of absence of attenuating power in, 199

Rabbit, the, in Australia, 265, 266, 267

Rabbit-rabies, rarity of a wholly convulsive element in, or in that of intensifiers, 233; cf. Normal rabbit-rabies

Rabbits, absence of rabies in countries without, 265

Rabic condition of saliva, an indication of implication of the sympathetic system, 210; of lymphatic fluid in later stages of incubation, 145; intermittent character, 12, 14

Rabic nerve-structures, comparative investigation of, 21—29

Rabies, of the cat and of the fox, 244; a germ-disease of the country rather than of cities, 262; absence of, in countries without rabbits, 265; centric, not peripheral, in cultivation, 133; in the connective-tissue of the cerebro-spinal axis, or the neuroglia, 154, 155; malady of the hunted rather than of the hunting class of animals, 236, 237; of intensifiers rather than attenuators, 222—235

Rabies, of the dog, convulsive, 205, 233; of the deer, convulso-paralytic, 224, 225, 226; the hen, intermittent and subacutely paralytic, 26; the rabbit, profoundly paralytic, 198, 222—235; the sympathetic system, always paralytic and infective, 50; characteristic of intensifiers, 28, 50—63

Rabies in cerebro-spinal axis, anatomical classification of, 28; disclosures of bulbar centres of germination, 46; rabies from various amounts and sites of infection, comparative investigation of the forms of, 29—35; prevalence of a special form of, in attenuators, no test of its stability, 207; summary ending of outbreak of, in attenuators and intensifiers, 227, but for opposite reasons, 227; of the Middle Ages, theory of, 205

Rabies or hydrophobia, analgesic or hyperæsthetic, its lesion of sensory system underlying all lesions, 38—49; a descending neuritis from cerebro-spinal centres, 45, 46; an intoxication of nervous system like acutest alcoholism, 107; considered, as a preventive germ-disease, 100—112, 177; as a prophylactic germ-disease, 100—106; whether convulsive or paralytic, not necessarily canine, 219, 220, 257; order of germ-diseases to which it belongs, 99—117; cf. also Acute, Ascending, Attenuation, Attenuators', Bulbar, Canine, Completely convulsive, Convulso-paralytic, Dispersal, Dumb, "Fixed," Furious, Idiopathic, Instability, Intensification, Intermittent, Paralytic, Spinal

Rabies-infection, external or peripheral sites of, the more important the nearer to bulkier sections of cord, 32—38; face and neck exceptionally dangerous sites of, 34

Rabies-micro-organism, a microbe of living not of dead tissue, 124, 169; of nerve-structure, exclusively, 20, 92; sensory rather than motor side of the cerebro-spinal axis, 38, 47; its deterioration in pre-incubation period, 95, 123, 124; its elaboration of virus, when and where, 125, 126; its extreme minuteness, 87, 202; its moribund or degenerating condition in rabic saliva, 8, 124; in bulb, 124; its multiform structure as a virus-germ, 86, 98; speciality of the multiform virus-germ, the cause of the speciality of the typical varieties of the disease, 86—98; extension or migration through nerves, 45, 92; when it occurs, 94; medium by which borne to central nervous axis, 93, 94, 96, 98; by what nerve-tracts, from cerebro-spinal to sympathetic system, 59; amount of, in central nervous substance in convulsive and in paralytic rabies, 21, 25, 28; amount of rabies-virus due to amount of rabies-microbe, 70, 82; amount of rabies-virus, an animal capable of tolerating, and how far it can tolerate it, 113, 114, 115, 116; constancy of, in bulb, as compared with salivary gland, 23, 24; difference in composition, form, and force of, 83; rabies-microbe, or that of any centric preventive germ-disease, why not destroyed by the phagocytes of the circulation, 120; cf. also Conveyance, Virus-germ, Normal tracts

Rabies-protection, graduated accumulation of rabies-virus, *sine quâ non* of, 109

Rabies-virus, or product of the specific micro-organism, deadliest of ferments, 110; causing the disease, and all morbid changes, 106, 125; occasioning protection or prevention, 90—96, 108—112; the protection or prevention, like that from the virus of every preventive germ-disease, being pathological, 175; unenduring, 112, 174; with the disease recurrent, 112; morbific results of, which prevents or protects, 114, 115; cf. also Duration

Rayleigh's, Lord, with Prof. Ramsay's, elimination of argon, 192

Recurrence, persistent, of malarial fever, 175; of the preventive order of germ-disease, 117; why, 141, 142, 151, 175

Red blood-cells, their possible origin, 149

Reinoculation, periodic, absolutely necessary for universal prevention, 112, 113, 114; why impracticable, 115, 116; its ultimate effect, 116—119

Repulsion from, with subsequent attraction towards irritants, of the amœboid order of cell, 163; of highest animals, 164; vital, not chemical or mechanical, 165

Restoration of an initial rabies, from a second transmission through rabbits of its fractional virus, 79, 84

Rheumatism, acute, as a centric preventive germ-disease, 141; its recurrence, 146

Richmond's, Duke of, Governor of Canada, hydrophobia from rabid fox-bite, 42; his dread of water, 44

Richmond Park epidemic of deer-rabies, 224, 225

Root-cells of plants, their absorptive power, 183

Roots of bulbar and lumbar sensory nerves the nidus of the rabies-microbe, 49

Ruffer on diphtheritic membrane, 136

Saliva of paralytic rabies, liquid condition of, 10

Salivary gland, considered as the specific seat of the rabies-microbe, 1—19

Salivary secretion, absorbable in paralytic rabies, copious in amount, and rabic, 5, 17, 56; churned in convulsive rabies, diminished in amount, non-absorbable, and frequently non-rabic, 5, 56; earliest involved of any secretion, and the most seriously, why, 57, 58, 62; main channel for elimination of the rabies-microbe, 19; its rabies-micro-organisms in every stage of degeneration, 8, 124; its effectiveness due to amount of paralysis in the case, 17, 219; its non-effectiveness to the sparse amount of rabies-microbe, and exclusively located in the bulbar sites, 15, 210, 219

Sanderson, Burdon, on fungoid spores and the leucocytes of *Daphne*, 134

Sciatic nerve, rabic, 93

Seat of germination, experimental determination of, in bulbar and lumbar substance, 24—29, in cerebro-spinal substance, 23—25, in sympathetic substance, 50—56

Secreting-organs implicated in paralytic, seldom or never in completely convulsive rabies, any more than in tetanus or strychnine-poisoning, 52, 53

Secreting-organs peculiarly characteristic of the animal organism, 195; rare in the extreme in the vegetable kingdom,

193, 195 ; attainment of, initial factor of evolution, 202

Secreting-structures in plants and animals, in relation to bacterial agency, 195

Secreting-tissues, fermenting foci ; their secretion, a fermentation, 200, 201 ; their specialised tissue habitually inhabited by a specific micro-organism, constituting it a specific secreting-organ, 201

Secretion of a secreting-organ, why unlimited in amount, and specific in character, 19, 60—64

Secretions, the so-called, of the plant organism, 188

Sensibility, disturbance of, fundamental feature of rabies, 37, 43

Sensory, junction of, with the ganglionic sympathetic system ; its importance in the production of acute, paralytic rabies, and in the implication of the glandular system, with infective forms of the disease, 52, 53, 55, 57, 62

Sensory centres of bulb primary and very special seats of germination, 43, 44

Sensory nerves, incorporation of, with sympathetic ganglia, 55—60

Serpent-venom, how it originated, and how it is maintained, 195, 196, 197

Serum, after a preventive germ-disease, bactericidal, 159 ; why, 168—177

Serum treatment ; cf. Anti-toxin

Sharpey, on serous spaces or the "anfractuous cavities" of the lymphatic system, 145 ; on structure, connective-tissue, of serous sacs, membranes and valves, 143

Sheep, clearing the gunwales of a steamboat, why, 243

Signs and symptoms of canine-rabies, however prevalent, no test of its typical stability, 207

Soil, the natural habitat of micro-organisms, 183 ; bacterial zone of, 186

Soil-life of the rabies-microbe, 271

Solidists, the, on germ-disease, 160

Sormani's discovery of the rabies-microbe, 89

Specialisation of germ-disease to milder forms, through transmission, 179, 180 ; of particular tissues for storing toxic products, characteristic of vegetable kingdom, 189

Spinal nerves rabic, 93

Spinal rabies, 29

Spleen, as a centre of the leucocytic system, 140 ; as the main seat of malarial fever, 150 ; softened and atrophied lymphoid element of, in malarial fever, 151, also of specific organs, infected with cancer, leprosy, tubercle, etc., 151

Spontaneous generation, no explanation, 204, 219, 267

Spontaneous protection, 130

Spores of "the paludal parasites," how they are so constantly conveyed to the intimate structure of the spleen, 120, 146, 150; of exclusively peripheral micro-organisms, occasionally conveyed to centric connective-tissue, 137, 146, 150

Spores in the ultimate tissue of the spleen found at the earliest stages of malarial fever, 150

Statistics of infective canine-rabies of Battersea Dogs' Home, and of the London police authorities, 255

Stelling, on the anatomical origin of the bulbar nerves, 46, 47

Sting of nettle ; its relation to habitual bacterial agency, 187, 190

Strain to the nervous system of the persistently hunted existence, 241, 244

Strychnine of nux vomica, as a product of bacterial agency, 190

Superinduced liability after any virus-protection, 116, 117

Suzor, on convulsive, 38, and paralytic canine-rabies, 40; on Hunter's historic "instance" of hydrophobia, 11, 12; on statistics of the Comité d'Hygiène, 33

Swallowing, act of, greatest agony of rabies or hydrophobia ; why, 44, 45

Sympathetic system, an important relic of the nervous system of the invertebrate kingdom, 60; less highly specialised than any part of the cerebro-spinal substance, 55, its relation to secretion and secreting-organs, 19, 55, 203

Taste and the other special senses exaggerated in convulsive, perverted in paralytic rabies, 38, 39

Terminal nerves, their rabic condition as compared with that of spinal substance, 94

Terrier's indomitable courage, 239

Terror, predominant feature of hydrophobia, 42

Tetanus and strychnine-poisoning, compared with convulsive and paralytic rabies, 37

Tetanus bacillary product and strychnine, 188

Tetanus, a germ-disease of the country rather than of cities, 91, 270; extremely rife in villages of India, 188; its bacillus of peripheral connective-tissue cultivation, 90, 91, 93, 135; its site of infection in no way determining the character of the disease, 31

Thirst in hydrophobia and convulsive rabies, excessive; why, 52

Tobacco, habitual use of, its results, 164, 166; its specific protection, 167

Toxic principles of a plant, fixed amount and unvarying strength, the special character of, 188, 191, 195; dearth of, in vegetable kingdom, where dearth of micro-organisms, 184

Toxic plant-products and the viruses of pathogenic micro-organisms, specially neurotic poisons, 182; how conveyed to the remotest structures, 183; primarily pathogenic, ultimately physiological, even in plants, 189, 190, 191; why incapable of being stored in animals, 182

Toxicytones, 161—168; from which prevention or protection, absolute, 109, 110, 174; chemical and pathological, not physiological, 168, 175; transient and evanescent, 175; with likewise, a condition of subsequent unprotection, also equally transient, 175

Transmission, serial, through the dog, of ordinary convulsive rabies, even of profound paralytic rabies, progressively attenuated to extinction, 218; of canine-rabies through rabbits, 198

Tubercle-bacillus, a micro-organism of peripheral and centric connective-tissue cultivation, 182; its latent stage, 131, 144

Umbelliferous plants, why some deadly, some harmless and nutritious, 185

Uniformity of symptoms, lesions, incubation and infective rate, characteristic only of the profoundest paralytic rabies, 219, 226, 230

Unit-microbe of preventive germ-disease, unmodifiable; of prophylactic germ-disease pre-eminently modifiable, and capable of being transmuted into a vaccination, 84

Vaccinal protection or prophylaxis due to phagocytosis, 156—162

Vaccine, the modified micro-organism of small-pox, 101, 105; the prophylactic property of the original micro-organism fully retained, 106; its virulent property reduced to a minimum, 88, 89, 105; "vaccinal matter," the, in rabies-inoculations, not the dead micro-organisms, 169; not the virus of the pathogenic micro-organism, 168, 169; what it is, 156, 160

Variability of rabies in attenuators; of incubation and pre-incubation periods, 211, 212, 213, 214; of infective rate, 210, 211; of lesions, 209, 210; of ordinary canine-rabies from even intracranial inoculation, 212—214

"Varieties" or modifications of ordinary canine-rabies of the streets, considerable, 214; from amount of infection rather than from innate difference of breed or race, 215

Venom of serpent, physiological, that of rabid animal, pathological, but both of bacterial agency, 197

Virus, elaborated at later stages of incubation-period proper, 127; outflow of, from incubating micro-organisms, a final series of phenomena, 128; eliminated, simultaneously and repeatedly, in sudden outbursts from the ripest germinating-sites, 130, 131; never in peripheral tissues, 67, 68; nor in itself bactericidal, 169; obtained, before Pasteur's research, exclusively in salivary gland, 7; action of, continuous or excessive, on specific tissues, as cause of the germicidal condition of serum or tissues, 174; effect of the secretion of, on the process of germination, 127; graduated course of, protects, 107, 108, of rabies-virus, the *sine quâ non* of prevention and protection, 108, 109, 110, 126; cf. Onsets

Virus-germ of rabies, also quantitative in infection, both in intensifiers and attenuators, 84, 85; various and varying in structure and composition, 85, 86; amorphous, 86; collective and multiform, 86; fragmentary and completed, 83, 86; fractional, 82, 83; restored to its completed virus-germ on a second transmission through an intensifier, 83; individually unvarying, collectively most varying, 82—85; compared with virus-germ of prophylactic and other germ-diseases, 85; units of special, how constituted, 80—87; cf. also Rabies-micro-organism

Whooping-cough, 166, 179
Wilfarth, on the micro-organisms of the root-nodules of Papilionaceous plants, 192

Yeast fermentation, analogous to virus-elaboration in germ-disease, 106, 107; and to the bacterial fermentation, occuring incessantly in the soil amidst plant-roots, 181—187
Youatt on the symptoms of canine-rabies, 60